Case Studies in Child and Adolescent Mental Health

MS Thambirajah FRCPsych
Consultant Child and Adolescent Psychiatrist
Walsall Teaching PCT

Radcliffe Publishing
Oxford • Seattle

Radcliffe Publishing Ltd
18 Marcham Road
Abingdon
Oxon OX14 1AA
United Kingdom

www.radcliffe-oxford.com
Electronic catalogue and worldwide online ordering facility.

British Library Cataloguing in Publication Data

A catalogue record for this book is available from the British Library.

ISBN-10: 1 85775 698 3
ISBN-13: 978 1 85775 698 2

Typeset by Anne Joshua & Associates, Oxford
Printed and bound by TJ International Ltd, Padstow, Cornwall

Contents

Preface

Whatever may be said, whoever may say it,
To determine the truth is wisdom.

Thiruvalluvar, 18th century Tamil poet

The aim of the book is threefold:

1 to provide a description of a variety of cases seen in specialist (Tier 2 and 3) Child and Adolescent Mental Health Services (CAMHS)
2 to discuss the knowledge base that informs our understanding of the clinical problems; and
3 to illustrate ways of managing cases based on available evidence of effectiveness of our interventions.

This book would interest the busy CAMHS practitioner and trainee whatever their background, training and persuasion: psychiatrists, psychologists, specialist child mental health nurses, social workers, and others working in core CAMHS. It will be especially useful for those starting a career in the field and for those following courses in child mental health across the country. For mature and senior clinicians, this book should help open up space so they can position themselves to think critically about the cases described. In addition to describing the presentation and management of the cases, each chapter also provides a brief subject review that summarises the present state of knowledge about each clinical condition and its treatment.

The cases portrayed in the book depict the 'bread and butter' cases that practitioners encounter in their day-to-day clinical practice. The number of cases has been limited to those commonly seen in CAMHS. Admittedly there are significant omissions because of consideration of space. The cases are authentic ones based on real cases seen by the author. Although no brief case description can capture all the complexities of real life cases, we have attempted to convey the essential elements of the case without sacrificing the core features. The case histories have been simplified to help achieve the learning objectives for each chapter. The cases were more complex than what has been described here. Thus, there is a simplicity reflected in these accounts that would not have been found in the work itself.

In each chapter the case is described in some detail. Information collection is necessary but not sufficient for setting out a management plan. The information obtained, however extensive, matters little unless it is integrated into a meaningful formulation. Without a conceptual map to guide management, psychological interventions are of little use. Treatment techniques are only tools to achieve an end. The section on formulation describes the process of the construction of meaning that ultimately determines the choice of treatment. Like most things in life, in CAMH work, how the problems, difficulties or predicaments are defined, described and understood determine the perceived solution or intervention. The formulation given here is only one way of thinking about the cases. There are myriad ways of making meaning of cases. Therefore, the aim is to promote critical thinking rather than to get the reader to agree with the formulation.

Over the past quarter century a massive database of effective interventions for a range of mental health difficulties in children has built up that obliges the clinician to use, as much as possible, validated, evidence-based methods of treatment. This compels CAMH practitioners to pay attention to research findings and train themselves in evidence-based methods of assessment and treatment. This is true for those clinicians who have had generic training as well as for those who have had more specialised forms of training. Although we are far from answering the question 'What works for whom, under what circumstances and delivered by whom?', the 'one hat fits all' approach is no longer tenable. As Peter Fonagy (1998), one of the foremost researchers in the field has said, 'The era of generic therapies is over. No treatment can be equally applicable without modification to every disorder . . . Treatment will need to be disorder specific.'

Despite the inevitable but not insurmountable gap between the map of clinical research and the territory of clinical practice, the challenge for clinicians is to successfully deliver empirically supported interventions in clinic settings that are cost effective and that achieve good outcomes. Hence, much attention has been paid in the chapters to evidence-based approaches and choice of treatments. But there is also a need to individualise treatment. Research is about generalisation whereas practice is about particularisation. This implies that the therapist has to be flexible, and utilise a variety of treatment approaches and options available, so that if one does not work or is not acceptable for the child or family, alternatives are available. Therapists need to have a 'tool box' of interventions that can be used in cases as and when necessary.

Most CAMH practitioners are aware of the heavy burden they carry on their shoulders and the profound effects their pronouncements have on the children and families for the rest of their lives. The ethical principle of beneficence obliges clinicians to treat their clients/patients in a way that produces maximum benefit to the child. The principle of non-maleficence, the duty to avoid harm (*'Primum no nocere'*), obliges the clinicians to be thoughtful of the possible harm their actions may cause. This can happen either because a diagnosis *has* been made or a diagnosis *has not* been made. Making a diagnosis is considered an essential part of the assessment, but the effect of it on the child and family needs careful attention. Moreover, it has to be recognised that not only medications and diagnoses, but *all* activities of the therapist including feedback to the client and psychological treatments offered, may harm the children and families.

It is important to declare the author's prejudices. The author unashamedly admits to his preference for psychological therapies and family-oriented approaches. He believes in normalising emotional and behavioural presentations of children and adolescents to the extent it is reasonable, possible and useful. Both abnormal reactions to normal situations (e.g. anxiety) and normal reactions to abnormal situations (e.g. attachment-seeking behaviour in cases of abuse or rejection) may present to the clinician as psychologically anomalous behaviour in the child. There are few adults who would want a psychiatric diagnosis inflicted upon them. Yet many parents (and professionals) would demand a psychiatric diagnosis as a way of explaining the behaviour of the child. The author's preference for family-based treatment approaches should also be apparent to anyone reading the book. It appears unreasonable that the children should be made to bear the sole responsibility for change in the name of therapy when the contributions to the difficulties by the family are substantial and significant.

The work described here was carried out in two localities with high levels of social deprivation. The deprivation was also unmistakably manifest in the educational, social and mental health services available to the families and children. As a matter of routine Tier 3 work was carried out by single-handed practitioners struggling to do their best for the children and families; co-therapy was a luxury and getting a Statement of Special Educational Needs was an ordeal. No doubt this is reflected in the cases seen, the treatments offered and their outcomes.

The author wishes to record his indebtedness to the children, young people and their families, the subjects of the chapters in the book. Thanks are also due to those children and families not mentioned in the book from whom the author has learnt everything he knows. The names of the children and families have been changed and the circumstances altered to maintain anonymity. The author wishes to express his deep gratitude for members of the CAMHS teams with whom he has worked. Special thanks are due to Susan Burns for typing the various versions of the manuscript and for putting up with the author's idiosyncrasies.

MS Thambirajah
September 2006

Reference

Fonagy P. Prevention: the appropriate target of infant psychotherapy. *Infant Mental Health Journal.* 1998; **19**(2): 124–60.

About the author

Dr MS Thambirajah is a Consultant Child and Adolescent Psychiatrist. He has been involved in teaching and training for a considerable period of time. His book *The Psychological Basis of Psychiatry* (Churchill Livingstone) has been 'highly commended' by the BMA book awards for books published in 2005 on mental health.

List of abbreviations

CAMH   Child and Adolescent Mental Health
CAMHS   Child and Adolescent Mental Health Services
CBT   Cognitive behaviour therapy
DSM-IV   *Diagnostic and Statistical Manual*, Fourth Edition (American Psychiatric Association. *Diagnostic and Statistical Manual of Mental Disorders*. 4th edn. Washington DC: AMA; 1994)
GP   General Practitioner
ICD-10   International Classification of Diseases, 10th Revision (WHO, Geneva, 1992)
LEA   Local Educational Authority
NICE   National Institute for Health and Clinical Excellence
SENCO   Special Educational Needs Coordinator

Author's note

Those references marked with an asterisk (*) are recommended for further reading.

Dedicated to Carmen,
our one-year-old granddaughter.

Chapter 1

Oppositional defiant behaviour

It was a routine referral from the GP. The parents had taken Adam to the GP to get help with his behaviour problems. The referral letter was brief: 'I would be grateful if you could see this 7 year old boy. His parents describe him as a defiant and angry child with a bad temper. He does not do what he is told. This is worse at meal times and when he gets ready to go to school in the mornings. He talks back to his parents, uses bad language and is aggressive especially towards his mother. Parents describe him as "hard work". Other problems: surgical repair of VSD and coarctation of aorta (congenital heart conditions) soon after birth. I would be much thankful if you could see him fairly soon because the problems at home have been getting worse recently.'

Clinical presentation and background

Adam and his family were offered a routine appointment. Adam and his parents, Mr and Mrs Jones, attended the first assessment session. According to his father, Adam's behaviour was causing a great deal of problems in the family. He refused to obey simple instructions and argued over every small thing. For example, when asked to do things like putting his toys away after playing with them in the drawing room he simply refused to comply. Getting him to obey day-to-day parental requests and commands was extremely difficult. He defied parental authority and every simple request was met with defiance. His parents were experiencing great difficulty in getting him to abide by house rules. For example, the back garden of the house was small and was considered unsafe, but Adam demanded that he be allowed to play in the garden. Any attempt to get him to abide by the rules resulted in arguments or temper tantrums. Mrs Jones summarised the problems as: 'He would not do as he is told'.

In addition to challenging his parents' authority, Adam wanted to have his way in most things. He dominated the household and fought with his older brother Lee over wanting to watch his favourite television programmes or to play on the computer. He took things from Lee's room without his permission and insisted that he had the right to keep them. On one occasion he had taken the remote control for the television with him to the toilet so that others could not watch the programmes they wanted. This had lead to a major incident in which he and his father got into a physical struggle to recover the TV remote control. Mr Jones felt that Adam deliberately annoyed everyone in the family. During family times he would push, elbow or prod his brothers and provoke them. This usually led to retaliation by them, resulting in physical fights.

What concerned parents most was his aggressiveness. He was easily provoked and when he lost his temper he would go into a rage, attack his brothers, kick doors and throw things. Temper tantrums were a daily occurrence; it could take two hours for the temper to subside. On one occasion he had urinated on the carpet when sent to his room. During family times he would play up over small matters and one of the parents would end up taking him away from the scene. Getting him ready for school in the morning was a hard task. He would delay, obstruct or quibble over going to the bathroom, brushing his teeth and getting dressed. His mother had to be behind him all the time to get even the simplest task seen through. He could not be taken out to the shops because he caused severe disruption by meddling with things in the shelves.

Developmental history: Adam was born full term and the delivery was normal. But 36 hours after the delivery he had difficulty in breathing and was placed in intensive care. He was later transferred to the regional children's hospital for investigations. He was diagnosed as having congenital heart disease (ventricular septal defect and coarctation of aorta). He underwent surgery soon after and was in hospital for four weeks. When he returned home he continued to cry at nights and took a long time to settle. He was followed up at the hospital till the age of five. His parents had been told that his heart defects had been completely corrected and that he had made a full recovery. He had no other medical problems.

Adam's developmental milestones were normal. He started walking at 14 months and he spoke his first word by his first birthday, He was described as a difficult baby; he cried a lot and was a very irritable child. Mrs Jones recalled that soon after his discharge from hospital he was very demanding and did not settle down for a long time. Parents attributed this to the surgery and hospitalisation. Mrs Jones felt tired all day and even confused through loss of sleep. He started having his first temper tantrums around the age of 2 years and, contrary to parent's experience with his older brother, the tantrums had got worse as he had grown older. They had tried to ignore the tantrums at the beginning but now he had about two to three tantrums a day.

Adam did not experience much difficulty when he started nursery. After some initial aggression directed towards other children he settled down, made friends and enjoyed going to school. In his present school he was good at games and was popular with peers. Asked about Adam's strengths, both parents were quick to say that in spite of all that they had said about him he was a caring and loving boy.

Family history: The family consisted of Mr Jones, a plumber, Mrs Jones, a part-time shop assistant, and three boys. Adam was 7½, his older brother Lee 9 and the younger brother Mathew was 5. The parents had been married for 13 years. Both sets of grandparents lived locally and were supportive. The maternal grandparents had offered to keep Adam with them over weekends to provide respite for the family. But, of late, they had found Adam very difficult to manage and were now making excuses not to have him. The family history was unremarkable. There was no psychiatric illness or learning disability in the family.

Examination: During the interview Adam was initially well behaved and pleasant but when parents were describing his difficult behaviours he began contesting their version of events, often saying 'it was not my fault' and blamed others for the problems. He disagreed that he was being difficult and often turned to his mother for support. Mrs Jones did not overtly take his side but appeared to be close to tears during these exchanges. Mr Jones said that he could manage Adam on his own but it was his mother who experienced difficulties. Mr Jones appeared to be in some physical pain at the time of interview and on enquiry he revealed that he had been suffering with low backache for some time. During the interview Mr Jones raised his voice several times to get Adam to stop arguing.

Adam was seen on his own later. He was a somewhat slim boy with a mischievous smile. He was cooperative and amiable. He liked school because it was fun. He talked a great deal about his friends and the birthday parties to which he had been invited. When asked about his difficulties at school he said, that his class teacher hated him and blamed him for things that other kids did. He said that his father shouted at him 'all the time' and he was 'always in trouble' meaning that he was 'always sent to his room' and he commented that 'it was unfair'. He agreed that he lost his temper often and threw things or punched holes in the door. As for the things that he would like to see changed, he said that he would like

1   his father not to shout at him
2   to be a good boy and
3   to get his older brother to share his computer games with him.

He was not sure why he had been brought to the clinic. He had thought he was coming to a clinic similar to the regional cardiac clinic but the clinician had been 'only just asking questions'. Later in the examination he asked, 'Are you a real doctor?'

Adam's drawings were colourful and detailed. In the draw-a-man test (Harris, 1963), a rough method of assessing cognitive development in children, he produced a detailed picture of a man with glasses wearing a tie. But his writing was rather poor; he just managed to write his name. He made numerous spelling mistakes and there were many lateral inversions (for example, he would confuse the letters b and d). A short reading test (Schonell graded word reading test) was administered to assess reading. The test consists of a list of words of increasing difficulty that the child is asked to read. The number of words the subject is able to read is compared with the 'norms' provided for each age group. Adam's could not read even one word in the list. This gave him a reading age of 6.0 minus (his chronological age was 7 years 6 months). In a later session Mrs Jones recollected that Adam had had difficulties naming colours till very recently. He could choose a red felt pen if asked to do so, but, if asked to name the colour of the pen, he could not do so.

Permission was obtained from parents to contact school and ask for a report. The school report arrived sometime later. Adam's level of general intelligence was reported to be above average, confirming the clinician's initial impression that he was sharp and witty. But it also confirmed the initial impression that Adam did indeed have significant difficulties in reading and writing. He was soon to be assessed by the educational psychologist.

Case conceptualisation and formulation

Conceptualisation of the case and making a formulation of the problem in a coherent and meaningful way is central to any therapeutic activity. This is especially so in child mental health where the problems have multiple dimensions and are complex both in their presentations and causations. Essentially a case formulation consists of answering two basic questions:

1 The *what* question: what is the problem and how is it best characterised? This involves describing the essential features of the clinical picture. It may consist of a brief description of the psychological presentation or a psychiatric diagnosis. It is important to remember that psychiatric diagnoses are purely descriptive and do not impute a biological dysfunction in the person nor do they ascribe any particular causation. Another necessary step in the assessment process is to consider the other possible reasons (not causations) for the clinical picture. In medical jargon this is called *differential diagnosis* but what it means is rather simple: the exclusion of other possibilities.

2 The *why* question: why is the problem occurring in this child and family at this particular time? This stage of assessment involves an attempt at explaining the causative or aetiological factors that may have lead to the problem including factors that maintain it. As a rule mental health problems in children and adolescents are caused by multiple factors and any adequate assessment involves the identification of factors in the child, family and environment that may be contributing to the causation and maintenance of the problem/s.

It is important to stress that the above two steps, describing the problem and ascribing causative and maintaining factors, necessarily involve the construction of hypotheses that need to be confirmed, changed or refuted from information gathered from subsequent sessions. The important point though is that these are only hypotheses and the clinician should be prepared to revise, modify and, at times, replace them with new ones and not 'fall in love' with their favourite hypothesis!

Thus, the formulation represents the essential links between aetiological factors and clinical picture; it connects theory and practice and encapsulates the idea of how we view the difficulties presented by the child and the family and, therefore, forms the basis of treatment planning and interventions. The approach adopted here is not associated with a particular (e.g. psychodynamic, cognitive behavioural or systemic) model of conceptualisation and treatment; rather it is empirically oriented and incorporates the following:

• Available research evidence.
• Making simple (but not simplistic) formulations that encompass aetiological factors in the child, family and environmental (especially school and peer) factors.
• A multi-level and multi-dimensional approach. Most of the problems referred to CAMHS are sufficiently complex and often warrant more than one form of intervention.

In the case of Adam, on the basis of the first assessment session, the main problem was described as follows: Adam showed a considerable degree of noncompliant and defiant behaviours; these behaviours occurred both at home and school but the situation at home was worse than that at school. At home the difficult behaviours were of high frequency and moderate intensity. This constellation of behaviours is commonly described as oppositional defiant behaviour. On the basis of the findings in the first interview it was felt that Adam's behaviours met the criteria for Oppositional Defiant Disorder (ODD).

Although Adam's case looks rather simple and straightforward, it was essential that the clinician considered other possible descriptions to the clinical picture and not bypass the stage of *differential diagnosis*. In Adam's case the other possibilities were:

1 conduct disorder
2 hyperkinetic disorder and
3 adjustment disorder.

The defining feature of conduct disorder (*see* Chapter 12) is the presence of rule-breaking behaviour, i.e. the behaviours that violate the law or basic rights of others; this includes behaviours such as theft, cruelty, bullying, fighting, assault and destructiveness. Adam's pattern of behaviour, as bad as it was, was confined to being negativistic, defiant and disobedient towards authority figures, rather than the violation of rights of others or societal norms. Hyperkinetic disorder (*see* Chapter 9) is characterised by impulsivity, lack of concentration and general over-activity occurring in various situations. There was little indication of these features in Adam. Lastly, some children react to difficulties in adjustment to change in life situations such as parental illness or divorce (*see* Chapter 5) with disturbance in behaviour. In the case of Adam there were no such major life events.

The next step was to consider the possibility of any *coexisting developmental problems*. The commonest developmental problems seen in children presenting to CAMHS are: general intellectual (learning) disability (*see* Chapter 4), specific developmental disorders (sLD) and autism spectrum disorder (ASD, *see* Chapter 7). In Adam's case he was judged to be a bright boy and there was no evidence of autistic features. However, he did show considerable difficulties in reading indicating he had specific reading disorder.

A number of aetiological factors were considered to be important in contributing to Adam's oppositional defiant behaviour:

1 Difficult temperament: Adam appears to have been a temperamentally difficult child from early infancy. Although the period of his early infancy was complicated because of his congenital heart problems and the surgical intervention, he had been a difficult baby with poor sleep, irregular biological rhythms and high levels of activity.
2 Specific reading retardation, sometimes known as dyslexia, has been shown to be consistently related to behaviour problems in children. Specific reading retardation refers to a condition in which there is significant impairment in the development of reading skills which is not solely accounted for by general (global) learning difficulties or other problems.
3 Significant parenting difficulties: By far the most important factor that contributed to and maintained Adam's oppositional behaviour was un-doubtedly the way the parents managed him. Adam's parents were considered to be caring and loving but they had very different styles of parenting. Mr Jones considered himself to be the disciplinarian in the family and had adopted an authoritarian style of parenting. He believed in strict discipline and attempted to exercise a high degree of demand and control while Mrs Jones was rather permissive in her parenting. She demonstrated a high degree of nurturance and warmth but was also overprotective of Adam and infanta-lised him. In addition to their markedly different parenting styles, both parents

were inconsistent in their management of Adam's behaviour, adhering to the rules that they had laid down at certain times and not at other times. It was highly likely that Mr Jones's backache made him less tolerant of Adam's misbehaviours.

Putting together the salient features that were known about Adam and his family's problems, a tentative case formulation or case conceptualisation was made as follows: Adam showed considerable oppositional defiant behaviour both at home and, to a lesser extent, at school. He was of average intelligence but appeared to have specific reading difficulties. The most striking feature in the presentation was the widely different parenting styles of Mr and Mrs Jones. The father's parenting style was authoritarian whereas the mother was more permissive. What's more, they were inconsistent in the way they dealt with Adam. Mr Jones suffered with a bad back that made him irritable and short-tempered, preventing him from being proactive in responding to Adam. Mrs Jones was overprotective, partly because of her experience with Adam soon after his heart operation that made her take extra care of him and partly to compensate for her husband's low frustration tolerance and authoritarian parenting. The distal cause/s of their parenting differences, such as their own parenting experiences as well as their current couple relationship, needed further exploration.

The initial formulation and the possible points of interventions are illustrated in Figure 1.1. No doubt the various elements in the formulation had to be tested in future sessions. More information about Adam's difficulties in reading and writing had to be gathered from school and the educational psychologist. A parents' only session was arranged with the aim of finding out more about the parents' styles of parenting and their roots. A note was made to inquire more about how dad's backache affected the way he managed Adam.

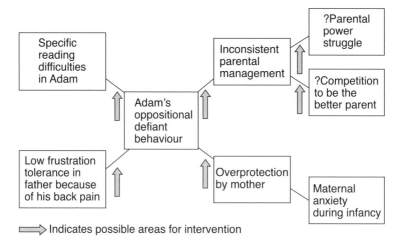

Figure 1.1 Aetiological factors contributing to Adam's oppositional defiant behaviour and the possible points for intervention.

Theoretical perspectives

The diagnostic category of ODD describes a group of behaviours shown by children who exhibit persistent, developmentally inappropriate levels of anger, irritability, defiance and oppositionality which cause functional impairment. Such children have been noted to show verbal aggression and some also display physically aggressive behaviour. Epidemiological studies have shown that the average age of onset of ODD is about 6 years and its overall prevalence is around 3% in boys and girls between the ages of 4 to 18 years (Lahey *et al.*, 1999). The main features of ODD are losing their temper often, arguing often with adults, actively defying or refusing to comply, deliberately annoying people, blaming others, being touchy and easily annoyed (*see* Box 1.1). Such children are often angry or resentful and spiteful or vindictive. In addition some children may show destructiveness such as destroying their toys, punching holes in doors and being deliberately spiteful.

Box 1.1 Key features of oppositional defiant disorder

- Markedly defiant, disobedient and provocative behaviour
- Active defiance of adult requests or rules
- Deliberately annoying people
- Angry, resentful and easily annoyed by other people
- Blaming other people for their mistakes or difficulties
- Lose temper readily

Conduct disorder, as described in DSM IV, is characterised by behaviours that violated the law or basic rights of others. This includes behaviours such as theft, cruelty, bullying, fighting, assault and destructiveness. The oppositional behaviour exhibited by Adam falls short of descriptions of conduct disorder (*see* Chapter 12). Although his aggression and destructiveness to his own toys may be construed as a manifestation of his aggressiveness, he showed no overt rule-breaking behaviours such as theft or fighting outside the home. The difference between ODD and CD appear to be one of degree and severity. An early history of ODD is often present in children later classified as conduct disorder. Many authorities feel that ODD and CD fall on the same continuum and that a significant proportion of children showing oppositional behaviour in early childhood progress on to exhibit the features of conduct disorder.

Disruptive behaviour disorders are determined by the reciprocal interplay of characteristics of the child and the quality of the environment in which he or she develops. The main aetiological factors for ODD have been grouped under child, family and environmental factors. In every case of ODD it is important that the clinician identifies the main risk factors that are relevant to the case.

Child factors: The main individual factors that have been found to be associated with disruptive behaviour disorders are: difficult temperament in the child, specific reading retardation and global learning disability.

Temperament: Temperament refers to the *style* of behaviour (the *how* of behaviour) of children. In what has become a landmark study in child development, Thomas and Chess (1986) identified a number of characteristics that constituted temperament in infants. This included infant attributes such as activity level, threshold for responsiveness and adaptability. From their studies of temperamental characteristics of infants Thomas and Chess identified three temperamental constellations: easy, slow-to-warm-up and difficult. The children in the difficult temperament group had irregularities in biological functions, negative withdrawal responses to new stimuli, non-adaptability or slow adaptability to change, and intense mood expressions that are frequently negative. In their research this group comprised approximately 10% of their sample. When these infants with difficult temperament were followed up over several years, 70% were found to have had behaviour disorders during childhood (Thomas and Chess, 1986). In Adam's case his early temperament is consistent with descriptions of difficult temperament.

Specific reading retardation (SRD), also known as dyslexia, is a relatively common developmental language disorder, with an estimated incidence of around 3–10% of the population. SRD refers to a condition in which there is a specific significant impairment in the development of reading skills which is not solely accounted for by general (global) learning difficulties or other problems. For a diagnosis of specific reading retardation a child's reading performance should be significantly below the level expected on the basis of age, general intelligence and school placement. The condition has a strong genetic basis and is associated with abnormalities at chromosome 15q and 6p but the psychosocial environment too is important as shown by the increased rates in deprived communities. Although the processes involved are not clear, the association between specific reading retardation and conduct problems appears to be a robust one, with one third of the children with specific reading retardation showing ODD.

Other developmental disorders: Intellectual disability, or learning disability and autistic spectrum disorders are associated with externalising problems in children and clinicians need to be skilled in identifying these conditions when making a generic assessment of a child with behaviour problems.

Parental factors: Research has repeatedly shown that a number of individual factors in parents are closely associated with behaviour problems in children. For example, depression in mothers, antisocial behaviour in parents, especially fathers, and high degrees of parental stress are others factors associated with childhood behaviour problems.

Attachment: The other important risk factor for development of behaviour problems in children is the security of parent–child attachment. Attachment refers to the quality of child–parent relationship and has to do with how available, sensitive and responsive the parent is to meet the child's emotional needs. Attachment difficulties in infancy predict behaviour problems in middle childhood. For example, mothers who are unresponsive to their infants have been found to have children with more significant levels of disruptive behaviour during their middle school years relative to mothers who are initially responsive to their infants (Wakschlag and Hans, 1999).

Parenting practices: It is well established that certain parenting practices play an important role in the development of behaviour problems. Empirical studies have shown that discipline that is inconsistent, erratic, harsh and ineffective is associated in the long term with behaviour difficulties in children, as is poor supervision, low warmth and rejection of the child. Patterson's (1982) seminal studies in the development of oppositional and defiant behaviour have identified the various processes involved. He points out that while parents try to train the child to behave better, the children too train their parents to behave in particular ways. Parenting a temperamentally difficult child is not an easy task and many parents unfortunately fall into parenting practices that are ineffective and unrewarding. Two such parenting traps have been described; both serve to exacerbate the child's problematic behaviour, particularly non-compliance.

The *negative reinforcement trap*, as described by Patterson (1982), occurs when a parent issues a direction to a noncompliant child, 'Ben, please pick up your toys'. The child is likely to respond by protesting, refusing to comply with the command and whining. The parent may give in or give up after some time to stop the child protesting or to complete the designated task in a more timely manner. However, doing so unintentionally reinforces the very behaviour that the parent is attempting to avoid. The child learns that loud protestations and defiance are effective in overcoming undesirable parental directions (negative reinforcement). Thus not only does non-compliance increase but so do other behaviours that are precursors of other defiant and oppositional behaviours.

At other times, the parent maybe so frustrated and try to be 'tougher' by shouting, yelling or even becoming physically aggressive with the child when he or she is noncompliant. In this case the child stops protesting and complies out of fear, thereby negatively reinforcing the *parent's* 'tough' behaviour. Over time both parent and child escalate their negative behaviour through the negative reinforcement processes. This results in a coercive and destructive cycle within the parent–child relationship.

Another factor contributing to the development of problem behaviour of children is the *positive reinforcement trap*. In such cases oppositional behaviour is reinforced because a parent responds with attention most frequently when the child misbehaves (spending time with the child talking about why he or she is not compliant). Although parental attention is a necessary feature of good parenting, using it in response to undesirable behaviour creates rather than solves problems. Given intermittently, parental attention to such behaviour becomes a powerful reward for difficult children. The net result of the positive and negative reinforcement traps described above is that the child comes to learn to overcome parental objections through undesirable means and, more importantly, trains the parent to use coercive means to attempt to control behaviour, albeit ineffectively.

Other parental factors associated with child behaviour problems are abuse or extreme forms of coercive parent–child interactions Physical abuse in young children has been found to predict antisocial behaviour, bullying and negative peer relationships.

Environmental factors: Families that experience social and economic deprivation and disadvantage are over-represented in clinical populations of children referred to child mental health services for behaviour problems. Overcrowding, poor neighbourhoods and poverty are important social factors that predispose children to the development of behaviour problems. School and peer influence become more important as the child grows up and his horizons expand.

Prognosis: Behaviour problems in children carry a poor prognosis. Contrary to popular belief, most children with early severe behaviour problems do not 'grow out' of it. This statement needs to be qualified by saying that not all children with disruptive behaviour problems become antisocial adolescents and adults.

Research findings provide strong and consistent evidence that in around 50 percent of preschool and primary school age children showing *clinically significant* behaviour difficulties the problems persist, if not get worse. A number of follow back studies show that in adolescents who are violent about half the group had exhibited aggressive and disruptive behaviour as children. Studies involving adults with antisocial behaviour show that in the vast majority the problems had started in childhood. Thus there is now abundant data to show that early severe behaviour problems tend to persist through middle childhood to adolescence and to adulthood. A number of studies have repeatedly shown that aggressive behaviour problems at age 7 predict conduct problems later.

Choice of treatment and management

Research into treatment of behaviour and conduct problems in children is unanimous in advocating parent training as the most effective form of intervention. The evidence base for parent management training (PMT) is substantial, with established long-term benefits. Individual treatment methods such as counselling and other forms of individual therapy have been shown to be singularly unhelpful in externalising disorders such as ODD and CD (Fonagy *et al.*, 2002). Available evidence favours parent training groups based on empirically validated models as the main form of intervention. PMT is based on principles of social learning theory and teaches parents new ways to manage the child. Most PMT programmes share several common or core elements:

- focusing more on parents rather than the child
- moving from a preoccupation with antisocial behaviour to an emphasis on prosocial behaviour
- teaching parents to identify, define and record child behaviour
- instructing parents in social learning principles
- teaching new parenting skills via didactic instruction, modelling, role playing
- where necessary, addressing parental (e.g. maternal depression), family (e.g marital conflict) and community (e.g. neighbourhood violence) risks, which may interfere with acquisition or maintenance of new parenting skills and adaptive child behaviour

Though these core elements are present in all parent training interventions, programmes differ in the emphasis on each component. There are no less than 10 well researched and validated parent training programmes are. Four of the best known are:

- Helping the noncompliant child (McMahon and Forehand, 2003): This is a popular programme for 3–8-year-olds that has been empirically validated in several studies over the last 30 years. It stressed the importance of teaching procedures and emphasises didactic instruction, modelling and role playing.
- The Oregon Social Learning Centre programme (Patterson and Forgatch, 1995) is targeted at 3–12-year-olds. It is one of the most widely used parent training programmes, having been researched and applied in a wide variety of settings. It is solidly based on the social leaning principles.
- Group Discussion Videotape Modelling programme (The incredible years: Early childhood BASIC parent training programme, Webster-Stratton, 1992): This

programme is used typically with children in the 4–8 year range and emphasises the demonstration of parenting skills through videotaped modelling of skills rather than therapist teaching. A standard set of 10 videotape programmes of modelled parenting skills are shown by the therapist to groups of parents.

- Triple P – Positive Parenting Program (Sanders *et al.*, 2000): Based on a sound behavioural family intervention model, this programme is unique in offering different levels of interventions tailored to the assessed needs of families ranging from telephone support to standard triple P to enhanced triple P.

All the above parent training programmes have been subjected to a number of rigorous studies and have been found to be useful in bringing about various degrees of long-term change in behaviour in children with conduct/oppositional behaviours. Of these, the Webster-Stratton model has been the most influential and has been adopted for use in a number of local authority, educational and CAMHS settings in the UK. A well conducted randomised controlled trial by Scott *et al.* (2001) using this model of parent training in an area of relatively high deprivation in London involving children referred with conduct problems showed a significant and clinically meaningful improvement in their antisocial behaviour and the gains were shown to hold up in follow-up studies conducted one year later.

Management plan for Adam

Considering Adam's treatment needs, it was clear that parent training was the most appropriate method of management. But a parent training group based on the validated models was not available in the local CAMHS or any of the other services. Hence it was decided that parent training be carried out individually with the Jones family. Before commencing the programme a parent-only session was arranged to find out more about their difficulties in parenting and attempt to address them.

Parent sessions

The purpose of the session was to explore with the parents their different ways of parenting, the beliefs behind them and how they viewed each other's attitude to parenting. Mr Jones came up with a long list of Adam's misbehaviours, often repeating himself and going into great detail. Mrs Jones appeared to agree with her husband. It is common for parents who are stressed out by children's behaviour difficulties to use the session to try to tell how terrible the child's behaviours are by giving example after example. Once the extent and nature of the problems are clear, it is more useful for the therapist to focus on other issues rather than engage in problem-saturated conversations. Realising that the session was not achieving any purpose apart from airing parent's unanimous concern about the Adam's bad behaviour, the therapist decided to intervene by finding out what beliefs each of them held about what was causing the problems:

> *Therapist*: What I would like to know at this stage is what ideas each of you has about why Adam behaves the way he does. I would like to do this by asking each of you in turn.

> *Mrs Jones*: I am not sure (hesitates) . . . I feel that Mathew (Mr Jones) expects too much of him. He is only a child . . . (Mr Jones shakes his head and starts to interrupt; therapist gestures at him to prevent him interrupting). He needs more love; I think Mathew is too harsh with him. It does not work. I agree that he needs to be disciplined but . . .'
>
> *Therapist*: You seem to feel that he could be a little more understanding and be a little less demanding of Adam (Mrs Mathew nods). Can you think of an example where Mr Jones has been a 'bit too harsh'?
>
> *Mr Jones*: (interrupting) When he is difficult and violent you have to do something. You can't just let him go on.
>
> *Therapist*: Let me hear what your wife has to say first. I will come to you later. (Addressing Mrs Jones) Can you think of an instance that made you feel he was being somewhat harsh and unreasonable?

Mrs Jones recollected a few occasions when her husband had shouted loud at Adam, lost his temper and sent Adam to his room for what she considered were trivial misbehaviours. Next the therapist addressed Mr Jones.

> *Therapist*: Can I ask you the same question, Mr Jones? What do you attribute Adam's misbehaviours to? Obviously you have very different views from those of your wife.
>
> *Mr Jones*: She is all for Adam. He can do no wrong. With her, he can get away with murder. The other two boys get their share of disciplining but when it comes to Adam, oh, (shakes his head) she is all soft and gives in. The moment she comes from work, he rushes to her with open arms and complaints about me, the boys and everyone. He knows that she will take his side no matter who is at fault.
>
> *Mrs Jones:* It is not fair by him. When others watch television and he has to spend most of the time in his room as punishment. Whatever you might say, Mathew, it is not fair (starts to weep).

This part of the session confirmed the initial hypothesis that there were considerable differences in the way the Jones's parented Adam. Mr Jones believed in an authoritarian style of parenting, delivering commands and wanting Adam to follow them without questioning. Mrs Jones had a very different style of parenting. She was permissive and, in fact, overprotective in the way she parented him. It was difficult to say whether her way of parenting was a way of compensating for Mr Jones' harsh disciplinarian attitudes or if she believed that he needed more love and care, as she put it, than punishment and coercion. It was also clear that the parents disagreed about how Adam should be managed and arguments between the parents on disciplinary issues were common. It was felt that disagreements about parenting ran much deeper in the family and was a reflection of a hidden power struggle between the husband and wife.

When this was addressed in the next parent-only session, Mr Jones openly admitted that he was quite jealous of his wife's successful career, which had made him feel that he had to take a one-down position in the family. This was reinforced by Mrs Jones' parents who had always thought that their daughter had married 'beneath her status'. Mr Jones, therefore, attempted to compensate by being the parent who was better at controlling Adam, thereby proving that he was, at least in one aspect, better than his wife. Mrs Jones was surprised to hear this and was in tears when she heard her husband discuss his perception of his position in the family in a very emotional tone. Another significant factor that emerged during the second interview was that Mr Jones' chronic back problems made him irritable and 'have a short fuse'. He was less tolerant of Adam's behaviour on the days when he had pain but he had not given serious thought to the effect of the pain on his management of Adam.

At this point, it appeared to the therapist that although the issues were clear and the parents were able to discuss their difficulties, it was important to find a way of reframing the problem in a way that could help parents to understand the issues from a different perspective. Reframing is a technique that comes from family therapy, in which the clinician offers the family a different perspective on the situation. Family therapy literature indicates that for reframing to be effective, it should

1 fit with the facts of the case
2 be credible to the family and not be too far-fetched and
3 capitalise on the family's strengths.

The therapist, therefore, put forward a hypothesis for consideration by both parents: 'It appears to me that Adam had been born with a heart defect which required major surgery and hospitalisation. After he was discharged from the hospital and during the time that he was recovering at home, it was Mrs Jones who was looking after him day and night and was, for understandable reasons, very anxious and worried about his recovery and, I am sure, she was quite concerned about Adam's frailty and wondered how he would make a good recovery.' At this point Mrs Jones started describing the period of time when she spent the post-operative period with Adam and how anxiety-provoking it was. She would look at the monitor all the time and wondered what would happen if his heart stopped beating. She could not stop worrying about him, even when he had completely recovered soon after the operation. Even now she would worry about his heart condition and although she had been reassured that the repair had been successful and there were no specific problems at the moment she continued to worry about his heart and his general wellbeing.

The therapist went on to say: 'It is highly likely that soon after the operation and the few years following it, Mrs Jones and Adam developed a very close and, in fact, too close a relationship with Adam. Because of this over-close relationship, Adam looked to her for security, protection and comfort much more than most children of his age would be expected to. As Adam has grown older, matured and become more independent, this relationship, which served an important purpose at the early stages, has become counterproductive. In fact Adam now takes her for granted and expects her to intervene whenever he is distressed, whether it was because of his quarrels with his siblings or being disciplined by Mr Jones.'

There was some discussion between the parents at this stage about how overprotective and over-close Mrs Jones had been and both agreed that it had not been helpful for Adam in the medium term. Although some degree of consensus has been arrived at by the parents about what the problems were, attributing all the problems or most problems to his mother's overprotection would have left her feeling guilty and the husband feeling vindicated ('I was right'). It was felt important, therefore, to address also issues associated with Mr Jones' need to feel in control and be seen in the family as an effective husband who was an equal in the family, rather than being put down by Mrs Jones and her family. Two more parent sessions were scheduled to discuss these issues.

In these sessions there was more information and more material that came to light about long-standing difficulties between the parenting couple and their family of origin experiences. Mr Jones had been brought up in a strict family with an authoritarian father but found himself to be in a powerless position in his current family. He found this very difficult to accept. Adam's defiant behaviour provided him with the opportunity to assert himself as a parent and a family member so that his authority would be respected and counted. The parents decided to work on the power issues and back each other up when it came to disciplining Adam.

As an initial task it was suggested that Mrs Jones, who found disciplining Adam difficult, should learn to do most of the disciplining herself. Her husband's role was to support her and teach her how to discipline Adam, after all he was the 'expert' at disciplining. Thereafter most, if not all, disciplining was to be done by Mrs Jones, and her husband's role would be to help her discipline Adam rather than taking on the role himself. He would provide support, encouragement and teach Mrs Jones how to control and discipline Adam. Two barriers to such course of action were identified. Mr Jones was warned he would find it very difficult to stay out of the disciplining process, his tendency would be to step in and take over, and that he should guard against such action. For Mrs Jones' part, she was bound to feel guilty when she implemented any disciplinary procedure because that would interfere with the special relationship that she had with Adam. Both parents agreed to work on those issues and discuss it amongst themselves and present a united front to the children. It was also agreed that they were not to discuss these issues with the children, especially Adam, and that as a parental couple they would observe boundaries between themselves and the children and implement what they had decided.

For her part Mrs Jones was to help her husband to be aware of his irritability and bad temper on the days that he was suffering with backache. She would 'take over' managing the children on the days he had pain. They were also to make an appointment with their GP to explore the possibility of Mr Jones attending the pain clinic.

During the next parent-only session, they reported that they had discussed the issues that arose out of the previous session and were able to put into practice some of the ideas. With some difficulty Mr Jones had held back and Mrs Jones did 'most of the telling off' of Adam while her husband stood by patiently observing Adam's reactions. They felt that they, as parents, acted together better as a couple.

Liaison with school: Although school did not have great concerns about Adam's behaviour, liaising with school was considered important. In a telephone conversation with the SENCO, the therapist explained the strategies that he was undertaking with the parents and it was agreed, as much as possible, the teachers would employ similar strategies (with advice from the educational psychologist) and also keep in contact with the parents. The individual education plan (IPA) devised by the educational psychologist had recommended special attention to his literacy skills and he was getting 6 hours of help with reading and writing in a small group.

Parent training programme: At this point a parent training programme individualised for the needs of the Jones' family was offered. Parents were seen weekly on their own for the next 10 sessions to discuss parenting skills. The sessions were based on, but not identical to, Barkley's model for management of defiant children (Barkley, 1997). The Barkley model of parent training is a well tested and tried method that has been manualised. It consists of 10 parent sessions and comes with convenient handouts for parents. The sessions are described below as discrete steps although in practice they were there was some overlap and variable amounts of discussion about other related issues.

1 Differential attention

One of the cardinal principles of parent training programmes is the emphasis on focusing on the positive aspects of the behaviour of the child *before* dealing with problematic behaviours. There is an apparent paradox here. While the therapist wants parents to focus on positive behaviours, the parents are interested in talking about (and getting rid of) the problem behaviours. Success at this stage depends on how well the therapist is able to control the session and not be overwhelmed by immediate parental concerns.

The main aim in this phase was to get parents to:

1   pay attention to good behaviours
2   reward good behaviour and
3   learn to ignore bad behaviours.

Mr and Mrs Jones were rather surprised that they were not being asked to target Adam's difficult behaviours. After all, that was the reason they had come to us in the first place. It was explained to them that although Adam's problematic behaviours were frequent, it did not mean that he was misbehaving 100% of the time and it was important to build on the positive behaviours first before concentrating on the bad behaviours. After a discussion about 'what he did right', they were set three tasks and asked to keep notes about their observations so that they could be discussed in the following session:

*   **Special play time:** They were to set aside 30 minutes each day to be their special time with Adam. If possible they would try to make this about the same time each day. Each parent would carry this out at a time of his or her choice. The activity would be chosen by Adam and the play would be led by him. The parent was not to take control of the game or direct it.
*   **Paying attention to desirable behaviour:** Hand in hand with the special playtime, they were asked to attend to Adam's desirable behaviours, praise him as well as show physical affection such as hugs. They were asked to 'catch him being good' and praise him for being well behaved (e.g. 'I am pleased that you did not interrupt me when I was on the phone; I really appreciate it').
*   **Ignoring bad behaviour:** They were to ignore inappropriate behaviours as much as possible by not responding to them verbally or physically and, if necessary, they were to move away from the scene.

At the subsequent session the parents reported that the special play times had gone well except for a few missed days, but Adam's behaviour was as bad as before, if not worse. Mr Jones reported that he was finding it most difficult to ignore bad behaviour but was managing OK. In the next two sessions parents reported some improvement in Adam, not so much in his bad behaviour but in his general attitude toward parents, especially his father. Mrs Jones observed that the relationship between Adam and his father had got better and that Adam appeared to be trying not to upset his dad as before.

2 Compliance training and promoting independent play

The next step was to get Adam to comply with parental requests. The therapist discussed four tasks for the parents to carry out:

- **Paying particular attention to compliance:** When they issued commands as they normally did they were to pay special attention to Adam's compliant behaviours. They were to remain near Adam when they gave him commands and, as in the previous exercise, provide positive attention by making appreciative comments about behaviour such as 'I like it when you put things away after playing with them'.
- **Giving effective commands:** The first rule in giving effective commands is to stop giving unnecessary commands. Adam's parents, especially his mother, was asked to make sure that when they gave commands they meant them, presented them as a single command and did so in a clear serious tone of voice. They were to make sure that distraction such as the TV, music or computer games be reduced or got rid of when they gave commands.
- **'No error' compliance training periods:** These are periods of training during which parents request the child to carry out simple behaviours that are within the child's repertoire. Parents were told to choose a convenient time and ask Adam to carry out a simple request that requires little effort. For example, his mother could ask him to get the tissues or the TV remote control. When such a request was well timed and chosen correctly Adam was bound to carry it out.
- **Promoting independent play and preventing interruptions:** One of Adam's behaviours that the parents resented most was his tendency to interrupt and disrupt parental activities such as talking on the telephone, speaking to visitors or when they did the cooking. Speaking on the telephone was chosen as the 'battle ground'. The strategy here was to (1) prepare him before the parent started speaking on the phone by saying that he or she was going to be on the phone for the next 10 minutes or so and that he was not to interrupt during this period and (2) assigning an activity he liked such as playing quietly with his toy cars. The crucial component of the exercise was for the parent to reinforce Adam's good behaviour by intermittently stopping the telephone conversion and praising him for not interrupting. At the beginning they were to praise him every minute and later after longer intervals. In behavioural terms this is a simple shaping procedure that is easy for the parents to carry out.

The following week the parents said they were just beginning to understand what the programme was designed to achieve. In spite of the various demands on them they had carried out the three tasks and felt that Adam was responding positively to them. They had decided to try out the same procedures with the other two children and found that it was working. Mr Jones felt that the relationship between him and Adam had improved and that they were doing lots of things together. But his bad behaviour, especially the temper tantrums and misbehaviour at mealtime, were not any better.

3 Daily behaviour chart and establishing a point system

In the next part of the training programme the concept of token economy was introduced. Parents were told that it was time to start a system of tangible rewards. Mr Jones was quick to point out that they had tried the method previously and found it to be useless. Adam would start arguing about the rewards and had thrown tantrums over getting the rewards anyway! It is not uncommon for parents to be demoralised by their previous failed attempts and feel less confident about carrying out another reward scheme. The therapist pointed out that most programmes fail because they are not designed properly and executed rigorously.

It was explained that the principle behind any rewards or privileges programme is to make it strictly contingent upon child compliance; the rewards need to be tangible and powerful; and they need to be administered consistently and systematically. To set up an effective point system, the parents should:

- decide which behaviours earn points; the behaviours should be defined precisely and in behavioural terms
- choose how many points will be awarded to each behaviour
- select a list of special treats or rewards
- determine how many points must be earned to receive a treat or reward
- monitor the child's behaviour and award points.

The parents were keen to target Adam's behaviours that they considered the most difficult. Following some discussion it was agreed that positive behaviours should be reinforced first and that the point system was not to be used primarily as punishment for bad behaviour. The parents felt Adam would be able to understand a 'smiling face' sticker rather than the abstract point system. One of the behaviours to be targeted was getting ready in the mornings. Since this is a composite behaviour consisting of several acts and because this had been a long-standing problem, it was decided to break the behaviour down into its component parts and focus initially on getting dressed in the mornings. It was agreed that the school clothes would be laid out on the bed and Adam would be expected to put them on. This would earn him one smiley face. He was perfectly capable of this and was more likely to carry it out rather than the chain of behaviours leading up to being ready for school. The second behaviour to be rewarded was *not* arguing with parents. (If the parents were wrong they were to own up immediately). Since arguing was a high frequency behaviour for Adam, it was agreed that he would be provided one smiling face each for not arguing between certain time periods such as getting up and breakfast, between lunch and dinner and for the period of time from dinner to bedtime. The third behaviour to be reinforced was putting his toys away after playing with them following one reminder by the parents. This was included so that Adam would find it easy to accomplish this and consequently earn points anyway. He would be awarded one smiley face for this task.

A list of rewards were to be agreed upon (*see* Box 1.2). Initially rewards would be awarded on a daily basis and once he was used to the system he might save up the smiling faces for larger rewards like going biking or fishing with his father, both of which he loved. Adam's behaviour and reward chart is shown in Figure 1.2.

Box 1.2 Reinforcement menu for Adam (7 years)

- Use of computer game for extra half hour (2 smiley faces)
- Special snack at bedtime (3 smiley faces)
- Bike riding with dad (8 smiley faces)
- Fishing with dad (10 smiley faces)
- Watching favourite video (4 smiley faces)
- Get a friend over for the day (12 smiley faces)
- Mystery reward (15 smiley faces)

Behaviour	Monday	Tuesday	Wednesday	Thursday	Friday
Getting dressed in the morning	☺	☺		☺	
Not arguing with parents (morning)	☺		☺	☺	☺
Putting toys away	☺	☺		☺	☺
☺ Total smiling faces	3	2	1	3	2

Daily reward: According to the reinforcement menu (*see* Box 1.2)

Figure 1.2 Adam's daily behaviour chart.

4 Using time out

When seen two weeks later the reward system appeared to have been successful and Adam had earned at least one reward each day. His morning behaviour in getting dressed had been achieved quite readily and the parents were hoping to extending it to include brushing his teeth and washing his face. However, his temper tantrums and rude behaviours when he got angry remained unchanged. At this stage the parents were introduced to the idea of using time out for discrete misbehaviours.

Time out from positive reinforcement (TO) is a well-tried and tested method that works exceptionally well as long as it is tailored for the specific family. Detailed descriptions of the procedure as well as handouts to parents are available in most behavioural manuals (e.g. Barkley, 1997; McMahon and Forehand, 2003). The basic principle in the time out procedure is to remove the child from all forms of reinforcement whenever the child exhibits the target behaviour. In Adam's case the parents identified his temper tantrums as one of the behaviours that they wanted to overcome. Since the word temper tantrums may mean different things to the parents and Adam, it was decided to use time out for certain defined aggressive behaviours. Initially they were to target the following:

1 being violent or threatening towards mother and
2 being destructive to toys, throwing or kicking things.

The basic principles of TO were explained to the parents in some detail. The key elements of the time-out procedure are:

* Giving a clear command ('Stop hitting'); count from 5 to 1.
* Give warning that you will use TO; count down from 5 to 1.
* Get child to the chair located in a boring area.
* Get child to stay in chair for 3–5 minutes plus 15 seconds of quiet period.
* Release from TO; no discussions, apologies etc.

In Adam's case, the parents were used to sending him to his room when he misbehaved. This was hardly effective because he had all his toys in his room and would happily play with them. Following discussion they agreed to use a chair placed at the bottom of the stairs for the TO procedure. Initially his father would be around when his mother used TO to ensure that she was able to carry it through. Siblings were to keep out of the scene as much as possible so that Adam did not feel humiliated. The parents were given a handout on TO. They were warned that Adam's behaviour may get worse before getting better because he was bound to test out their resolve to carry out the procedure. They were encouraged to keep a record of the circumstances in which they used TO. They were warned that of all the skills they had learned TO was by far the most difficult to implement, especially for his mother.

When reviewed two weeks later the record indicated that they had used TO only five times (they had expected to use it several times a day) and, more importantly, Mrs Jones had been able to implement it without much difficulty. Asked what they had learned from all this they said they felt that, after all, the problems were not that bad and that they were getting better at being assertive, consistent and acting as a parental couple.

5 Using the daily school behaviour report card

The next step in the programme was the introduction of a home-based reinforcement procedure for school behaviours. The aim was to target behaviour problems Adam was exhibiting at school. They were asked to discuss with his teacher the sort of behaviours that the school wanted changed and design a special school report card. Having identified the target behaviours the teacher would fill in the card each day and sign it (Figure 1.3). The parents would review the card each day, find out from the child what happened and reward good behaviours as before according to an agreed system of points. Mr Jones was to meet the teacher every fortnight and discuss the reports.

The school report card system turned out to be a remarkable success. In two weeks Adam had stopped fighting with his classmates and his school card showed that he was behaving well in class and at break times.

Behaviour	Period					
	1	2	3	4	5	6
Keeps seated in class						
Keeps to rules at break times						
Gets along with peers						
Cooperates in class work						

Please rate each of the child's behaviour indicated above from 0 to 4.
(4 = excellent, 3 = good, 2 = fair, 1 = poor and 0 = bad)

Comments and teacher's initials:

Figure 1.3 Daily school behaviour report.

Up to this point in time the programme was working well and Adam was responding positively. His behaviour had shown vast improvement and his parents were quite pleased with themselves and Adam's behaviour. At this juncture an incident occurred that had the potential to throw the whole programme into doubt and disarray. On a Saturday morning when everyone was in bed Adam had come down to the kitchen, taken the bread knife and chopped off the kitchen tabletop and smashed the shelves. When Mrs Jones came down the kitchen was like a war zone. She found Adam in the living room watching television. The other children were in bed and Mr Jones had gone to work early in the morning. There was no doubt that Adam was the culprit. When questioned he completely denied any knowledge of it and continued to watch television. Her first impulse was to telephone her husband at work or telephone the therapist for advice. After overcoming the shock and after some calm reflection she decided to confront Adam. He vehemently held onto his initial position that he did not know anything about it. She resolved to act decidedly. She emptied his room of all the toys and the computer, asked him to go to his room and be there until he was ready to accept that he had carried out the 'attack'.

About noon she asked him to come down and get dressed. Adam was surprised and asked 'Why?' She firmly replied that the two of them were going to the police station. She had wrapped the knife that Adam had used in polythene and was taking it to be tested for fingerprints. The police would be able to say who had used it and take necessary action. At this point Adam started crying and admitted he had done it. She told him that he would be punished for it and proceeded to carry on with her duties. Although she had pretended to be in control and acted with certainty, she was deeply troubled by what had happened and was at a loss as to why Adam had behaved so appallingly.

Mrs Jones turned up at the next session with the kitchen knife wrapped up in a bag and talked about the above incident. She was particularly worried about the meaning of the act. She wondered whether the destruction wrecked on the kitchen represented an attack on her and wanted to know where all this anger against her came from. Mr Jones got back to his familiar theme that 'something must be wrong with him'. They started doubting the recent improvements in Adam and felt it was just a temporary phase and that there was some deep-seated problem in Adam that had to be addressed.

It was clear to the therapist that the incident had undermined their confidence and made them revert back to their default mode of thinking leading to catastrophic thinking and doubting the effectiveness of the programme. After listening to them the therapist pointed out that, in spite of her current concerns, Mrs Jones had acted most appropriately; she had dealt with Adam calmly, she had not panicked nor she called her husband, but acted with firmness and determination. Whatever her doubts were, she had not allowed them to interfere with the way she handled him. She was commended for the way she kept her cool and called Adam's bluff – something that she would have not done just a month ago. Her husband readily agreed and said that he was surprised that she had acted so firmly and resolutely. The therapist then went on to explain that since parents were now becoming good at taking control rather than giving in to Adam, he must have wondered what was going on and decided to test it out, albeit unconsciously. They were reminded about the discussion about how things may get worse before getting better. The incident, they were told, is best treated as a temporary set-back, a blip, rather than a disaster. It was proof that they were getting better at managing him.

As it happened, this incident turned out to be the turning point in the programme. The parents returned to implementing the programme and never looked back. They were more confident than ever before about their ability to deal with Adam's misbehaviours. There were no further critical incidents. The next step, according to the original plan, was to manage Adam's behaviour outside home.

6 Managing behaviour outside home

Some of Adam's disruptive behaviours occurred when he was taken to shops, public places or when travelling by car. A review of such typical scenarios occurring outside home indicated that the parents were not proactive in planning for such eventualities. Rather, they responded to them as and when they arose, leading to an escalation of coercive behaviour on the part of both the child and the parents. A new strategy was devised that involved the following:

- Preparing Adam for the event and telling him what was expected of him once outside (e.g. going to the store) and repeating it before entering the place.
- Establishing a reward system for good behaviour in the store such as points or smiling faces.
- Designating an activity for Adam to perform while in the store. This would usually take the form of helping in shopping such as finding certain items. While travelling by car he was to help find the route or read the signposts to 'assist' dad.

- The parents were to make sure that the time that they would spend with Adam in public places or travelling was initially as short as possible so that he would not get bored. Also the parents were not to change their mind on these occasions and prolong the time they spent on the task.

During the next week the parents were to practice applying the above principles by arranging two fake trips, one with each parent, to stores or other public places with the explicit purpose of trying out the above steps.

Toward the end of the programme, the parents were successful in carrying out most of the tasks assigned to them in the sessions and were seeing significant change in Adam's behaviour. The point system was in operation, the daily school report card was being implemented, the parents were spending special time with Adam and were using TO when necessary. It had taken 12 sessions over a period of 30 weeks to achieve results. They reported that they were finding it rewarding to spend time with Adam. The last session was about what they had learned from the programme and how they could apply the principles to any future behaviour problems.

Course and outcome

The family was seen six weeks later for a routine follow-up. The improvement in Adam's behaviour had been maintained apart from minor setbacks. The parents felt that they were managing Adam better. Adam was seen on his own to say goodbye. He was happy that his behaviour was better and was pleased his father was not shouting at him. Everyone, including his teacher, had been telling him what a good boy he had become. He attributed all the improvements to the fact that he was growing up, becoming a 'big boy'. At this stage his three magic wishes now were:

1 to become a football player
2 to catch a large fish next time he went fishing with dad and
3 to have any wish he wanted!

After discharge from the clinic there was no contact from the family but in a casual conversation with the GP about a year later the therapist learned that he had seen the family recently and Adam was 'fine'.

Comments

The management of Adam's behaviour difficulties illustrates some of the principles that underpin the treatment of children with ODD. Before embarking on parent training (in groups or individually) issues that pertain to the parent level of organisation need to be addressed. Invariably these involve possible parental conflicts, depression or physical illness in either parent or other problems associated with the family.

Many well intentioned parent training programmes fail because the therapist does not anticipate barriers and prepare parents adequately. Structuring each session is important in order to avoid parents going back to the 'complaining mode'. Some parents complain a lot about the child's behaviour but do little to change it. The therapist should start the session by reviewing homework and outline the plan of the current session rather than going back on what the child's last misbehaviour was.

Parent training involves a degree of commitment and motivation on the part of parents. While the effectiveness of parent training programmes is well established in research trials, in practice, this effectiveness is reduced by high attrition; it is estimated that between 40% and 60% of families do not complete treatment. Many low income families with multiple family and social problems find the demands of the programme too onerous and often drop out of treatment. Studies comparing group with individual parent training programmes show that the former achieves better levels of change and are more effective. Moreover, they are more economical, provide support to families, especially isolated families, and enhance their self-confidence (Richardson and Joughin, 2002)

Sadly, parent training groups based on validated models mentioned above are not available in some, if not many, areas of the country. It would be hard to deny the public access to a drug that has been repeatedly shown to be effective for a particular condition. Yet, in child mental health, parenting programmes (the treatment) is not available in many parts of the country. No doubt there are numerous 'parenting groups' run by a number of services including social services, voluntary agencies and youth offending services. But many services continue to use ineffective, non-empirically supported parent training methods or non-evaluated parenting and family support programmes. The NICE guidelines on parent training for conduct disorder reinforces this message (NICE, 2006).

Box 1.3 Research on Oppositional Defiant Disorder (ODD) in children shows that . . .

- ODD occurs in about 3% of children and is one of the most common reasons for referral to CAMHS.
- Parent training is the treatment of choice and is best carried out in groups and based on empirically validated methods such as the Webster-Stratton model.
- Parental and family issues may have to be addressed before embarking on parent training.
- Non-specific, poorly structured individual forms of treatments such as generic counselling, dynamic therapy, and individual work are ineffective.
- The majority of children with ODD do not 'grow out' of it; ODD is often a precursor to the development of conduct problems in adolescents and antisocial behaviour in adults.

References

* Barkley RA. *Defiant Children: a clinician's manual for assessment and parent training*. 2nd edn. New York: Guilford Press; 1997.

Fonagy P, Target M, Cottrell D *et al. What Works For Whom? A critical review of treatments for children and adolescents* (Chapter 5). New York: Guilford Press; 2002.

Harris DB. *Children's Drawings as a Measure of Intellectual Maturity: a revision and extension of Goodenough draw-a-man test*. New York: Harcourt, Brace & World; 1963.

Lahey B, Miller B, Gordon TL *et al*. Developmental epidemiology of disruptive behaviour disorders. In: Quay HC, Hogan A, editors. *Handbook of Disruptive Behaviour Disorders*. New York: Plenum Press; 1999.

* McMahon RJ, Forehand RL. *Helping the Noncompliant Child: family-based treatment for oppositional behaviour*. 2nd edn. New York: Guilford Press; 2003.

National Institute for Health and Clinical Excellence and Social Care Institute for Excellence. *Parent-Training/Education Programmes in the Management of Children with Conduct Disorders* (Number 102). London: Department of Health; 2006. Available at: www.nice.org.uk/TA102

Patterson GR, Forgatch MS. Predicting future clinical adjustment from treatment outcome and process variables. *Psychological Assessment*. 1995; **7**: 275–85.

Patterson GR. *Coercive Family Process*. Eugene, OR: Castalia Press; 1982.

* Richardson J, Joughin C. *Parent Training Programmes for the Management of Young Children with Conduct Disorder: Findings from research*. London: Gaskell; 2002.

Sanders MR, Markie-Dadds C, Turner KMT *et al*. *Triple P – Positive Parenting Program. A guide to the system*. Brisbane, QLD: Families International Publishing; 2000.

Scott S, Spender Q, Doolan M *et al*. Multicentre controlled trial of parenting groups for childhood antisocial behaviour. *British Medical Journal* 2001; **323**: 194–8.

Thomas A, Chess S. *Temperament in Clinical Practice*. New York: Guilford Press; 1986.

Wakschlag LS, Hans SL. Relation of maternal responsiveness during infancy to the development of behaviour problems in high risk youth. *Developmental Psychology*. 1999; **35**: 569–79.

* Webster-Stratton C. *The Incredible Years*. Toronto: Umbrella Press; 1992.

Chapter 2

Adolescent depression

A worried and concerned GP telephoned CAMHS to say that he had just seen a 16-year-old girl, who he thought was depressed and suicidal. He wanted her to be seen as soon as possible. During the telephone discussion the GP said that he had known the family for some time and that both parents were teachers and he was not aware of any particular family issues that may have a bearing on Sarah's current depression. The parents had been extremely concerned about Sarah's recent behaviour. Although she had been attending school, she had been keeping herself away from the rest of the family and refused to talk to them. She would withdraw herself to her room and play her music and come down only for meals. She was said to be irritable and snappy and be 'nasty' to all members of the family. She broke into tears at the slightest provocation and said things like, 'Nobody loves me; nobody cares for me'. No amount of reassurance by parents had made her feel any better. Parents had noticed this change in her behaviour over the last 8 months or so but could not identify any particular precipitant or event that may have caused the problem.

The parents had initially attributed her behaviour to normal adolescent moodiness and hoped that Sarah would eventually grow out of it. However, the previous day the mother had discovered a letter under Sarah's pillow. The mother had brought the letter to show the GP. It read as follows:

> Dear Mum & Dad
>
> I feel so terrible that life does not mean anything to me. The mental pain that I go through day in day out is so severe that I do not think life is worth living any more. You may not understand the mental torture that I have been going through over the last few months. It is difficult to explain what these experiences are to someone who had never known it. I am fed up with the struggle and I do not want to live any more. I want you to know I love you.
>
> Love
>
> Sarah

Sarah had been at school on the day her mother discovered the letter. After reading the letter, the parents had spoken to Sarah. She had broken down and cried her heart out. Both Sarah and her parents were unable to understand why Sarah should be so depressed. The GP wanted Sarah to be seen urgently.

Clinical presentation and background

Sarah and her family were offered an appointment the next day. The parents appeared quite worried and anxious as they outlined Sarah's problems. They described Sarah as a bright and conscientious girl. She was particularly good in English and was good at creative writing. She had a good group of friends but often kept changing her friends. They had considered Sarah's irritability and mood fluctuations to be part of normal growing up and felt that it was 'the effect of hormones'. She liked school and had been attending school regularly. Of late she had dropped out of sports and her grades too had been slipping recently. The parents attributed this to the increasing demands that were placed upon her because of the oncoming exams. She did go out with one or two of her friends and there were no problems about coming home late, as was the usual case with teenagers.

Her mother said that she was shocked to have discovered Sarah's letter under the pillow. After reading it she had called her husband at work in a state of great distress. She admitted she had not realised how troubled Sarah had been over the last few months. She was in tears when she said that she had had a close relationship with Sarah but had become out of touch with Sarah's feelings more recently. At this point Sarah too was in tears but said very little. Sarah's father was concerned about the situation but he felt that Sarah was full of self-pity and should 'shake herself out of the depression'.

The family consisted of the parents, Mr and Mrs Wood, both of whom were teachers; the mother was head teacher at a primary school and the father taught science in a local secondary school. They had been married for the last 18 years. Sarah was the elder of the two children; her younger sister was 13 years of age and was described as a lively and outgoing. There were no particular family stressors, except for her maternal grandmother who had been admitted to hospital recently for what was later diagnosed as cancer of the bowel. She was reasonably well at the time of the interview, having had surgery but required frequent visits by Sarah's mother to check on her.

Sarah was preparing for her GCSE examinations and the parents felt that she was under considerable pressure to achieve high grades but they felt that the pressure came from Sarah, rather than from them. They described Sarah as a competitive person who wanted to excel in all the activities that she undertook, including schoolwork. Sarah had been a good violinist and had been taking regular lessons but had given them up recently and the parents felt that this was because of the increasing demands of her schoolwork. She was described as a voracious reader and a good writer.

When asked about any family history of depression or 'nerves', initially the family denied any such history. It later transpired, in the following sessions, that the grandmother had suffered from depression and been on antidepressants on a number of occasions. There had been a recurrence of her depression after surgery and she was taking antidepressants again. The mother described herself as an anxious person who had experienced panic attacks in the past and been scared of being in enclosed spaces but had largely overcome these difficulties without any help. It also became clear in later sessions with the family that the father had suffered a severe episode of depression soon after the birth of Sarah that lasted almost a year. The mother described this as a reaction to becoming a father, a role that he had been unprepared for. He had been seen by a psychiatrist and been on antidepressants during this period. These were closely held family secrets about which the children had little knowledge.

Sarah's developmental history was unremarkable. Apart from the usual minor infections of childhood, Sarah had not had any particular medical illness. She was described generally as a healthy child. Academically she was described as clever. She had taken to school quite well both in nursery and primary school. There were no particular separation problems when she started school. She had always had few friends and preferred to have one or two close friends, rather than a crowd. However, she fell out with her friends frequently and then felt rejected by her peers. Her parents described her as a girl who had intense feelings towards people; either she liked them or hated them. She was also described as somebody who was quite judgemental in her assessment of other people. She had strong moral values and was very critical most of her peers. Recently she had become very sceptical about the media and the adult world in general. She had refused to watch television news because she felt it was quite biased and 'manufactured'. She was keen to please both her parents and teachers. She was an accomplished musician and although somewhat shy, she could give a good performance in school events.

Examination: When seen individually, Sarah appeared eager to talk about her problems. She was assured of confidentiality but with the caveat that where her safety is concerned, it would be important for the clinician to discuss it with her parents and make sure that she was kept safe. In order to encourage rapport and 'break the ice', the initial part of the conversation was about neutral topics, like school and friends and her writing. Sarah said that she liked school and the schoolwork; she got on reasonably well with the teachers but she had few friends. She had fallen out with one of her friends and felt betrayed by her. She went into some detail about what happened.

When asked how she would describe her personality, Sarah thought for a while and then described herself as a quiet and shy person who lacked confidence, especially in the presence of young people of her age. She said that she was good with young children and adults but sometimes found it difficult to manage the demands placed on her by her peers. She described herself as ambitious and wanting to be a career woman. She had a good knowledge of world affairs and was particularly concerned about poverty in Africa and the state of children in Third World countries. She was an avid reader and read both fiction and non-fiction. She also wrote short stories and poems but had not shown them to anyone. She had taken music lessons from a young age and was good at the violin. She described her relationship with her parents in non-specific terms. She felt that recently she had been withdrawing herself from the family. She found it difficult to confide in her mother or father. The last occasion in which she had discussed her problems with her mother was when she was 12 years of age. She felt she should keep some of her experiences and thoughts private.

She said she found it difficult to understand some of the kids in her class because, in her view, they put up a front and wanted to be somebody else. She hated the pop culture and the celebrity-oriented discussions that went on in school. She said that she was not a 'Barbie' but a 'Bratz'. She explained this to mean that she did not fit the feminine stereotype but wanted to have her own personality. She felt that most of her peers lacked depth and were 'silly'. She was somewhat derogative of her female peers and said, 'All that they are interested in is how many inches their skirts are above the knees'. She was particularly irritated by her younger sister, whom she described as outgoing, extroverted and having a large number of friends. But she said such people are shallow and although they appear happy they were not, they are only putting up a front. When asked about whether she puts up a front, Sarah said she hides her inner feelings and tries to appear as if everything was normal but it was getting increasingly difficult to be 'play acting all the time'. Sarah was close to tears when talking about this.

Mental state examination: A mental state examination was carried out and is given below in the conventional order, although the information was collected through an open-ended interview.

Appearance: For someone of her age Sarah appeared somewhat carelessly dressed. She was in a pair of jeans, a top and trainers. She had not taken the trouble to put on any make-up. She was somewhat plump though not obese. During the family interview she had appeared withdrawn and said very little. But when seen on her own, after some initial reluctance, she appeared animated and lively.

Behaviour: During the interview with the family Sarah said very little and allowed her parents to tell the story. She avoided eye contact, preferring to look at the floor or outside the window and on many occasions she came very close to tears, especially when parents were taking about how worried they were about her and how much they loved her. Sarah slumped in to the chair and during the whole course of the interview there was very little spontaneous movement. However, during the individual interview, she was a little more animated and maintained good eye contact and tried her best to express herself clearly. On a number of occasions Sarah broke down and had to be given a box of tissues. There were long periods of silences and the interview had to be paced according to her emotional state.

Speech: Sarah spoke in a monotonous, low-toned voice but expressed herself clearly and coherently. She often paused to think about the question and gave thoughtful answers.

Mood: Sarah said that (subjectively) her mood had been quite depressed over the last 12–18 months; she was unclear as to when it started. She said it crept on her like a dark cloud and engulfed her. It was worse when she was on her own, especially when she was at home. She felt a little better when she was with friends and this was one of the reasons why she continued to attend school. She said that she found it difficult to talk to friends, even on topics of mutual interest, because she found the effort tiring. It was as if she could not be bothered to talk to people or explain her view or experiences. She said she felt exhausted most of the time; she called it 'mental exhaustion'. Objectively she appeared depressed, with furrows in her forehead and drawn down angle of the mouth. During the entire individual interview, which lasted about 40 minutes, Sarah did not smile even once. She did not appear to brighten up even when talking about her friends and her music or writing. She said her mood was somewhat better in the morning, especially when she was at school, but on returning home she felt depressed and lonely and unloved.

In the past she had enjoyed both playing music and listening to music but more recently she had found this more of an effort. She did not like noise. She avoided watching the television or listening to the radio and often kept the window blinds drawn in her room. She admitted she cried to herself quite a lot for no particular reason. She had not been eating very well but was not sure whether she had lost any weight. She said she did not care the way she looked. She fell asleep quite late at night and her sleep was disturbed throughout the night. She had lost enjoyment in life and did not even enjoy the food she ate. She said she ate to please her parents. She said it felt as if something had been taken away from her and that there was a large hole in her. She felt empty and drained of anything worthwhile. She felt that her friends did not like her and were talking behind her back. Asked about her parents, she said 'I don't think anybody loves me but I know my parents love me'. She paused at his point as she appeared to be aware of the contradiction in the statement. She said she felt lonely and alone in the world and was fighting her battles on her own. She said she felt like a tired soldier who was giving up in mid-battle. It was better for her to lie down and die rather than carry on the struggle. Life itself had become a burden and even the efforts by others to help her were more of a burden. Describing it in poetic terms she said, 'It is as if the oars themselves have become too heavy to paddle.' She admitted that she had lost interest in the things that she liked previously, such as playing the violin and listening to music. Previously she used to telephone her friends and that used to have an uplifting effect but now she had stopped doing it because she was not sure whether she was bothering friends with her problems. She had become irritable and snappy with her parents and shouted back at them at the slightest provocation but regretted this later. She did not know why she felt angry about minor things. She said, 'I don't like the way I am.'

Thoughts: Sarah was convinced that she was never going to improve and that things would only get worse. She was pessimistic about the past, present and the future. She said she had the feeling that she was going to die when she was 17 and went on to say that many people died young and that it did not matter. On a number of occasions she had had thoughts of killing herself. The following is an excerpt from the interview:

> *Clinician*: When did you first notice such thoughts?
>
> *Sarah*: I am not sure . . . it was probably about eight months ago when I began to feel badly down and depressed
>
> *Clinician*: What sort of things usually lead up to these thoughts?
>
> *Sarah*: I remember at the beginning it happened soon after I fell out with Helen (her friend). I thought nobody really liked me or wanted to be friends with me. It was awful . . . (starts crying).
>
> *Clinician*: When Helen and you fell out you felt rejected and upset (nods her head). How often have the thoughts of dying been occurring recently?
>
> *Sarah*: Almost everyday, usually in the evenings when I am on my own; some days are worse than others.
>
> *Clinician*: How close have you come to acting upon those thoughts?
>
> *Sarah*: I don't think I have the courage to harm myself; I am a coward, I think. I keep thinking about it but never do anything about it.

Clinician: How likely do you think you will act upon them in the future?

Sarah: I am not sure. It is getting more and more difficult and one day I may not be able to stop myself.

Clinician: Have you ever made any specific plan to harm or kill yourself? If so, what did it include?

Sarah: Not really. I write a letter or something like that. It helps to get it out. But I keep crying after writing and imagine all sorts of things.

Clinician: Such as . . .

Sarah: Scenes of my death. I get pictures of my funeral in my mind . . . I think I am weird (laughs impassively).

Clinician: We have been discussing the reasons for why you feel like harming yourself. Can you tell me what reasons do you think you have for living?

Sarah brought out a smile and said that her parents loved her, her teachers liked her, especially her form teacher; she was hoping to be a journalist, and perhaps become a writer of fiction. The conversation then took a turn towards discussion of positive aspects of her life and her strengths.

She appeared also to feel helpless and thought that nobody or anything in the world could help her to overcome her sense of desperation. She felt guilty that she was letting her parents down and if she were to die, her family would grieve her death. She said she had visions of her funeral and kept imagining as to who and who would attend the funeral, where it would be held and how others would behave during the funeral. She said that the school would send a wreath, which would be carried by two of her best friends, but everyone would forget about her as soon as the funeral was over. She said that she often thought about death and dying and found it difficult to get rid of these thoughts from her mind.

Perceptual abnormalities: Sarah had denied hearing voices or seeing things that were not there.

Cognitive functions: Sarah said that her concentration was poor and often she was not paying attention to what went on in class. Many of her friends had commented on how she had become ill-tempered, which was unusual for her. Sarah came across as academically average, if not above average. Her memory was good but appeared to be selective for negative events.

Insight: Sarah knew that she was depressed but was not sure what caused it or the nature of it. All she could say was that a dark cloud had descended on her and she found it difficult to get rid of it. She blamed herself for her problems and attributed it to her 'weakness of character' and lack of confidence in herself. 'Somehow I fell that I am not as good as the other kids,' she said.

Risk assessment: Sarah had thoughts of self-harm and was actively suicidal. She had not made specific attempts to harm herself or act upon her suicidal thinking partly because of the depth of her depression and the lack of motivation to do 'anything'. It was noted that the level of risk could be expected to increase when she started recovering from the depression and her mental state began to improve.

Case conceptualisation and formulation

It was clear from the mental state examination that Sarah was severely depressed. Her mood was persistently low and had been so for the last 12 months or so. The onset had been insidious, so much so that her parents had taken it seriously. She was withdrawn and had been avoiding social interaction both with her family and with her friends; she had been having frequent thoughts of harming herself; she had a pervading sense of hopelessness and pessimism; she was preoccupied with thoughts of death, her funeral etc. and had a sense of a foreshortened future. A key feature of Sarah's mental state was anhedonia, i.e. lack of enjoyment. Sarah was not able to enjoy playing or listening to music, something she had liked intensely in the past. Her anhedonia was so severe that she was not even enjoying the food she ate. The most significant finding on mental state examination was the degree of suicidal ideation and hopelessness present in Sarah. Although she had not made any specific plans or attempts to harm herself, she was preoccupied with the thought of killing herself. It appeared that she was so sucked of mental energy that she did not have the will or volition even to make a suicide attempt. It was obvious that Sarah exhibited features of severe and extreme clinical depression with suicidal ideation. Sarah's presentation fulfils the criteria for diagnosis of clinical depression. The main features of clinical depression are given in Box 2.1 at the end of this chapter.

The possibility that the current depressive episode might have been part of a bipolar disorder (manic depression) had to be considered. Bipolar disorder is characterised by episodes of depression and mania or hypomania.

The factors that contributed to her depression were unclear. There was a strong family history of depression; her father and her grandmother appear to have suffered from episodic depression. In Sarah's case there did not appear to be any particular life events or losses that may have accounted for the depression. The loss of friendship with her classmate was significant for Sarah and in later sessions she spoke of it at some length. The lack of any immediate or remote precipitating factors made it all the more significant, for the depression appeared to be endogenous in nature rather than reactive. Although she was managing to attend school, she was otherwise hardly functioning. A particular area of Sarah's difficulties appeared to be around peer relationships. She had very few friends and appeared to be moving from one group of friends to another and had not yet found a suitable friendship group. Based on the above understanding of Sarah's difficulties the following formulation was made:

> Sarah is a 16-year-old teenager who had been experiencing severe clinical depression over the last 12 months with suicidal ideation. The onset had been insidious and there did not appear to be major precipitants. There was a strong family history of depression and her father was depressed at the time, although he was functioning reasonably well. It was hypothesised that parents were also experiencing difficulties in understanding and adjusting to the developmental needs of their teenage daughter. Sarah was considered to be an intelligent girl with varied interests and good pre-morbid functioning. However, she had significant difficulties in making and sustaining satisfactory peer relationships, which may have contributed to continuing feelings

of poor self-concept, lack of self-confidence and low self-esteem. She was considered to be at high risk of harming herself.

Theoretical perspectives

The identification of clinical depression in adolescents is made difficult by the fact that mood swings are common during teens ('the moody teenager'). Sometimes such mood swings can last for months and have a depressive quality making it difficult to distinguish between intense misery and depressive disorders. In the Isle of Wight study of adolescents, where more than 2000 14- and 15-year-olds were surveyed, Rutter *et al.* (1976) found that on self-reported measures more than 40% reported misery.

The term 'depression' has a range of meanings from a description of normal unhappiness, through persistent and pervasive ways of feeling, to depressive psychosis. As Richard Harrington (2002) has put it, 'Defining the boundaries between extremes of normal behaviour and psychopathology is a dilemma that pervades all of psychiatry. It is especially problematic to establish the limits of depressive disorder in young people because of the cognitive and physical changes that take place during this time'. Like most emotional disorder, depression falls along a continuum from normal adolescent mood swings, described above, at one end of the spectrum to clinical depression or depressive disorder at the other end (*see* Figure 2.1).

Depressive reactions to minor events and transient depressive states are quite common in adolescents. It has been estimated that about one third of the adolescents who present with typical features of clinical depression remit within 3 months or so. Although such transient states are short-lived and respond to simple family or individual interventions, it has also been shown that about one-third of them relapse within the next few years.

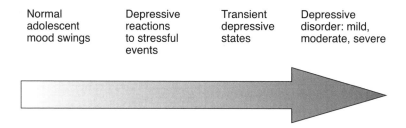

| Normal adolescent mood swings | Depressive reactions to stressful events | Transient depressive states | Depressive disorder: mild, moderate, severe |

Figure 2.1 The spectrum of mood variation and depression in adolescents.

In cases of depressive disorders that meet the criteria for clinical depression, the condition is thought to be no different from adult depressive disorders. In clinical depression the symptoms are more numerous and more severe and are frequently accompanied by social, family and educational impairments. Psychotic symptoms (delusions and hallucinations) are uncommon in adolescent depression. For a diagnosis of clinical depression to be made there should be evidence of:

1 significant symptoms of depression
2 personal suffering or distress and
3 significant impairment in educational, social and other areas of functioning.

The core features of clinical depression are pervasive and enduring low mood, markedly diminished interest in previously pleasurable activities, loss of capacity for enjoyment (anhedonia) and reduced activities or social withdrawal. These may be accompanied other somatic features such as sleep and appetite disturbance. A sense of hopelessness and helpless are cardinal cognitive features of depression. The emotional, behavioural cognitive and somatic features of depression are shown in Table 2.1. Both the diagnostic systems, DSM-IV and ICD-10, make a distinction between mild, moderate and severe episodes of depression.

Table 2.1 Features of clinical depression (* indicates core features)

Emotional	Cognitive	Behavioural	Somatic
Pervasive low mood*	Concentration difficulties	Reduced activity*	Sleep disturbance
Irritability or irritable anger	Hopelessness/helplessness Pessimism	Social withdrawal	Fatigue or lack of energy*
Diminished enjoyment (anhedonia)*	Negative view of past, present and future	Agitation	Other somatic complaints (e.g. headaches)
Loss of interest	Suicidal ideation	Tearfulness	Appetite increase or decrease
Guilt and worthlessness	Lack of motivation	Decreased school performance	
	Poor self-esteem worthlessness and low self-confidence	Deliberate self-harm	

Several rating scales, such as Children's Depression Inventory (CDI, Kovacs, 1992), and Mood and Feelings Questionnaire (Angold *et al.*, 1995), have been designed to assess depressive symptoms in children and adolescents. The CDI is a self-rating scale consisting of 24 items marked on a Likert Scale, ranging from 'Never' to 'All the time'. It should be noted that high scores on these scales do not necessarily indicate that the young person has clinical depression. Because of their low specificity, these scales are not useful for diagnosing clinical depression but can be used to screen for symptoms, to assess the severity of depressive symptoms and to monitor clinical improvement.

A sub-type of depression is *dysthymic disorder*. Dysthymic disorder is diagnosed when there is depressed mood that lasts a year or longer, with symptom-free intervals lasting for no more than 2 months. The condition is chronic and many adolescents who have dysthymia subsequently develop a major depressive episode (double depression). However, longitudinal studies have shown that in children there is much overlap of major depression and dysthymia.

Another affective disorder that may present as depression is *bipolar affective disorder* or manic depressive psychosis. Studies show at least 20% of those with early onset depressive disorders are at risk for bipolar disorder, particularly if they have a family history of bipolar disorder. Bipolar disorder is characterised by depressive episodes that alternate with periods of mania, characterised by a decreased need for sleep, increased energy, grandiosity, euphoria and an increased propensity for risk taking behaviour. Often in children and adolescents mania and depression occur as 'mixed states' in which the liability for mania is combined with depression or there is rapid cycling between depression and mania over a period of days or even hours.

Clinical depression is very uncommon in pre-adolescent children but rates show a steep increase during adolescence. Recent studies show that among adolescents the one-year prevalence of major depressive disorder associated with impairment is around 1%. Depressive disorders are equally frequent in boys and girls until adolescence and from the age of 14 there is a predominance of girls, with a 2 to 1 preponderance (similar to the gender gap seen among adults).

The aetiology of depressive disorders in young people is not fully understood but available evidence suggests that depression arises from a combination of predisposing factors in the individual (genetic vulnerability, chronic stress and adverse early experience) and precipitating stressful life events (family, peer or school problems).

There is robust body of evidence from genetic studies of depressed adults suggesting a strong genetic component to the aetiology of depressive illness. Several studies of depressed adolescents show that a significant proportion of their parents (about 20%) suffer with depressive disorders.

There is also considerable evidence to show that early adversity, such as poor social economic conditions, social deprivation, child abuse and neglect, are associated with later depressive illness. These aetiological risk factors seem to result in psychological (negative thinking) and biological (neuro-chemical imbalances) changes in the individual making them vulnerable to later depression through individual, familial or environmental maintaining factors.

The course of adolescent depression shows an episodic nature characterised by high rates of recovery from episodes but with high rates of relapse and continuity into adulthood. Adolescent depression carries a poor prognosis in the long term. All follow-up studies show that adolescent depression continues into adulthood. One of the largest follow-up studies of adolescent depression is that of Weissman and colleagues. In a prospective case control study of 73 subjects with adolescent depression over a period of 10–15 years they found that two thirds had a further depressive episode in adulthood (but no other psychiatric disorder), half the sample had at least one suicide attempt and 8% committed suicide. They conclude that 'there is substantial continuity, specificity, morbidity and potential mortality from suicide into adulthood in adolescent onset major depressive disorder patients' (Weissman *et al.*, 1999).

Treatment choice and management

The management of depressive disorder in adolescence consists of four inter-related steps.

1   treatment of the symptoms of depression
2   reducing the risk of complications especially risk of suicide
3   management of risk and maintaining factors
4   prevention of relapse.

Management of depressive disorder depends on the degree and severity of the condition. Where the depression is mild and there are few risk factors involved, simple measures to identify and reduce stress and ensure support to the young person by parents, teachers and others in the network is all that is necessary. Around one third of mild or moderately depressed adolescents will remit following this kind of brief, non-specific intervention. Depression that is severe or persistent will require specific forms of treatment. It is now generally agreed that the first-line treatment for mild or moderate depression causing moderate social impairment should be psychological therapies. Antidepressant medication is reserved for the more severe cases or for those who do not respond to or who only respond partially to psychological therapies.

Psychosocial treatments

Two forms of specific psychosocial treatments have been studied in adolescent depression, namely cognitive behaviour therapy and interpersonal therapy.

Cognitive behaviour therapy (CBT) for adolescent depression: A number of studies and reviews attest to the efficacy of CBT in adolescent depression. In this approach, the patient learns to increase pleasurable activities, acquire skills to improve interpersonal effectiveness and identify and modify dysfunctional and self-defeating patterns of cognitions that can lead to depressed mood. The general consensus is that CBT appears to be effective in reducing symptoms of depression and accompanying social impairments. Most studies on the application of CBT to adolescents with depression have been carried out with mild to moderately impaired adolescents, rather than with severe cases.

In a systemic review of efficacy of cognitive behaviour therapies in childhood and adolescent depressive disorder carried out, Harrington and colleagues (1998) came to similar conclusions. They found six randomised trials comparing the efficacy of CBT with inactive interventions in subjects aged 8–19 years with depressive disorder. Analysis of their results showed that cognitive behaviour therapy was an effective therapy for depressive disorder of moderate severity. The rate of remission from depressive disorder was higher in the therapy group (62%) than in the comparison group (36%). They conclude that 'cognitive behaviour therapy may be beneficial for mild or moderate depressive disorder in young people'.

Cognitive Behavioural Group Treatment for Adolescent Depression: Group therapy based on broad CBT principles has been shown to be an effective and economical way of alleviating adolescent depression. The Coping With Depression course for Adolescents (CWD-A) developed by Clarke et al. (1990) is one such manual-based programme that employs a psycho-educational approach to treating youth depression in a group or class like setting. Typically the course is delivered twice a week over 8 weeks and consists of 16 sessions, each lasting 2 hours. Group membership is between 6 and 10 depressed adolescents, aged 13 to 18. Although the results of the CWDA programme has been impressive, it is likely that the population of depressed adolescents treated by the authors may be different from those seen in clinics and represent the milder end of the spectrum of adolescent depression.

Interpersonal psychotherapy (IPT) for adolescent depression: interpersonal psychotherapy is a brief treatment approach developed by Klerman and colleagues for adult patients, which focuses on a number of interpersonal problems that may underlie the individual's depressed state. The approach has been adapted for adolescents by Mufson *et al.* (1991) and has been called IPT-A. The focus of IPT treatment is on the patient's depressive symptoms and their current interpersonal context, regardless of the aetiology of the disorder. The main goals of IPT-A are to decrease depressive symptoms and to improve interpersonal functioning. A more detailed discussion of each area is given in the IPTA manual (Mufson *et al.*, 1993) Randomised controlled trials using IPT have shown promising results.

Medication

A more recent introduction to the medical treatment of depression in adults has been the group of drugs called Selective Serotonin Reuptake Inhibitors (SSRIs) typified by the drug fluoxetine ('Prozac'). Other SSRIs commonly used in depression are fluvoxamine, paroxetine and sertraline. SSRIs have been the drugs of choice for adult depression because of their relatively high efficacy and low toxicity in overdoses. These findings have been replicated in drug trials with adolescent depression and were initially received with much enthusiasm. A number of randomised trials in children and adolescent depression have found SSRIs to be effective. Encouraged by these findings and extrapolating from adult experiences with the use of SSRIs, the rates of prescriptions for children and adolescents increased dramatically in the US and, to a lesser extent, in Europe.

The optimism generated by the first trials of SSRI in adolescent depression was soon undermined by the findings that adolescents taking many SSRIs reported more suicidal ideation and deliberate self-harm. A FDA review of studies for antidepressant drugs in children and adolescents found 20 placebo-controlled studies of 4100 paediatric patients for 8 SSRI drugs noted that there was an excess of suicidal ideation and suicide attempts when receiving certain SSRIs, although there were no suicides. In the context of increasing rates of prescriptions for SSRIs, drug regulatory authorities and user groups were alarmed by the findings.

Over the years serious concerns have been raised about the benefit to harm ratio of all antidepressants for children, leading to limits on the use of some drugs and warning statements on drug labelling. In response to concerns raised about suicidal behaviour and withdrawal effects, the UK Committee on Safety of Medicines (CSM) established an expert panel in 2002 to review paroxetine and other SSRIs. In December 2003 the CSM declared that all SSRIs, except fluoxetine, were contraindicated for use in patients under 18 years old.

TADS: Given the controversies surrounding the use of SSRIs in children and adolescents, the National Institute of Mental Health in the US undertook a publicly funded study of the various available treatments for adolescent depression. The Treatment for Adolescent Depression Study (TADS, 2004) was a multi-site research study comparing short- and long-term effectiveness of medication and CBT for depression in adolescents aged 12–17. Federally funded, it was a randomised controlled trial involving 439 participants. It was designed to test the best practice for care for adolescent depression. It compared the effectiveness of

1   fluoxetine alone (10–40 mg/day)
2   CBT alone

3 CBT plus fluoxetine (10–40 mg/day) and
4 placebo.

Placebo and fluoxetine were administered double-blind; CBT and CBT with fluoxetine were administered unblind. Following an initiation phase of 12 weeks, responders were allocated to 6 weeks of maintenance therapy. A further 18 weeks of treatment maintenance phase for teenagers who continued to respond well was provided. At 12 months follow-up the main findings were as follows:

1 Compared with placebo, the combination of fluoxetine with CBT produced statistically significant effects.
2 Compared with fluoxetine alone or CBT alone, combined treatment with fluoxetine and CBT was superior.
3 Fluoxetine alone was superior to treatment with CBT alone. More specifically the response rates were: fluoxetine with CBT: 71.0%; fluoxetine alone: 60.6%; CBT alone: 43.2%; placebo: 34.8%.

Particular attention was paid in TADS to the risk involved in the use of fluoxetine. The data from TADS indicate that there is a favourable balance between risks and benefits, especially when used in conjunction with CBT. The TADS team concluded that 'the combination of fluoxetine with CBT offered the most favourable trade-off between benefit and risk for adolescents with major depressive disorder'. TADS is thus far the largest and best designed trials of treatment of adolescent depression. The methodology and results of the study have been subjected to close scrutiny by the protagonists and critics of drug treatment in children and adolescents. (NIMH is currently funding two further studies, Treatment of Resistant Depression in Adolescents (TORIDA) and Treatment of Adolescent Suicide Attempters (TASA).) Information on these trials is available at the NIMH website (www.nimh.gov/studies/index.cfm).

Taken together there is little doubt that SSRIs are effective in the treatment of adolescent depression but the risks of suicidal ideation and attempts have to be weighed against the benefits of drug treatments, and decisions about treatment be based on a case-by-case basis depending on the severity of depression and preferences by adolescents and their parents. Currently the only SSRI recommended for use with children and adolescents is fluoxetine. Once an adequate clinical response has been achieved, treatment should be continued for at least six months to one year, to reduce the risk of relapse.

Current consensus: It is now generally agreed that given the high rates of remission among children with depressive disorder, that the first line of treatment should be supportive therapy. As mentioned before, about one third of the children improve with reassurance, psycho-education and simple strategies to cope with their problems. When such interventions do not result in improvement, psychosocial interventions including either CBT or IPT-A can be considered as the first line of psychological therapies. Medication is indicated in those with severe symptoms or when CBT does not achieve clinically significant improvement. It is now felt that patients should be followed up for at least 2 years because of the relapsing and remitting nature of the condition. Antidepressant medications as first line interventions may be indicated in the following circumstances: depression with severe symptoms that prevent effective psychotherapy; psychotic depression; rapid cycling bipolar depression; and depression that fails to respond to adequate trial of CBT.

Reflecting the current status of the various therapies available for adolescent depression, NICE guidelines (2005) state that, 'Children and young people with moderate to severe depression should be offered, as first-line treatment, a specific psychological therapy (individual CBT, interpersonal therapy or short-term family therapy) for a period of at least three months. Antidepressants should not be offered to a child or young person with moderate to severe depression except in combination with a concurrent psychological therapy. Specific arrangements should be made for careful monitoring of adverse drug reactions, as well as reviewing the mental state and general progress; for example, weekly contact with the family or young person for the first 4 weeks of treatment . . .The drug of choice for young people with depression is fluoxetine and is continued for 6 months after remission. If treatment with fluoxetine is unsuccessful or is not tolerated, consideration should be given to the use of another antidepressant such as sertraline or citalopram as second-line drugs.'

It should be noted that 40–50% of treated subjects, across trials of both medication and psychosocial interventions, do not respond and remain depressed. This clearly shows that we need to continue to develop more effective models of treatment, and that meanwhile a range of alternative approaches needs to be retained.

Management plan for Sarah

Coming back to Sarah, her immediate management centred around issues of risk of a suicide attempt. Given that she had recurrent thoughts of self-harm and preoccupation with death, the risk of suicide in her case was considered to be quite high. A request was made for admission to a regional adolescent psychiatric unit. Unfortunately, beds were not available at the time of the request. The clinician was left with two alternatives. One was to admit her to an adult psychiatric ward, the other was to manage the risk at home. Sarah was unwilling to be admitted to an adult psychiatric ward (and the clinician agreed with this decision) and, therefore, plans were made to manage her as an outpatient in the community. This involved two important steps.

First, both Sarah and her parents were told she had to be kept safe both at home and at school. Since the risk appeared to be greater while she was at home, parents were advised to keep all tablets or medications under lock and key and keep Sarah under close observation. Parents were to knock on her door if she was spending more than 30 minutes in her room on her own. They were also to keep sharp instruments, such as blades, knives etc, away from her. She and her parents were asked to contact the service if emergencies arose. Sarah was given a telephone number to contact. The clinician agreed to telephone them over the next few days to find out how Sarah was progressing.

The second step involved discussions with Sarah about how she could manage the thoughts of self-harm. In the individual session, Sarah admitted that the thoughts were worse when she came back from school and was on her own. Under the clinician's direction, Sarah was encouraged to talk of her suicidal thoughts as something external to her and was enabled to consider ways and means of stopping the thoughts 'getting hold of her'. There had been a number of occasions in which she had been close to harming herself by taking an overdose but had prevented herself from doing so. This provided the opportunity to discuss with her how she had been successful in such attempts and, based on previous experience, Sarah and the clinician were able to work out a number of manoeuvres that she could use to keep the thoughts away. Sarah constructed a list of actions she could undertake when the thoughts of self-harm entered her mind. These included speaking to a friend on the telephone, coming down from her room and joining the family, watching television or going out for a walk. It was agreed that the parents make allowance for such behaviours and not be too alarmed by what Sarah did.

As a last resort, she agreed to talk to her mother if she felt the thoughts were persistent. (Her parents had agreed to be at home when Sarah came back from school for the initial period and take time off work, if necessary.) In the past Sarah had found it helpful to write down her feelings in a letter and found it helped her to gain some mastery over her feelings. Since Sarah was a good storywriter, she agreed to write the story about herself and the suicidal thoughts but give the character a different name so that it appeared as if the thoughts were happening to someone else. Sarah was particularly interested in using this manoeuvre to overcome her feelings of hopelessness and desperation. An appointment was made to see her again during the week.

Given the severity of depression in Sarah, it was felt that she needed medication in addition to psychotherapy. She was prescribed fluoxetine 20 mg in the morning, starting with half the dose. She and her parents were given the leaflet by the Royal College of Psychiatrists on depression (Royal College of Psychiatrists, 2004) and also a leaflet on fluoxetine. The purpose and side effects of the medication were discussed in some detail. It was emphasised that the medication would take about two weeks to produce its beneficial effects. Sarah or her parents were to contact the clinician if there were any untoward side effects. The clinician also discussed the plan of future management with Sarah and her parents. In particular the principles of cognitive behaviour therapy were discussed. The clinician outlined to them the evidence for the effectiveness of medication and cognitive behaviour therapy and the need to use both treatments. Altogether four parents-only sessions were arranged interspersed with Sarah's individual sessions.

Parent sessions: The purpose of sessions with parents were to:

1 get them understand the effects of depression on Sarah and support her and
2 address the impact of her father's depression on how he dealt with Sarah and her difficulties.

In the very first session with the parents it became clear that Mr Wood had had three episodes of depression in the past. He had been off work for six months on one occasion. Although he had never been admitted to hospital, the episode was severe and he had been on medication and been under the care of a psychiatrist. On account of this he had been overlooked for promotion as deputy head of the school. He had been bitterly disappointed. Mrs Wood felt that he never overcame the blow he suffered and was a bitter man. He continually brought up the subject in conversations with his colleagues and blamed the authorities. In her view, he had not overcome the depression and he was difficult to live with, particularly after Sarah's difficulties came to light. Following this discussion they agreed to seek more help for Mr Wood through their GP.

Cognitive behaviour therapy for Sarah: At the very beginning the format of the sessions was discussed and Sarah's responsibilities in maintaining her side of the contract were outlined. This would include carrying out tasks that were agreed in sessions, practicing them regularly, homework assignments including diary keeping; and her commitment to attend all sessions and discuss her difficulties during sessions. Although it is presented here under eight headings, the sessions did not follow the discrete pattern described below, rather there was some overlap and it is mentioned here separately for the sake of clarity, i.e. in practice a modular flexible approach was used.

I Introducing cognitive behaviour therapy to Sarah and her parents

Sarah was seen again the same week, together with her parents. She had started taking the medication and was tolerating it quite well. The main aims of therapy, it was explained, was targeted at the symptoms of depression that Sarah was showing such as a sense of hopelessness, and a lack of control over her emotions, thoughts and behaviour. Relationship of thoughts to mood was explained using simple examples. Sarah was able to identify minor incidents that happened in the past when a negative thought, such as not doing well in an exam two years ago, had produced short-lived feelings of depression and incompetence. Using such examples, the clinician was able to illustrate how thoughts often determined one's mood. They were also told that realistically it would take several weeks before Sarah felt better and even longer for her to be her usual self. Sarah was then seen individually. She was asked what she wanted to see changed. She said that she wanted to overcome the painful mental state that she was in and get rid of the 'cloud of depression that descended on her'. Following a discussion of the various domains that the depression affected, including affective, cognitive, behavioural and motivational aspects of depression, an agreement was reached on three goals for treatment.

1 To feel less depressed (current severity: 9 out of 10).
2 To be able to make friends and maintain friendships (current severity: 7 out of 10).
3 To be able to continue with violin and music (current difficulty: 9 out of 10).

She was given a diary and asked to record her mood (on a scale of 0 to 10), activities and the most troublesome thoughts.

2 Emotional education

At the second session the next week her diary was reviewed. Sarah had kept a good diary. In fact it was somewhat exhaustive and described her moods in graphic detail:

> Today has been horrible. I did well at school but on my way back everything came crumbling down. For no reason I was thinking about how useless I was and started crying in the bus. I think some girls noticed it and gave me funny looks. On reaching home I threw the school bag, shouted at mum and went upstairs and fell on my bed and started sobbing. Mum came upstairs and tapped on the door and when

I did not answer she opened the door and wanted to know whether everything was all right. She then said she would give me 10 minutes for me to finish crying and wanted me downstairs. I think this helped me and when I went downstairs I felt much better. She had prepared my tea but did not ask me too many questions. I am not sure why I feel this way. My emotions seem to be out of control and getting me down.

The main aim of the session was to define different emotions to be able to teach self-monitoring and later in the session to link emotions with cognitions and behaviours.

Following a general discussion of what emotions are, Sarah was asked to name as many emotions as possible and these were written down. The list included happy, sad, hurt, lonely, angry, unhappy, scared, upset, frustrated, excited, confused or mixed up, guilty and ashamed. Sarah had difficulty distinguishing between frustration, feeling angry, irritated and feeling sad: she said it was difficult to distinguish between them because often she felt confused by her experiences and usually acted upon them rather than think about them.

Next, the idea of self-monitoring was introduced. Sarah agreed to watch herself and be aware of the various feelings and moods that she experienced and record them in a diary for discussion in future sessions. Emotional monitoring was compared to the monitoring of the weather, where the temperature, pressure, humidity, pollen count and so on are monitored throughout the day. Sarah's task was to constantly be aware of her emotions as if she was a second person watching Sarah's moods.

Sarah was asked to think about the differences between emotional states and thoughts. She was asked to give a running commentary of the thoughts that went through her mind when she felt depressed. The clinician raised the issue that thoughts most often produced feelings and that identifying the thought is the key to cognitive therapy. The three-way relationship between thoughts, moods and activities were set out on paper for Sarah to have a graphic representation of what was being discussed.

3 Self-monitoring and basic cognitive techniques

Sarah had kept a good diary but it was rather long and verbose. Although it gave a good idea of how Sarah was struggling to distinguish between moods, thoughts and actions and a picture of her 'internal world', the recording was unstructured and haphazard. Sarah was complimented on keeping such a detailed diary. Several instances of the times she had felt depressed were taken up for discussion. One of these included being ignored by her friend in school.

One of her thoughts was the other girl (Mary) did not want to be a friend with her because Sarah was not good enough and not fit to be a friend. Sarah said that she was irritated by this thought and was unsure as to whether what she was experiencing in terms of feelings were those of depression or anger. On further discussion it transpired that the predominant feeling was one of anger rather than depression. It was clear that when Sarah felt a negative emotion (she called it feeling upset) she had difficulties identifying accurately the emotion she was experiencing. On this occasion the emotion was one of intense anger at her friend, rather than depression.

The next question was what she was to do with the anger. The clinician discussed a number of options open to her. On reflection Sarah said that keeping the anger to herself was one of the things that made her feel depressed later on. She said she felt that she had done nothing about being unfairly dealt with by Mary and that made her feel incompetent, inadequate and depressed. She said she would indicate to Mary in the nicest possible way that she was not pleased about what had happened, although she had never done this in the past,

The conversation then shifted to her behaviour following this event. Sarah said that after the event she had not spoken to anybody as the thoughts went round and round in her mind. She had not been paying attention to class, she had avoided conversations with others and on returning home she went straight into her room and broke down into tears. Recounting the incident as she did, it was felt that Sarah was becoming aware of the ruminative self-denigrating thoughts ('I am worthless') that were so powerful in determining her emotional state. The therapist felt that discussing negative thoughts alone was bound to concentrate the session on pathology and, therefore, the conversation was shifted to discussing positive thoughts that Sarah may have had during the course of the previous week.

She was asked to identify some positive thoughts and emotions that she had experienced. Sarah remembered getting a telephone call from one of her mates who she thought was no more a friend. She said she was surprised by the call. The girl had invited her to go to a movie but Sarah had excused herself because she did not feel 'up to it'. But she was quite pleased that the girl had remembered her and had felt that Sarah should join them at the movies. This opened up a number of questions. The first was how Sarah was dependent on other people's actions to feel good about herself. The second one was why Sarah had not taken up the offer and let the opportunity slip. These were discussed in some detail (not given here). Sarah was also taught simple cognitive techniques to overcome negative thoughts. After identifying the predominant negative thought, Sarah was to use distraction techniques, (e.g. thinking about a happy event) and thought postponement (e.g. telling herself that she will suspend the thought for the next six hours).

4 Pleasant activity scheduling and self-reinforcement

Sarah had recorded the pleasant and unpleasant events that had occurred in the previous week, as well as the thoughts that accompanied the events. There were two pleasant activities, which were then discussed in some detail. Sarah had recorded that she had had a good conversation over the telephone with her friend, Mary. It was pleasant and after the telephone call Sarah felt happy and contented. She had marked the level of depression as zero and on further enquiry said that after the conversation she felt that her friend had valued her enough to listen to her and she had felt buoyed up by this thought. The other thought that accompanied the conversation was that she felt that she had a contribution to make and was not that useless. The diary was reviewed with respect to unpleasant events as well (not given here).

The main tasks for the session were twofold: pleasant activity scheduling and self-reinforcement. The therapist described her mood state at any one time as a balance between pleasant activities and thoughts on one hand and difficulties, problems and bad thoughts on the other. Building on her satisfaction with the conversation with her friend, it was pointed out that pleasant activities led to pleasant thoughts, which in turn kept depressive thoughts away. She was then asked, 'What did you do for fun before you started getting depressed?' After a lengthy conversation she was able to recall a number of things that she enjoyed in the past and these included talking to friends, watching wildlife programmes on the TV, reading books by her favourite author, writing an inspiring piece of prose and helping other people with their schoolwork. Sarah then made a list of activities that she could engage in during the following weeks. With the help of the therapist Sarah drew an 'emotional see-saw' to represent how she felt at any given time (*see* Fig. 2.2).

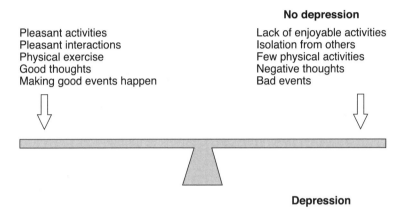

Figure 2.2 The 'emotional see-saw'.

She was then introduced to the concept of self-reinforcement; these included material rewards, as well as positive cognitions as self-rewards. She made a list of statements that she would repeat to herself once she had achieved a pleasant task activity. These included statements such as, 'I am getting there', 'I am pleased with myself' and 'Well done'. The parents were to encourage her and provide her with opportunity for self-reinforcement such as taking her to her friend, to a movie or for a special treat. She was to maintain her diary of activities, including the level of satisfaction and methods of self-reinforcement she used.

5 Communication and interpersonal skills

Because Sarah was thought to be somewhat short in interpersonal skills, considerable time was spent discussing her difficulties with her peers. Like most adolescents, Sarah started by blaming her peers for their meanness and lack of consideration. The therapist pointed out to her that one did not have to like the others in order be friends with them; moreover, interaction with others, such as having a pleasant conversation or helping another person, often produced in oneself a feeling of wellbeing, and thoughts of being worthwhile and helpful. The question, then, for Sarah, was to think about how she could communicate with others and suspend judgement, albeit temporarily, about her peers. Lack of contact or interaction with others, it was pointed out, led to a sense of being left out and feeling lonely. It was in her interest, therefore, to take a step back and think about how she could communicate with others, even if it be for selfish purposes.

It had been noted in the previous sessions that Sarah was a good listener. She was to make it a point to devote some time to listen to what her classmates were saying, even if it did not interest her. Using examples, the therapist and Sarah explored other domains of communication and interpersonal skills. These included starting a conversation, keeping a conversation going, joining in a conversation, sharing, complimenting and helping others. Sarah was particularly keen on helping others. For example, she was reminded of a girl in her class who was somewhat behind in her maths and who had many times sought help from various friends. Sarah felt that she would be able to set aside some time to help her. Sarah admitted that she found complimenting others most difficult.

6 Cognitive restructuring

In subsequent sessions she reported remarkable success on listening and felt that, as a result of her patient listening, she had found that others were talking to her more than before and had, in fact, started confiding about themselves and their difficulties to her. This was particularly so with three of her female friends with whom she had had a frosty relationship in the past.

The sessions involved observing and monitoring thoughts and evaluating them to find out whether they were valid or not. The first stage involved discovering the automatic thoughts and the associated emotions. A number of examples from the past were discussed in which Sarah was helped to identify the specific, automatic thoughts, the associated emotions that occurred in certain situations. An example was when one of her friends called her and said that she would not be able to come to see her over that weekend. Sarah said her immediate thought was that the friend did not like her any more. When asked to rate how much she believed the thought, Sarah said it was almost 90%. Then she was asked for the emotions that followed it and she said she felt terribly depressed and gave a score of 8 out of 10 on the depression scale. Sarah mentioned a number of instances when she had had negative thoughts about herself and consequently felt depressed. These included instances where one of her friends moved away from her during assembly, one occasion when she could not submit her home-work in time, and another where the teacher had made a remark about her slacking in mathematics. She was asked to keep a record of dysfunctional thoughts and the circumstances in which these occurred. She was also to record the feelings that accompanied them on a scale of 0 to 10.

At the next session the therapist helped her to question automatic thoughts, with the purpose of changing the negative cognitions and understanding her negative styles of thinking. Sarah found this quite difficult. Taking examples from her diary, the thoughts and beliefs were challenged. She was asked to think about her belief that she was a worthless person. She was asked what made her describe herself as a worthless person and to write down everything that came to her mind. This included being unpopular, not pretty and being somewhat clumsy. She was then asked to describe a person whom she felt was completely worthy. She described Mary as one who was good-looking, good in her schoolwork, had a lot of interests and lots of friends. Next she was asked to rate her friend Mary on the same dimensions that she rated herself. Further questioning elicited that, after all, the scores that she gave herself and Mary were not too far apart, she was good in some subjects and, in fact, better than Mary in some subjects, she was better liked by teachers than Mary, that Mary had sometimes got into arguments with peers and was often described as ill-tempered. The general conclusion that Sarah drew from this dialogue was that the descriptions that she used, such as worthlessness, were too general and that everyone had some worthless qualities.

Towards the end of the session she felt that having some worthless qualities was normal but she had exaggerated them in the past. She was helped to examine evidence supporting and refuting her statements about her unworthiness. Sarah was quite imaginative and could think of alternative interpretations and explanations for her thoughts. She was particularly intrigued when the therapist mentioned that one need not always believe one's thoughts but be able to question them if necessary.

7 Dealing with spontaneous imagery

One of Sarah's presenting problems was experiencing distressing images of herself and her mother. These images usually consisted of her funeral or her mother in an accident. Sarah was described by the therapist as somebody who had vivid imagination and one who thought in 'pictures'. The therapist discussed with Sarah a way of dealing with images, and the exercise for Sarah was to give the story a good ending every time she experienced distressing imagery. For example, if she saw herself in a coffin she could imagine that she got up from it and got her life back and surprised her friends. Similarly, if she had visions of her mother in an accident, she would imagine that the ambulance arrived and took her to hospital and her mother then makes a good recovery. Sarah was fascinated by the various possibilities for the story endings. She had a number of thoughts herself as to how the stories could end.

8 Ending cognitive therapy

During this session all Sarah had achieved was summarised. She had been particularly successful in the imagery tasks, where she had been able to give happy endings to the images that came to her mind. Some of these were hilarious. She said she had imagined herself being like Dracula, getting up from the coffin and marauding the vicinity looking for things to do. The activity scheduling was reviewed and it was found that Sarah was doing more activities than ever before. She had been invited by friends to their places and she had gone to the cinema with her friends. She was able to link her thoughts with moods and also challenge her thoughts. Her general mood rating had improved and although she did have low moods, especially when she was on her own, Sarah had been able to identify this and make a connection with being alone and low moods and timetable her day accordingly. She also described herself as having more strength to fight the thoughts and felt all the more good about it. She reported that she did not have any suicidal thoughts any more and that she was looking forward to sitting for the exams and was treating it as a challenge. Intriguingly, she had stopped writing stories. She said she will continue this after her exams. The parents, too, reported that Sarah was much happier. She was more involved with the family and participated in family activities. The parents felt that they had got their original Sarah back.

Progress and outcome

After the CBT course was completed Sarah was followed up fortnightly, although the sessions were much shorter. Her mood showed progressive improvement and her hopelessness and pessimism gradually lifted. She was interacting better with her friends and socialising more than before. The images of death and dying disappeared very quickly after specific interventions targeted at them, making the therapist feel that it should have been done earlier in the course of CBT. Although clinically she was thought to have recovered from the depressive episode, it was felt that in view of the pressure of preparing and sitting for her examination that medication should be continued until the examination was over. Medication was withdrawn gradually after 10 months. She was followed up for four months after stopping medication, at which point she was doing well and was symptom-free. She was doing her A-levels and aspiring to do a degree in English literature. Her father did not follow through the suggestion of getting help for himself.

Comments

Treatment of depression in adolescents is challenging but gratifying. Most adolescents improve in the short term. In the case of Sarah, in spite of the severity of depression and her initial passivity, she was motivated to continue with treatment. She carried out the suggestions and homework assignments reasonably well. However, she found cognitive work difficult and found it hard to think about thinking. Her diary records were poor. Usually they consisted of long-winded descriptions of her feelings and mental state rather than thoughts that accompanied them. However, she was good at carrying out behavioural tasks once she understood the principle behind them. She found the idea of the 'emotional see-saw' appealing. Thereafter the therapist employed diagrams and figures more and more to get her to understand the concepts they discussed.

What, or which elements, in the treatment programme worked? One could argue that it was medication that brought about the change and that the CBT only helped marginally. Others may point out the limited evidence for the effectiveness of SSRIs in depression and consider the agent of change to be CBT. When two methods of treatment are used concurrently, it is almost impossible to be sure which of the two was the main source of help. When this was discussed with the family at the end of therapy, Sarah remarked, 'What does it matter if the cat is white or black, as long as it catches the mice?' In Sarah's case it was thought that the severity of the condition required both forms of treatment. If the results of TADS are anything to go by, simultaneous use of CBT and medication has a cumulative beneficial effect.

Unfortunately there were no groups for adolescents with depression in the service. Given the excellent results reported by group CBT therapy, many services may want to consider this form of treatment being made available. The lack of inpatient beds for young people with severe depression and suicidal ideation is a cause for concern. In the case of Sarah this was a particular problem. Clinicians working with this group of young people have to resort to unsafe practices, take chances and run risks when treating suicidal young people in the community.

Box 2.1 Research on adolescent depression shows that . . .

- Adolescent depression occurs in about 1% of the population; it is more common in females than males.
- The majority of adolescents with major depressive illness recover within 2 years but the rates of relapse are high and extend into adulthood.
- Rates of completed suicide are six times higher than in the general population.
- In randomised controlled trials two methods of treatment are shown to be effective: antidepressant medication and cognitive behaviour therapy/ interpersonal psychotherapy.
- Combined treatment with fluoxetine and CBT has been found to be more effective than CBT or pharmacotherapy alone.

References

Angold Al, Costello EJ, Messer SC *et al*. The development of a short questionnaire for use in epidemiological studies in depression in children and adolescents. *International Journal of Methods in Psychiatric Research*. 1995; **5**: 237–49.

Clarke GN, Lewinsohn PM, Hops H. *Adolescent Coping with Depression Course: Leader's manual for the adolescent groups*. Eugene, OR: Castalia; 1990.

*Harrington R. Affective disorders. In: Rutter M, Taylor E, editors. *Child & Adolescent Psychiatry*. 4th edn. London: Blackwell Science; 2002. (A masterly account of adolescent depression by late Prof. Harrington.)

Harrington R, Whittaker J, Shoebridge P *et al*. Systemic review of efficacy of cognitive behaviour therapies in childhood and adolescent depressive disorder. *British Medical Journal*. 1998; **316**: 1559–63.

Kovacs M. *Children's Depression Inventory Manual*. New York: Multi-Health Systems Incorporated; 1992.

Mufson L, Moreau D, Weissman MN *et al*. *Interpersonal Psychotherapy for Depressed Adolescents*. New York: Guildford Press; 1993.

NICE. *Depression in Children and Young People: identification and management in primary, community and secondary care*. Clinical Guideline 28. London: Department of Health; 2005.

Royal College of Psychiatrists. *Mental Health and Growing Up*. 3rd edn. Depression in children and young people, Fact sheet 34, for young people. London: Royal College of Psychiatrists; 2004.

Rutter M, Graham P, Chadwick O *et al*. Adolescent turmoil: fact or fiction? *Journal of Child Psychology and Psychiatry*. 1976; **17**: 35–56.

*Treatment for Adolescents with Depression Study (TADS) Team. Fluoxetine, cognitive-behavioral therapy, and their combination for adolescents with depression. *Journal of the American Medical Association*. 2004; **292**: 807–20.

Weissman MM, Wolk S, Goldstein B *et al*. Depressed adolescents grow up. *Journal of the American Medical Association*. 1999; **281**: 1707–13.

Chapter 3

School refusal

The Education Welfare Officer (EWO) was very concerned about Richard, a 12-year-old boy, who had not been attending school for some time. He brought up the case in the monthly 'consultation clinic' with CAMHS. The local CAMHS and Education Welfare Services held a regular 'consultation clinic' in which the EWOs brought up those cases of children with a variety of problems for discussion. The 'consultation clinic' had been found to be a useful platform for the discussion of cases that were of particular concern to either party.

The school had informed the EWO about Richard's prolonged absence from school. The EWO had visited the school and found that Richard had started attending the secondary school from the previous year and was now in Year 7. No problems had been evident when he started in the school. His form teacher described him as a well-behaved boy with above average academic performance. He was well liked by the teachers and peers. But during the past term his school attendance had become poor. On going through the attendance register the EWO had discovered that Richard's school attendance had been rather erratic with several episodes of unauthorised absences lasting up to four to five days. He had also had a number of days off sick supported by sick notes from the GP for minor illnesses. He had stopped attending altogether for the past eight weeks. The EWO had made inquiries about possible bullying at school, but Richard and his teachers had assured him that there had been no bullying.

The EWO had visited the family a number of times to discuss the problems and offer help. On his most recent visit they had revealed to him that they had been experiencing considerable problems with Richard for some time. He had always been reluctant to attend school and, even when he was at the primary school, had made excuses to keep away from school. The problem had got worse after he started at the secondary school. He had been complaining that he had not been feeling well and was experiencing headaches, tummy pains and feeling sick. He had been taken to the GP numerous times. The GP had examined him and ordered some blood tests but she could not find anything specifically wrong with him. The GP had felt that he may have had a minor viral infection and recommended that he stay away from school for a few days. When the sick note ran out he managed to attend a few days of school but soon started being defiant and difficult in the mornings.

There had been a crisis recently. A few weeks ago his mother had taken him to the school bus herself and, as agreed with school, had then telephoned school to make sure that he was at school. She was surprised when she learned that he was not at school. She had telephoned his grandmother next. He was not with her either. She had gone looking for him in the neighbourhood and called friends and family. He was nowhere to be found. She telephoned her husband at work in a state of panic. Police were informed and they set up a search. As time passed and he was nowhere to be found police mounted a helicopter search with no results.

Later that evening Richard had turned up at home in a rather distraught and dishevelled state. He was cold and hungry. They were shocked to see a mark around his neck and on questioning he had told them that instead of going to school he had gone into the chase, a wooded area in the locality, and wandered around. He had been scared to come home and face his parents who, he was sure, would have found out that he was not at school. In desperation he had tried to hang himself with a vine. After this incident his parents had become reluctant to force Richard to attend school and started taking a more lenient attitude towards him. For the sake of peace, Richard was allowed to stay at home. They felt that Richard, previously an affectionate and well-behaved boy, was turning into a problem child. They were convinced he had undergone a 'personality change'.

The EWO was puzzled by Richard's behaviour and wondered whether the CAMHS team could assess him and his family to get to the bottom of the problem.

Clinical presentation and background

Family interview: Richard and his family were seen in the clinic the following week. Richard appeared somewhat quiet and subdued when his parents spoke about their concerns. They felt defeated in their attempts to get him to school. They were at a loss to understand why Richard, who was good in his schoolwork, was stubbornly refusing to attend school. During the family interview Richard spoke very little apart from saying that he liked school but found getting there difficult. At one point he became weepy and was comforted by his mother.

His mother described a typical school day as follows: Richard would start getting restless and uptight the night before. He would keep asking her if he could keep off school 'just for one day'. He lost sleep and could be heard going to the toilet several times that night. In the morning he delayed getting up from bed and later refused to get ready. He complained of feeling sick and would usually refuse to have his breakfast. He would then pace the hallway and become agitated and restless. When the time came to leave the house he would be in tears and start pleading with his mother to let him stay at home. She found him to be such 'an emotional wreck' in the morning that she had started to give in to him very much against her better judgement. Asked about weekends they said that on Fridays and Saturdays he was back to his usual self, happy and playful. He enjoyed playing on the computer, watching television and being helpful at home. But on the Sunday night he would start getting upset and emotional. During school holidays he was relaxed and carefree.

Although Richard was upset and fought any attempts to get him into school, once he was in school (on the days that the parents managed to get him to school) he settled down within a short time and joined in class work enthusiastically. He could spend the rest of the time in school without much distress and even enjoy it. But the next morning the problems would begin again

Richard's difficulties in attending school had begun when he started nursery. He would not leave his mother and clung to her 'like a leech'. He cried a lot and was inconsolable in class. His mother would hide herself and watch over him till he settled down. It took him more than six months to settle in the nursery. He experienced similar difficulties when he stared primary school; this time it took him only several weeks and when he did settle down his parents felt that he was getting over the problem. When he stared secondary school at 11 years of age, at first he had managed rather well. He liked the teacher, he had a good group of friends and his academic performance was above average. But one term into the second school year in the secondary school, he had started to refuse to go to school again, only it was worse this time round. At the time of the interview, in addition to sporadic previous absences, Richard had not been to school for more than eight continuous weeks. The school was sending work home and he completed this promptly and looked forward to the next batch. He was, however, losing touch with his friends and had started feeling that they were losing interest in him. The parents felt he had become almost homebound and was quite happy to be at home playing on his computer and watching television.

Richard's developmental history was uneventful. His mother described him as an easy baby. He had 'abdominal colics' until the age of three and had been admitted to hospital several times for investigation but all tests had been normal. His developmental milestones had been normal. The parents felt that he was somewhat a shy boy who liked to be inconspicuous while with a group of his peers. Unlike his brother, he was reserved and not very venturesome. But he had a few friends who liked him and invited him to their birthday parties. He had not spent any nights away from home. He had refused to join a school trip because he wanted to be at home. The parents felt that he was not yet ready to spend nights away from home.

The family consisted of Richard, 12 years, his younger brother, Kevin, 10 years and the parents. Richard's father worked as an engineer for a company and had to work long hours. The firm was making redundancies and was placing extra demands on him. He left home early in the morning before the children were ready to go to school. The two boys were loving and caring and the parents were proud of them. The mother had worked as a secretary to a well known firm but had given up work after to look after the children. The family did not have any particular stresses and there had been no recent changes in the family. Mrs Jones described herself as an anxious person and had been treated for panic attacks in the past. She had been seen by a psychiatrist and had been on medication for nine months.

Individual examination: During the family interview, Richard had said very little. The therapist had observed that when he had been asked questions, he looked at his mother before answering and many times she answered for him. When the therapist mentioned that he wanted to see him individually, Richard became quite distressed and did not want his mother to leave the room. The therapist told him that he saw lots of young people of his age and he wanted to talk to him about his difficulties and assured confidentiality. It took some persuasion before he reluctantly agreed to be seen on his own. He found it easy to talk about non-school related subjects. When he did talk about school and his friends, he did so in fond terms. He liked maths and was better at it than most of his friends. He was particularly good at mental arithmetic. He was keen to do well in studies. He said he wanted to be a mathematician. His said that he wanted to attend school but found it difficult. He did not want his parents to be taken to court because of him.

At this point the therapist asked him to describe his experiences in the morning in some detail. Richard said that usually he started worrying about going to school the previous night. When he woke up in the morning a chill would run through him as he thought of getting ready to go to school. He would lie in bed pretending to be sleeping but kept worrying. As he managed to get up and get ready there developed a feeling of dread as if something terrible was going to happen. He felt sick, he had to go to the toilet several times and at times he had tummy pains and diarrhoea. As the time for leaving home neared these feelings would get unbearable and it was at times like this he became angry. As Richard related his morning experiences, he started to become weepy and upset. He said, 'I like my friends and the lessons but just thinking of school makes me feel sick and my legs go wobbly'. At this point he was getting red in the face and his legs were shaking noticeably.

Next the therapist gave a list of bodily symptoms of anxiety and asked Richard which of these he had experienced in the mornings. 'When a person is very upset or feels scared, he may feel that he is going to be sick, have pain in the tummy, experience a tightness in the chest or find it difficult to breath and may feel hot and flushed or have sweaty palms. Do you go through any of these in the mornings?' Richard appeared to have most of the somatic features of anxiety. He had nausea, diarrhoea, sweating, shaking, abdominal cramps, palpitations and dizziness when attempting to leave home to go to school. Richard also agreed that when he managed to get to school and once he was in the class his 'problems were over' and the feelings of dread and nausea got better and he could join in and even enjoy school. It was becoming clear that Richard's anxiety was about leaving home and not about things at school.

When asked about other situations that brought about anxiety, Richard said that he found crowded places somewhat daunting. He found school assemblies, crowded lifts and buses overwhelming and made him feel sick and dizzy, especially if he was on his own without friends or family. He could not go to the local shop on his own and would take his brother with him if he had to. Unknown to the parents, he had been bribing his brother with promises of buying him sweets if he came with Richard to the shops. He was good at music and used to go for music lessons two days a week, but lately he stopped going because he felt sick.

Richard said that when in school he would worry about 'home' and call his mother several times. On further discussion he said that he worried about his mother quite a lot especially when he was at school. 'When I am at school I get scared that something will happen to her,' he said. His mother had bought him a mobile phone so that he could contact her whenever he felt worried or upset. He remembered one occasion on which he could not contact her and he had panicked and was taken to the clinic room at school. He was breathing heavily, sweating profusely and feeling faint. He was given a paper bag to breathe into.

Case conceptualisation and formulation

Richard's difficulties in attending school and his behaviours and experiences are consistent with the descriptions of anxious school refusal. He showed both the features of anxious distress and avoidance behaviour. Anxiety about going to school resulted in symptoms that were physical (abdominal pain, diarrhoea, sweating and so on), emotional (extreme distress, fear, anxiety, panic) and cognitive (thoughts of harm to his mother). These were relieved by avoidance of school. When permitted to stay away from school and during weekends he was symptom-free. In order to avoid the distress and anxiety, he fought with his mother in the morning, absconded from school and, on one occasion, tried to harm himself.

Richard's school refusal stemmed from anxieties related to separation from his mother rather than from anxieties or fears related to school situations. His constant worry about the safety of his mother when at school and telephoning her from school to check if she was alright indicated a severe degree of separation anxiety. It is obvious that he refused to go to school in order to be with her. In functional terms he was avoiding the distress and anxiety of separation from his mother with whom he felt safe and secure. It is worth noting that, in addition to separation anxiety he showed other anxiety features when in crowds, buses and going to the shops. What started as separation anxiety appears to have generalised to other situations and there are indications that he was rapidly becoming more anxious and almost homebound. He had lost most of his friends and become socially isolated. The vicious cycle of separation anxiety and its (negative) reinforcement by school avoidance is shown in Figure 3.1.

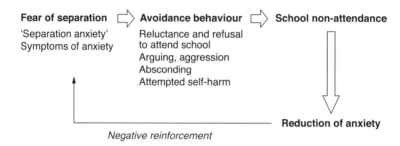

Figure 3.1 The vicious cycle of separation anxiety and avoidance behaviour.

Several factors seem to have contributed to produce separation anxiety in Richard, the most prominent of which was the over-close and age-inappropriate emotional closeness between him and his mother (this became more clear later). His mother appeared to have problems separating from Richard as much as he did from her. The normal process of separation and age-appropriate individuation seem to have been hindered by the overprotectiveness of his mother. For whatever reasons (these became apparent in later sessions, see below), the message that she had given Richard was that the world was a dangerous place and only she could protect him from the catastrophe that awaited him if he dared to venture into it. Thus he had become overdependent and failed to move away from the secure base and experiment and find his own way of coping with the minor stress of life. He had managed reasonably well in primary school (after a shaky start) and had been able to develop an exclusive relationship with the teacher because primary schools are more child-friendly, with small classes, and children get personalised attention from teachers. Secondary schools have large classes and typically children move from one class to another for different subjects.

Skynner has likened primary schools to 'one parent' families and the situation in secondary schools to that of a 'multiparent' environment (Skynner, 1974). From a developmental perspective, the mother's over-close emotional relationship with Richard had prevented the normal age-appropriate separation–individuation process. The other factors that contributed to the problem were his mother's own anxiety and the lack of support she received from the husband. The marital relationship appeared weak. The hypothesised aetiological factors that contributed to Richard's separation anxiety are shown in Figure 3.2.

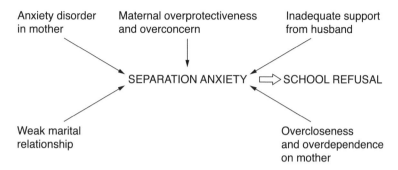

Figure 3.2 Hypothesised factors contributing to separation anxiety in Richard.

Theoretical perspectives

School non-attendance, or school absenteeism as it is known in educational circles, is common: about 10 percent of children and young people are absent from school at any one time. In countries where schooling is compulsory, absence from school is taken seriously and often there are systems in place to notify authorities of unauthorised absences. Children do not attend school for a variety of reasons, not all of which are related to mental health issues. The causes of *school non-attendance* are as follows:

- **Physical illness:** This is one of the commonest causes for a child to be away from school and should be fairly straightforward. But when the child or young person presents repeatedly to the medical practitioner with physical symptoms of anxiety such as abdominal pain or other somatic complaints it may be more difficult to unravel and may take time.
- **Parental withholding:** Sometimes parents may deliberately keep the child at home. It is not uncommon for a depressed or agoraphobic parent to withhold the child from attending school to provide help or company for the parent.
- **Truanting:** Truanting is said to occur when the young person keeps away from school without the knowledge of parents; neither the parents or school know about his or her whereabouts. Often it reflects lack of interest in schoolwork, defiance of adult authority and a desire to engage in more attractive pastimes in the company of peers with similar interests. Frequently they show other externalising behaviours such as antisocial behaviour; indeed, truancy may be part of wider problem such as conduct disorder.
- **School refusal:** School refusal is defined by most authorities as difficulty attending school associated with emotional distress, especially anxiety. Anxiety about attending school and resultant school avoidance can stem from a variety of anxiety-related problems. Richard's difficulties in attending school belong to the category.

- **Wilful or deliberate non-attendance:** Many young persons especially adolescents decline to attend on their own volition because of lack of motivation and that they find school uninteresting or aversive. They usually have no mental health problems. Parents may collude with the young person's behaviour or feel helpless and defeated in their attempts to get him or her to school.

It should be pointed out that although the above classification of school non-attendance appears easy and simple in clinical practice it is not uncommon to see 'mixed' pictures. Recent studies have examined the prevalence of school refusal and truancy in normal school populations and come to the conclusion that there was a 'mixed' group that showed features of both anxiety and truancy. A study from the US (Egger *et al.*, 2003) of a sample of 4500 children from the age of 9 to 16 showed that they fell into three subgroups: pure anxious school refusal (1.6%), pure truancy (5.8%) and 'mixed school refusal' (0.5%).

Clinicians and researchers have commonly divided children who fail to go to school into two groups: those who stay at home because of fear or anxiety, and those who skip school because of a lack of interest in school and/or defiance of adult authority. The behaviour of the first group has been called school refusal while the behaviour of the second group has been called truancy. Hersov (1960a, b) conducted one of the first studies to use descriptive, rather than aetiologically derived, definitions of 'school refusers' and 'truants'. He concluded that truancy was an indication of problems of conduct, while school refusal was a manifestation of an emotional disorder, with anxiety more prominent than depressive symptoms. These findings have been broadly replicated by subsequent studies. Table 3.1 shows the main features of school refusal and truancy.

Table 3.1 Features distinguishing school refusal and truancy

School refusal	Truancy
Severe emotional distress about attending school; may include anxiety, somatic symptoms or temper tantrums	Lack of excessive anxiety or fear about attending school
Parents are aware of the absence; child often tries to persuade parents to allow him or her stay at home	Child often attempts to conceal absence from school; parents are usually unaware of the young person's whereabouts
Absence of significant antisocial behaviours such as fighting and offending	Frequently shows behaviour problems such as disruptive acts (e.g. stealing, fighting, lying), often in the company of antisocial peers
During school hours, the child stays at home because it is considered a safe and secure environment	During school hours, the child usually does not stay at home
Child expresses willingness to do schoolwork and complies with completing work at home	Lacks interest in schoolwork and is unwilling to conform to academic and behaviour expectations

Several diagnostic studies have examined the prevalence of various psychiatric disorders among school refusers. A study by Berg *et al.* (1993) helps to put the problem in perspective. They carried out a study of 80 youths, aged 13–15 years, who had not attended school (unauthorised absences) for at least 40% of a school term. This study is remarkable for the reason that, unlike previous studies which examined populations referred to clinics, the sample was drawn from a normal school population. The results showed that half the sample had no psychiatric disorder, a third had a disruptive behaviour disorder and a fifth had an anxiety or mood disorder. A similar study by Bools *et al.* (1990) assessed 100 children with severe school attendance problems and found that only half met criteria for a psychiatric disorder, with truants more likely to have conduct disorder and the school refusers more likely to have anxiety disorders. Thus, overall, about 50% of school non-attenders have a diagnosable mental health disorder.

School refusal

In the literature on the subject this behaviour has been variously called 'school refusal', 'school phobia' and 'school avoidance'. It is now generally agreed that the term 'school phobia' be restricted to situations that describe refusal to attend school due to circumscribed or specific phobias (unreasonable and excessive fear) related to school such as a phobia for assembly or heights. It is now customary to use the generic term 'school refusal' to refer to the group of children who persistently refuse to attend school because of emotional problems.

School refusal is characterised by the following:

1   Severe difficulty in attending school, often resulting in prolonged absence.
2   Severe emotional upset at the time of going to school, which may involve such symptoms as excessive fearfulness, misery and features of anxiety; the child is symptom-free during weekends and school holidays.
3   During school hours the child remains at home with the knowledge of parents.
4   Absence of significant antisocial behaviours such as other rule-breaking behaviour and delinquency.
5   Child expresses willingness to do schoolwork and complies with completing work at home.

Typically two constellations of behaviours are associated with school refusal:

1   **Features of anxiety:** When the time comes to go to school the child experiences extreme anxiety that manifests as physical and psychological symptoms; these swiftly disappear when the child is allowed to stay at home and are usually absent during weekends and holidays.
2   **Avoidance behaviour:** In order to escape from the distress and emotional pain the child may fight the parent, go into a temper, run away or even threaten self-harm. It is not uncommon for the avoidance behaviour to be seen as the primary problem and the underlying anxiety to go unrecognised.

School refusal is not a psychiatric diagnosis; rather it is a description of behaviour. School refusal as defined above occurs approximately in 5% of all school children, although the rates of school absenteeism are much higher. Most studies suggest that school refusal tends to be equally common in boys and girls. School refusal can occur throughout the entire range of school years, but tends to peak at key transition times, i.e. at ages 5–6 (school entry) and 10–11 (transfer to secondary school) and 14 (adolescence).

Several diagnostic studies have examined the prevalence of various psychiatric disorders among school refusers. Although theoretically any severe psychiatric disorder may be associated with school refusal, the commonest disorders encountered are separation anxiety and social phobia. Based on a review of studies over the previous 10 years, King and Bernstein (2001) concluded that although the school refusal (as defined above) is heterogeneous with variable presentation, it comprises three primary diagnostic subgroups:

- **Separation anxiety:** This was the most common disorder in school refusers and occurred more commonly in the younger age group. The mean age of onset for this group is 8–9 years.
- **Social phobia or simple phobia:** This group is somewhat older, the mean age of onset is 12–13 years and have more severe school refusal.
- **Other anxiety disorders (e.g. generalised anxiety disorder) or depression:** Seen mostly in adolescents.

Separation anxiety disorder

Developmentally 'normal' separation anxiety occurs around the age of one year, during which the child experiences anxiety when separated from the main attachment figure. Separation anxiety peaks between one to three years and gradually declines, and by the time the child starts nursery and later the reception class, the child learns to be away from the parents over longer and longer periods of time. By the time the child enters school he has sufficiently internalised the mother to enable him to manage his anxieties at school until he returns home.

Separation anxiety disorder is characterised by developmentally inappropriate and excessive anxiety upon separation or anticipation of separation from home or those to whom the child is attached. The hallmark of the disorder is extreme fear and distress at the time (or in anticipation) of separation from the mother. School refusal is a prominent feature of the disorder in middle childhood. In young children with the disorder clingy behaviour is common. Often they follow the mother everywhere in the house ('shadowing'). They have a fear of sleeping alone and come up with various excuses to sleep in the parent's bed or get the mother to come to their room. In middle childhood they are unwilling to sleep away from home. They may express fears of getting kidnapped or getting killed. They worry about the safety of the mother or some harm befalling her. When anticipating separation from the mother, they may plead, throw tantrums, threaten self-harm or become aggressive. The main features of the disorder are summarised in Box 3.1.

Box 3.1 Features of separation anxiety disorder

- Unrealistic worry about the major attachment figure (e.g. some harm befalling the mother).
- Unrealistic and excessive worry that some thing catastrophic may happen to self resulting in separation from the attachment fear (e.g. kidnapping, getting lost, being killed).
- Persistent fear of being alone, clinginess, reluctance to sleep unless close to the mother.

- Excessive distress during (or in anticipation of) separation from the major attachment figure.
- Somatic symptoms of anxiety (e.g. nausea, vomiting, abdominal pain) on separation from attachment figure.

The onset of the disorder is most common during childhood (7–12 years) with marked decline during adolescence and young adulthood. Difficulties in separation–individuation may occur for a number of reasons and these may not be evident initially. Parents do not volunteer such information and in many instances they may be consciously unaware of them. Problems in separation may occur in one or more of the following circumstances:

- mother's adverse childhood experiences including maternal overprotection, abuse or punitive parenting
- unmet needs of the mother during childhood (e.g. parental neglect)
- early life-threatening illnesses in the child
- a previous miscarriage
- amplification of the motherhood role
- anxiety disorder in one of the parents
- reversed parenting (e.g. in parental depression).

Typically in families that have a child with separation anxiety, the fathers play a peripheral role in the family and are emotionally distant. Some mothers feel emotionally deserted by the husband and find themselves burdened with family day-to-day decision-making. In the separation–individuation process the father feels unable to intrude in the mother/child relationship and support both through the pain of separation. Often there are marital problems, with either a conflictual or distant emotional relationship between the parents. In such circumstances it is essential that the role of the father in the dynamics of separation anxiety be addressed.

The psychodynamic conceptualisation of separation anxiety holds that the mothers have not relinquished the intense and exclusive relationship they had developed with the newborn infant (termed 'primary maternal preoccupation' by Winnicott). As a result, what comes to exist is a symbiotic relationship between the overprotective mother and the overdependent child. The mothers themselves have not achieved separation from their mothers, while the couple relationship between the parents is weak taking only a second place to the pathological tie between the mother and child. Overindulged and lacking containment, the child fails to develop a system of inner controls. His narcissism and omnipotence are enhanced and he comes to resent his dependence on the mother. He comes to completely dominate and possess the mother.

Behavioural model of school refusal: An alternative conceptualisation of school refusal is to approach it from a behavioural perspective and examine the motivation and function of the behaviour. Kearney and colleagues (Kearney and Albano, 2000) have been the foremost proponents of the approach. According to this model a functional analysis of the school refusing behaviour yields four possible reasons:

1   avoidance of negative emotions (e.g. anxiety, distress, depression)
2   escape from aversive social situations (e.g. bullying) or evaluative situations (e.g. peer interaction in social anxiety/phobia)
3   obtaining attention from significant others (e.g. parents)
4   seeking tangible reinforcement or rewards (e.g. watching television, sleeping).

In behavioural terms the first two of the above conditions provide negative reinforcement or avoidance of something aversive and the latter two situations are positively reinforcing. Kearney and Silverman (1993) have devised a questionnaire, The School Refusal Assessment Scale, to measure the relative strengths of the four functional conditions for a particular case of school refusal behaviour. However, they clearly state that their method of assessment and interventions may not be effective in those meeting the criteria for a psychiatric diagnosis.

Treatment choice and management

In the past the choice of treatment for anxious school refusal was made on the basis of single case studies and clinical experience. There is now overwhelming evidence that behavioural–cognitive approaches based primarily on exposure-based interventions drawing upon systemic desensitisation techniques are the mainstay of treatment. Two well-designed studies attest to the efficacy of behavioural–cognitive interventions for school refusers. King *et al*'s (1998) study involved 34 school refusers aged 5–15 years. Diagnostic evaluation showed that 84% experienced a current anxiety or phobic disorder. They were randomly assigned to a four-week cognitive-behavioural intervention involving gradual return to school and CBT involving six sessions with the child and five with the family; one session was held with the teacher to explain the strategy and enlist corporation. The control group was placed on the waiting list. Relative to controls, the treatment group demonstrated significant improvement in school attendance (90%), anxiety, fear and coping. Treatment gains were maintained at follow-up three months later.

   In the second study, Last *et al*. (1998) randomly allocated 56 school-refusing children to either twelve weeks of CBT or an 'educational and support treatment' group. The CBT treatment consisted of gradual return to school (exposure) and CBT while the latter consisted of manual based group sessions in which, in addition to providing information to help themselves, children were encouraged to talk about their fears and anxieties and maintain daily diaries. Both treatment groups showed clinically and statistically significant levels of improvement and the gains were maintained 2 weeks into the next school year. Two conclusions may be drawn from these studies:

1   that CBT is an effective form of intervention in anxiety based school refusal and
2   educational supportive measures may be equally effective; the 'active ingredient' in the latter group remains unknown.

Management plan for Richard

There is general agreement that for optimal outcomes the treatment of anxiety disorders in children be mutimodal. It has been pointed out that in the treatment of anxiety based school refusal the involvement of the parents and school is essential in order to derive the maximum benefits of treatment. In keeping with this view, a three-pronged approach was employed in the case of Richard:

1 Liaison and consultation with the school to implement gradual reintroduction to school.
2 Individual interventions based on behavioural or cognitive-behavioural strategies.
3 Family work to address specific family issues and assist the family cope with a developmental challenge they have previously failed to transcend.

Consultation – liaison with school: the exposure programme

The EWO acted as co-therapist and undertook the work with school. In the meetings with Richard a fear and avoidance hierarchy was constructed by the therapists and rated on a 10-point scale, containing items covering situations that he feared or avoided. An abbreviated version of Richard's fear ratings were as follows:

- Leaving home in the morning (10/10)
- Entering school through the school gates (10/10)
- Taking part in PE (8/10)
- Entering the classroom (6/10)
- Break times (4/10)
- Spending time in the library once at school (2/10).

The EWO held a meeting (after school hours) with Richard, his parents, Richard's form teacher and the special needs coordinator to explain Richard's problems. The issue was framed as a temporary setback brought about by Richard's 'sensitivity' and a graded reintroduction to school was outlined. Richard was to attend school immediately but begin with after-school hours and spend time in the library and the sports hall. These were considered warm-up exercises before starting the programme.

Next, he was allowed to choose three days in the week during which he would be brought to school by his parents, the EWO would receive him at school and, on the first day he would spend some time in the library and be taught by a teaching assistant. The next day, he would be accompanied by one of his friends to the classroom to attend the maths lesson (his favourite subject) and the lesson following it. After the lessons if he wished he could decide to leave school or continue to attend the other lessons. Since Richard's difficulties were separation from home rather than remaining at school, it was expected that he would choose to remain in school after the maths lesson. This procedure was to be repeated every other day in the first three weeks and increased to four days the next three weeks; thereafter on he would attend all days of the week. This would be followed by full attendance of all lessons. As a reward for implementing the programme he would be temporarily excused from PE. Although the desensitisation procedure did not strictly follow the hierarchy from the least difficult to the most difficult, it was felt that rapid introduction to school (with the help of CBT) was crucial to the success of the programme.

The EWO arranged with the school that, in case Richard experienced difficulties in the class, such as feeling very dizzy or sick, he would indicate to the teacher and would be allowed to go the 'clinic' room or spend the time in the library until he was ready to go into the class again. On such occasions the SENCO would be available to talk to him and reassure him. But it was made clear to him and his parents that on no account was he to go back home, even if he had to spend the whole time in the library or 'clinic' room.

Individual behavioural-cognitive work

Richard was seen in the clinic for individual work twice weekly initially. Appointments were scheduled after school hours so that attendance at the clinic did not interfere with the school attendance programme. The therapist discussed with him and his parents the nature of anxiety and the principle behind the plan of treatment by exposure. Individual treatment consisted of four main elements:

1 instruction about the nature of anxiety including its four components (cognitive, physiological, emotional and behavioural)
2 relaxation training
3 coping self-statement training and
4 cognitive restructuring.

Richard's anxiety appeared to follow a particular pattern. Initially it manifested as somatic symptoms, especially nausea, followed by 'butterflies in the stomach', sweating and feeling hot. This would trigger thoughts of fainting, collapsing and making a fool of himself. Escalation of the somatic and cognitive symptoms peaked at the time of leaving home, then getting out of the bus or car followed by entering the school.

Richard was taught relaxation exercises using controlled breathing and muscle relaxation to overcome the physiological effects of anxiety. He practiced it with the therapist several times, was given a tape recording of the session and was instructed to use it twice a day. He was told about the early signs of anxiety and asked to use controlled breathing and relaxation when leaving home and entering school. At the second session he was taught to identify his maladaptive thoughts (e.g. 'I am going to faint') and replace them with more adaptive coping self-statements. Together with the therapist he wrote down a menu of six self-statements (e.g. 'I will not allow anxiety to get into me', 'I have overcome these thoughts before and can manage these thoughts now', 'It will be over soon if I hold on for some time') that he could use during the exposure sessions. He was told that to get better at using self-statements he needed to practise and it was no different from practising his music. Richard could identify with this and in the sessions he practised making self-statements after imagining situations in which he left home or entered school. He was asked to maintain a record of his anxiety levels and the strategies he employed during the exposure exercises so that it could be discussed during the succeeding session. He was encouraged to have 'trial runs' using the techniques he had learned while attending the music lessons and going to the local shops.

The first stage of cognitive restructuring involved discussions about the link between feelings and thoughts. Beginning with examples of normal situations such as taking a test, the therapist discussed the connection between thoughts and feelings. He was taught to answer the questions, 'What what was I feeling?' and 'What was I thinking?' Later he was asked to describe the bodily sensations when getting ready for school and the thoughts that came to his mind at the time. He was encouraged to come up with the negative thoughts (e.g. 'I am going to faint') that made him avoid going to school. Next, he was asked to think of a neutral or positive thought ('I have never passed out', 'It will not last'). Following the discussion of the relationship between thoughts and feelings, the homework task was set for him to practise 'catching himself thinking anxious thoughts' and linking and rating the feelings accompanying them on a scale of 0 to 10. The second part of the cognitive restructuring programme was to get him to replace the 'worrying thoughts' ('I am going to be sick and make a fool of myself' with 'calming thought' ('I can manage. I have never been sick'). In the course of the session he was asked to think about evidence supporting his 'worrying thoughts' and think of as many alternative explanations as possible. He was asked to keep a 'thought and feeling' diary for discussion in subsequent sessions.

Parent work: Work with the family proved to be vital because the parents were at the point of giving up trying to get Richard to attend school because they, especially the mother, could not tolerate witnessing the extreme state of distress in him. In his mother's words, 'It was too painful for me to see him turn out to be such a nervous wreck.' Her catastrophic thinking had to be dealt with before the programme of return to school was begun. Fortunately her experience with anxiety and panic attacks were a potent reminder that confronting the anxiety-provoking situation does no great harm.

Weekly parent-only sessions were held in which the hypothesis about maternal overprotection was tested. His mother agreed that her own anxiety had stood on the way of dealing with Richard's difficulties. She had overcome the panic attacks and anxiety but found that when it came to Richard she worried too much. She said she had been a secretary prior to having the children and with the arrival of the children her career aspirations had been forgotten. In a moment of extra-ordinary insight she wondered whether she was clinging on to Richard because she had nothing else to do now that the children were growing up. Her husband agreed and suggested that she should explore the possibilities of contacting her former friends and co-workers.

In the sessions there was some discussion about how unsupported she felt by her husband, especially when it came to dealing with Richard's school problems. She complained that it was left to her to deal with the school most of the time and that her husband had been making his work an excuse for not playing his part in addressing the school problems. Generally Richard was more compliant when he was with his father. The therapist chose this opportunity to emphasise the need to get it right when Richard's reintroduction programme started. As a demonstration of his commitment to the programme and the family, Mr Jones agreed to take time off work for the first two weeks of the programme and take Richard to school himself, if that is what was required to overcome the problem.

In the subsequent parent session they were able to talk more about how they functioned as a family. They described themselves as a close family and their marriage as stable and satisfactory. Her husband described his wife as a 'worrier' and a 'bundle of nerves'. He felt that she worried about Richard unnecessarily. When he started nursery, and later, schools, she would be very upset after

Richard left home and had volunteered to assist the teachers at school so that she could attend to him if he had any problems.

At this point in the interview she became very tearful and said that her husband did not understand the 'bond' between her and Richard. She said that Richard was 'only a child' and, unlike his younger brother, he was sensitive and weak. He needed more love, not less. Asked about why she felt that the older boy was seen as weak and vulnerable rather than the younger one, she said that she had always felt that Richard was her special son, probably, she added, because he was the first child. Her husband agreed that she treated Richard as if he was the only child and treated him like a younger child. She had not allowed him to learn to cycle or go and play with the kids in the neighbourhood. She continued to wash and dress him. She would constantly check him to see whether he had a temperature. When he came back from school he first comment was 'you don't look so well'. She took him to the GP for the slightest sniffle or cold. At this point she retorted by saying, 'you never mentioned these before' but agreed that she worried too much about Richard.

She agreed that she had never stopped worrying about Richard and felt lonely without him. 'When he started school it was as if my right arm had been cut off,' she said. Asked why it was the right arm, she said, 'It is the right arm that carried him.' Sending him to school was an ordeal for her. Around this time she started getting panic attacks and was treated by a psychiatrist. She also developed a fear of going out and became almost homebound for a period of time. She could understand Richard's difficulties better than her husband because she had experienced them herself. In the family, she said, Richard had her temperament and Kevin was more like his father. She wondered whether Richard would need some form of medication.

In one of the parents-only sessions they described themselves as a well-adjusted couple, but later it became clear that father was somewhat peripheral and the main tasks of parenting fell on the mother. He intervened in family affairs only when problems reached a crisis point and took little part in the routine upbringing of the children. Moreover, the couple described themselves as not being intimate. The father felt that his wife was overinvolved with the children, Richard in particular. He commented angrily that he was highly dissatisfied with the present relationship although he had not complained about it for fear of upsetting his wife. He felt that she had little emotional investment in the couple relationship and he was being taken for granted. Mrs Jones retorted, saying that she had always wanted his support but he was never available and she had to make all the decisions. They were asked to think about how they wanted to reorganise their lives so that the mother could reinvest her emotional energies in the couple relationship and herself instead of the need to identify with her son.

Richard's mother indicated that she wanted to discuss some of her issues with the therapist on her own. In the individual sessions with his Mrs Jones, the therapist wondered what had made her become so overprotective of Richard. This opened up a long discussion during which she said that she had not really wanted to have Richard and that she had not been ready to be a mother. This left her feeling guilty. 'I think I overcompensate for the way I felt about him', she said. She was relieved to hear that it was not unusual for mothers to have hateful feelings towards their children. The therapist pointed out that all intimate relationships had in them an element of anger and hate. What she had done by overcompensation was a typical example of the defence mechanism of reaction formation, turning an emotion into its opposite. The main issue was, now that she had come to realise it, what she wanted to do about it. This was followed by a discussion of dealing with ambivalence in her relationship with Richard.

Altogether Richard had eight individual sessions, the parents were seen in six parent sessions and the mother had two individual sessions. Both parents and Richard worked hard and the family proved to be resourceful in trying new ways of organising their lives and relating to each other. Once the school attendance problem had been addressed, separation from home on visits to friends, staying over night and going on school trips were arranged.

Progress and outcome

What helped Richard most was the behavioural aspect of the intervention. He was taken to school on the first day by his father about midday for the maths lesson. By previous arrangement his mother was not at home that morning and chose to go see relatives. In spite of mounting anxiety he was able to leave home. He practiced positive self-statements while in the car and was relieved to find his anxiety was getting better. He found the sight of the school somewhat over-whelming but managed to shift his gaze away and practice controlled breathing. He met with the EWO at the school who put him at ease by discussing his success with music lessons. Unknown to Richard, the EWO had arranged two of his friends to meet him. Richard felt quite moved when he met his friends and his anxiety levels dropped considerably.

He spent some time in the library with the EWO and a teacher and then went into the maths lesson. He was surprised at his own performance and decided to spend the whole day in school. The rest of the programme proceeded uneventfully over the next three weeks and by the fifth week he was attending school full-time. He did experience some anxiety (4 out of 10) in the mornings while leaving home with his father but it was manageable. Every Friday he telephoned the therapist at a prearranged time to report his progress and ratings of anxiety during the exposure exercises. There were two occasions on which he became sick at the time of leaving home and he and his father were inclined to give up for the day, but on telephoning the therapist they were persuaded to go back to school later in the day. It had already been agreed that in the unlikely event of Richard being unable to attend school, he would not be permitted to watch television, his mother would not provide company to him and that he would be asked to do the schoolwork according to a prearranged timetable.

With encouragement from his parents, Richard was able to get back to the music lessons without much difficulty. He found this and going to the local shop rather easy and became adept at using self-statements. But he experienced some difficulties using relaxation techniques during times of high anxiety. Richard initially found himself overwhelmed by feelings of anxiety and was unable to analyse the thoughts preceding his feelings of anxiety. With encouragement and over time he was able to identify the catastrophic thoughts but was only partially successful in replacing them with positive thoughts.

His mother felt happy that her husband took part in the programme and was relieved to be away from home at the beginning of the programme at the time

Richard left for school. She was determined not to let Richard sense her anxiety. She said initially she was 'worried sick' about how Richard was coping at school. By the second week she managed to take Richard to school herself. It took Richard six weeks to get to school by bus with his friends.

At the time of discharge six weeks after the initial assessment session, the parents were told to expect setbacks after school holidays or long weekends and be prepared to persevere with the management plan. Booster sessions and telephone support were offered, if necessary. Apart from one telephone call, the parents managed to keep Richard in school. They were seen as a family again at the beginning of the succeeding term. Richard was attending school full-time and not experiencing any significant anxiety. He was going out with friends and had even spent a night away from home. Around this time his mother had decided to take up a part-time secretarial job. She said that the nature of secretarial work had changed, wordprocessing had become the norm in her work and she felt initially discouraged by it, but later decided to take a course in wordprocessing. At the time of discharge from clinic she was doing a course in computing and hoping to get into full-time employment. Routine checking by the EWO over the next two years showed that Richard was attending school regularly; he had been on camping trips and was doing well in his schoolwork. He greeted the EWO enthusiastically whenever they happened to meet in school.

Comments

In many ways Richard's treatment was rather straightforward. The extent of the difficulties in the family were not evident at the beginning. In the beginning the Jones family appeared to be like any other family and Richard was seen as the main problem. It would have been easy to put the entire responsibility for improvement on Richard's shoulders. During the course of the sessions it became clear that family issues, especially his mother's overprotection, contributed significantly to his anxieties. Moreover, the reasons for his mother's overclose relationship with Richard were deep-seated and had to be addressed.

At times parents with school non-attenders come to CAMHS to prevent being taken to court by the Education Welfare Services for their child's failure to attend school. In such instances, assessment of the child for mental health problems is crucial; if no such problems are identified, parents need to be told so. The early detection of anxious school refusal is of utmost importance in order to achieve successful outcomes. The longer the young person is allowed to stay away from school, the more the symptoms get entrenched and more difficult it will be to get the child back to school. The chances of return to school are inversely proportional to the length of period away from school.

When anxiety is severe and pervasive or when the problem has lasted for a long time, the young person may be seriously disabled and even be crippled by it, and a gradual return to school programme may not be feasible. In such cases attendance at small group teaching units, sometimes called pupil referral units, may be a necessary step before reintroduction to school. As a rule, home tutoring is counterproductive in anxious school refusal and should be considered only as a last resort and with a clear plan of attendance at pupil referral units and, if possible, ultimate reintegration into school. In such cases one to one tuition at the unit may be more appropriate than being taught at home. In some instances, it may have to be accepted that the 15- and 16-year-old adolescent school refusers may never be able to attend school and may need alternative education in less stressful environments such as colleges. It is important to emphasise that anxious school refusers require a range of services to meet their needs and clinicians must be prepared to act as advocates for their cause.

The long-term outcome for this group is rather poor: they drop out of education, suffer long-term mental health, social and relationship problems; about a third continue to experience anxiety or depression into adulthood. A Swedish follow-up study (Flakierska-Praquin *et al*, 1997) of a group of 35 anxious school refusers over a period of 20–29 years found that as adults they needed more psychiatric help than the general population.

Finally, it is worth remembering that there are two outcomes for this population: one is educational or return to school and the other is mental health related. The latter involves treatments designed to overcome anxiety and may have to be carried out independent of educational interventions, if the latter do not materialise.

Box 3.2 Research on school refusal says that . . .

- School non-attenders fall into three groups: truants, school refusers and those who are withheld by parents.
- School refusal occurs in about 5% of children.
- Among school refusers the commonest disorders are separation anxiety (in the younger children) and social phobia (in the older children).
- The treatment of choice is gradual reintroduction to school together with cognitive therapy with the child; work with parents is often essential.
- Close working with school is crucial to obtain good results.
- In those with severe anxiety or long lasting school refusal, a range of facilities such as pupil referral units may be necessary.

Note

The author wishes to thank Carl Hobson, EWO, who was the co-therapist in this case.

References

* Berg I, Butler A, Franklin J *et al*. DSM-III-R disorders, social factors and management of school attendance problems in the normal population. *Journal of Child Psychology and Psychiatry*. 1993; **34**: 1187–203.

Bools C, Foster J, Brown I *et al*. The identification of psychiatric disorders in children who fail to attend school: a cluster analysis of a non-clinical population. *Psychological Medicine*. 1990; **20**: 171–81.

Egger HL, Costello EJ, Angold A. School refusal and psychiatric disorders: a community study. *Journal of the American Academy of Child and Adolescent Psychiatry*. 2003; **42**: 797–807.

Flakierska-Praquin N, Lindstrom M, Gillberg C. School phobia with separation anxiety disorder: A comparative 20–29 year follow-up study of 35 school refusers. *Comparative Psychiatry*. 1997; **38**: 17–22.

Hersov LA. Persistent non-attendance at school. *Journal of Child Psychology and Psychiatry*. 1960a; 1: 130–6.

Hersov LA. Refusal to go to school. *Journal of Child Psychology and Psychiatry*. 1960b; 1: 702–11.

* Kearney CA, Albano AM. *Therapist Guide to School Refusal Behaviour*. San Antonio, TX: Psychological Corporation; 2000.

Kearney CA, Silverman WK. Measuring the function of school refusal behaviour: the School Refusal Assessment Scale. *Journal of Clinical Child Psychology*. 1993; **22**: 85–96.

King NJ, Tonge BJ, Heyne BJ *et al*. Cognitive-behavioural treatment of school-refusing children: A controlled evaluation. *Journal of the American Academy of Child and Adolescent Psychiatry*. 1998; **37**: 395–403.

King NJ, Bernstein GA. School refusal in children and adolescents: a review of past 10 years. *Journal of the American Academy of Child and Adolescent Psychiatry*. 2001; **40**: 197–205.

Last CG, Hansen MS, Franco N. Cognitive–Behavioral treatment of school phobia. *Journal of the American Academy of Child and Adolescent Psychiatry*. 1998; **37**(4): 404–411.

Skynner ACR. School phobia: A reappraisal. *British Journal of Medical Psychology*. 1974; **4**: 1–16.

Chapter 4

Intellectual (learning) disability

A worried GP telephoned the local CAMHS asking for an urgent assessment of Ashley, a 15-year-old boy. The GP knew the family well. He was concerned about the sudden change in Ashley's behaviour. Ashley had left home two days ago for no apparent reason. He had been found sleeping under a bridge a day later. The circumstances as to why he left home were not clear and Ashley had been unable to tell why he had left home apart from saying that he felt confused. He had been experiencing some difficulties at school but his behaviour over the past two days had been quite extreme and out of character. The GP considered the parents to be caring and was not sure why this crisis had occurred at this particular time. At the time of examination, Ashley had been unable to provide an adequate explanation for his behaviour. On examination the GP had found it difficult to follow the line of Ashley's thinking. Although well oriented in time, place and person, Ashley's conversation did not quite make sense at times. After speaking to Ashley for 10 minutes the GP was left confused and did not know what to make of Ashley's presentation. The GP could not find anything physically wrong with him and he wondered whether Ashley was psychotic.

An appointment was made for Ashley and his family to be seen later that day.

Clinical presentation and background

Ashley, his sister and his parents attended the appointment. The family was seen together initially and Ashley was seen individually later. Ashley was a rather tall boy and was somewhat anxious about coming to the clinic. His parents too were in quite a distressed state. His mother said that they had not slept for two nights and were very worried about Ashley. Ashley, for his part, kept reassuring his mother that it was 'daft' of him to have left home and that he would not do it again. He told her that he loved his family and kept apologising for what he had done.

Over the past year Ashley had been getting progressively unhappier and even tearful at times. He usually came home from school in a highly distraught state and would throw his school bag down and lock himself in the bedroom. He refused to talk about school and what went on in school. He was particularly upset on every Sunday evening when he could no longer postpone the thought of going to school the next morning. He had confided to his sister once that he would rather kill himself than go to school but she had not told this to her parents until now. He had few friends and had recently fallen out with them. He was also desperate to make friends. The previous Sunday he had gone missing from home. They had telephoned friends and family and when he was nowhere to be found they had informed police. The next day the police found him sleeping under a bridge. He had been confused and incoherent but was able to give the parents' address.

When reunited with the family, Ashley was glad to see his parents and sister. He was in a dreadful state, cold and dirty. He found it difficult to recount what had happened that Sunday evening. His thinking was muddled and he appeared mixed up. All he could say was that he was sorry for having put them through the ordeal and he could not stop crying and apologising. They reassured him that they were not angry with him and took him home and, after a warm meal, he had slept for 12 hours. The parents too were in a state of shock. They were not sure what had gone wrong and, although they knew that Ashley was unhappy with school and friends, they had not realised how grave the situation had been from Ashley's perspective. They felt that they needed professional help and had taken him to the GP the next morning.

Developmental history: When pregnant with Ashley, his mother had pre-eclampsic toxaemia. She went into labour at 41 weeks and Ashley was born by Caesarean section on account of foetal distress. At birth he presented as floppy with a weak cry. However, there was no early feeding or other complications. His motor milestones were delayed. Ashley crawled by 12 months and walked at approximately 24 months. No difficulties were experienced with toilet training. His speech was also delayed: his first words did not emerge till 2 years of age and he began to combine words together into simple phrases around 3½ years. He was seen by a speech and language therapist but no therapy was offered.

Ashley received occupational therapy on account of his difficulties in motor coordination. He had been identified as having dyspraxia. He had always had problems with balance and was late to hop and jump. He was unable to pedal a bicycle till he was about 10 years of age. He could not use a pair of scissors until he was 11 years. His self-help skills were also poor. He could not dress himself independently till 12 years; he tended to put his clothes the wrong way round. His mother remembered that at that stage if he was left unsupervised to dress he became frustrated and screamed. Now at the age of 15½, he would not choose his clothes appropriately according to the weather conditions. He was known to go out in winter clothes during summer. Parents described his organisational skills as poor. His school bag had to be packed by his mother; he often lost pens, pencils and school books.

From the age of one year Ashley attended a private nursery part-time for two days a week. He transferred easily to the primary school. He was difficult to manage at school and the teacher complained that he ran around the classroom most of the time and did not do as told. In particular, he was 'rough' with other children and pushed them and pulled their hair. In Year 2 in the primary school he had a new teacher who took a personal interest in him. He liked her and did everything to please her. His behaviour showed remarkable improvement and his attention and concentration got better in due course and, in the next few years, he made considerable progress. He took part in group activities and was compliant. He liked to play with other children but his peers tended to reject him. He was behind in literacy and numeracy but the teachers felt he was improving and would 'catch up' with his peers eventually.

When he started secondary school Ashley found schoolwork difficult. He was in the bottom group in all subjects. In literacy he could do the work if the work was individually explained and if questions were put in plain words. The parents were aware that work at school was difficult for him. Teacher reports had commented that he had limited skills in independent work strategies and needed a lot of help with most tasks. He would not remember more than two instructions given at any one time and sometimes did not manage to follow even one. He had difficulties comprehending or recalling what he had read. His handwriting was poor and he had problems vocalising a sentence before he wrote it. He found number work difficult. Teacher reports at this time indicated difficulties even with very simple numerical problems. He would attain simple computation after much support but did not understand the basic principles involved. When a similar problem was presented he would not know what he was expected to do. He had consistently failed to join in class discussions or question/answer sessions in other subjects but when he did attempt to answer questions his input was at a tangent to what was being discussed. He produced a fairly small quantity of work whatever the subject or task. Ashley had been placed on the special educational register and later had a Statement of Special Educational Needs when he was 12 years. He had been assessed by an educational psychologist and an Individual Education Plan (IEP) had been drawn up. He was given two half sessions a week for literacy in a small group.

Ashley's difficulties got worse when he had to start doing French. Learning to read and write in English was bad enough, but French was something he could not cope with. His parents felt that, although school had identified Ashley's difficulties, he was not receiving the help he should. Ashley became reluctant to attend school and the parents had to resort to coaxing, cajoling and bribing him to get him to attend school. Certainly, he was not enjoying school. Teachers complained that he had developed the habit of wanting to go to the toilet especially during French and maths lessons to avoid being asked questions.

Current functioning: Ashley's difficulties were not just those of learning. They found him to be quite immature for his age. They had observed that his sister who was four years younger than him was more advanced than Ashley in most things. The toys he played with and the television programmes that he was interested in were more suitable for much younger children than him. While his sister was interested in science fiction programmes on TV, Ashley's favourite programmes were Scooby Doo and Tom and Jerry. He was found to have limited knowledge of how things worked in the real world. 'Every ordinary thing had to be explained to Ashley, sometimes again and again,' they said, 'and he would keep arguing about them'. For example, at 14 years he could not understand how airline tickets could be bought at a travel agent. According to Ashley, one has to go to the airport to buy them. When this was explained to him he had not believed his parents and kept asking the same question for several days. His sister had laughed at this and he had got angry and not spoken to her for days. None of these, on their own, seemed unusual to his parents and they felt he was being 'silly'.

Another of Ashley's problem was his relationship with his peers. He had had some friends when he was at the primary school. In the secondary school he had one friend with whom he walked around during break times. The parents felt that his peers in secondary school had not actively included him in their games and Ashley felt rejected by them. Ashley preferred the company of younger children and adults and found it difficult to fit in with children of his age group. He did not share their interests, and whatever he did to join them, he found that they were ahead of him. For a brief period he had tried to show some interest in pop music but his choice of music was considered 'uncool'. He had great difficulty joining the others in conversation on topics of mutual interest like football teams, as he was invariably less knowledgeable than his peers. In fact, this strategy had backfired on him as they started ridiculing him for his poor grasp of the knowledge of football clubs. They also had made fun of his lack of knowledge of 'facts of life'. They had got him to ask awkward questions from girls and then laughed at him.

For a short period Ashley had enjoyed being the class clown but things came to a head when he had unknowingly betrayed his friends. A group of his classmates had taken things from the school laboratory 'to do experiments' on their own at home. The mastermind behind the plot had asked Ashley to 'take' some chemicals from the laboratory and bring them to his house. The form teacher had noticed that Ashley was acting suspiciously and questioned him. Ashley gave the game away and told the truth. Thereupon the whole group set upon Ashley and beat him up. Upon learning about it, his parents had taken up the matter with the headteacher and Ashley was not punished. But the damage had been done. Ashley was ostracised and excluded by his peers. He was called a traitor and a coward. Some boys had turned up at home and threatened him; on one occasion rubbish was thrown through the letterbox. Thereafter Ashley could never have any friends in his class.

Meanwhile he was struggling with his schoolwork. Teachers complained that he was not doing his homework. His parents had to closely monitor the work he brought home. Often Ashley claimed he had no homework for the day while, in fact, he had destroyed the homework diary. The parents had to be constantly in touch with the teachers to find out what work Ashley was expected to do. At this stage his father decided to take a personal interest in his schoolwork and tried to help with his lessons. To his surprise he found that Ashley was very much behind in almost all the academic subjects. More worryingly, his ability to grasp basic concepts was limited. Every time Ashley had to do an arithmetic problem his father had to go back to the basic principles of the subject. For example, when he was helping Ashley with problems involving percentages his father had realised that Ashley did not know the six times multiplication tables!

At this stage, Ashley's difficulties were attributed to lack of motivation and want of application. The reports from school had consistently said that he 'had the potential' and 'could do better'. His parents had taken up the matter with school and wanted them to reconsider the choice of subjects, taking his academic difficulties into consideration. It had been recognised that PE, cooking and sporting activities were Ashley's strong points. A revised timetable was drawn up, but, unfortunately, it was never implemented. Consequently Ashley found himself having to do French and science, two of his worst subjects.

His parents described Ashley as a well-behaved boy and, after he had got over the temper tantrums and disruptive behaviour during the primary school days, there had not had any behaviour problems. He had always been loving and caring. He liked animals and pets. He was involved with the cadets for some time and received several commendations. He had enjoyed camping out with them. The family was involved with the local church and Ashley was well liked by their church friends and some of them had offered to take him under their wings. He had been involved in some voluntary work with them in a nursery. They had remarked that he had a flair for getting on with small children. Ashley was considering a career in nursery nursing or joining the army!

The parents described Ashley as naïve and not streetwise. He had been known to do daring things such as stealing things or talking back to teachers in order to please his friends and be part of the group. Compared to other young people, he was quite dependent on his parents and his sister. Although he would go to the local shops and visit his friend who lived in the neighbourhood, he could not travel by bus on his own. On the one occasion he had been adventurous enough to take a bus, he got lost.

Family history: The family consisted of Mr and Mrs Clerk, Ashley (15½ years) and Karen (11 years). Mr Clerk was a driving instructor and the mother worked as a secretary to a local firm. There was no significant family history of psychiatric problems, intellectual disability or epilepsy. The family had moved into the area when Ashley was 11 years old, at the time Ashley transferred to secondary school. His grandparents and the extended family lived not far away. He got on well with one of his 10-year-old nephews and they played computer games together.

Examination: At the time of examination Ashley was not confused or disoriented. He answered the questions reasonably well and without hesitation. He could tell the date, the day and the time. When asked about why he had decided to leave home, he said that when he left home he was not sure where he was going or what he would do; he just wanted to get away from home. He did not want to face another day of school and his parents had not understood how much he hated going to school. He had felt that his parents did not love him because they forced him to attend school even though they knew he hated it. He had wanted to get away from the house and had packed a bag and left home. He had sat in a park for a while and as it got dark he wandered aimlessly. A man had approached him and asked him if he was alright. He had got scared and quickly walked away. He could not remember how he came to be sleeping under the bridge. He was happy that he was back at home with his family. But he was not at all happy to go back to school, especially so because he had to sit for mock exams. He said he was so far behind in schoolwork that he would certainly fail the examination and his parents would be terribly disappointed with him. Moreover, he had no friends at school and felt isolated. He felt that his classmates ridiculed him and made fun of him.

Asked about his scholastic abilities, he said his reading and writing were reasonably good but he was poor in numbers. He was not good at managing money. For example, he was never sure, after paying for an article, how much money he should be getting back. To avoid embarrassment, he would either not count the money or get his sister to deal with it. For a boy of 15, Ashley's general knowledge was rather poor. When asked to name three cities in Europe he had great difficulty thinking of even one. When the same was asked of the UK he managed to name one city – London. Although he was a curious boy and was interested in watching the Discovery Channel on television, he could not name the continents of the world or the capitals of well-known countries. He did not know who the Prime Minister of the country was at the time of the interview, nor could he name any of the past Prime Ministers. He said he had watched programmes about the Second World War and found it interesting, yet he could not name the British prime minister at that time, let alone explain what the war was about. He was unaware of current happenings in the country and the world. While it may be considered normative for adolescents to be somewhat unaware or be uninformed about current affairs through lack of interest, Ashley's deficiency in general know-ledge was considerable and significant.

His abilities in abstract thinking too were limited. He could answer questions on similarities, for example between simple objects such as that pear and a banana or chair and table, but he could not tell the similarities between two conceptually linked abstract items such as poem and statue (works of art), praise and punish-ment (consequences of actions). On one occasion he had been sent to do carpentry and he was surprised he had to do woodwork! He had thought that carpentry meant working with carpets. In general, his verbal skills were poor. His accounts of incidents and happenings were very brief indeed. This was confirmed by his parents who described him as a 'poor historian'. He was quite poor at interpreting simple proverbs like, 'a stitch in time saves nine' or 'still waters run deep'. But Ashley could identify emotions and other people's intentions and thoughts when given common scenarios.

His self-care skills too were poor. He needed prompting to get himself washed and his clothes had to be laid out in the morning for him to get ready to go to school. While these may have been due to parental responses to his difficulties, he agreed that he did not always remember to get his schoolbooks and kits ready in morning. By the end of the week he had lost 90% of his pens, pencils and school paraphernalia. He also had difficulties with route finding. Until recently he had had difficulties finding his friend's house in their housing estate and had got lost many a time.

Ashley had many strengths. He was good at repairing things and constructing models. He described himself as a one who liked to do things rather than think about or read about them. He was good at jigsaw puzzles and construction toys (this was not formally tested, but his parents agreed that he was clever with his hands). He liked to find out how mechanical gadgets worked. His mother said he was good at dismantling things in the house rather than repairing them. He had one or two friends outside school whom he visited often. He admitted to having smoked cannabis with them on a few occasions, but he had not liked the experience. He denied taking any drugs on the day he had left the home.

At the time of examination there was no thought disorder, hallucinations or delusions. There was no evidence of unusual preoccupations, routines or obsessions. The contents of his speech were sometimes silly and his thinking was unrealistic. He wanted to leave home and lead an independent life, he said. He was not sure how he would pay the bills. He was sure his parents would meet all the expenses. When asked about how he would look after himself, he said that he will live on takeaway foods.

It was difficult to assess his capacity for moral judgement. The following is an excerpt from an interview held in a subsequent session.

Q: What would you do if you saw a purse in the street?

A: I'll take it.

Q: What would you do if you saw a person drop the purse?

A: I would take it.

Q: Is it not wrong to take someone else's money?

A: It is wrong; but I like the money. I can buy loads of games.

A school report was requested and he was referred to the child psychologist for formal testing of his cognitive abilities. He was referred to the paediatrician for medical tests to exclude any organic causes for his difficulties. The school report confirmed that he was of low academic abilities and was in the bottom set for all subjects. He was described as not being interested in schoolwork and lacking in effort. The report said that he liked to be the class clown and other children took advantage of him. His behaviour at school, apart from a few occasional incidents, was described as good. The teachers felt that he was out of step with his peers but was keen to be seen as part of a group. Hence he was easily led and got into trouble. He was known to act silly in class. For example, he would sneeze very loud in the library. This made others laugh and he would go on sneezing till he was asked to leave the library.

The paediatrician did not find any medical causes for his problems; chromosome analysis was normal. The clinical psychologist carried out the Wechsler Intelligence Scale for Children (WISC), one of the best known tests of intelligence (see later), on him and reported that his IQ was 66, i.e. in the 'extremely low' range, placing him on the 1st centile. Ashley's test scores are shown in Table 4.1. These results confirmed the clinical findings that Ashley's general intelligence was in the mild intellectual disability range and his verbal abilities were poorer than performance abilities.

Table 4.1 Ashley's scores on the Wechsler Intelligence Scale for Children – Third Edition UK (WISC – III^{UK})

Chronological age: 15 years 9 months 17 days	IQ	Percentile
Verbal	59	0.3
Performance	78	7
Full scale	66	1
		Index
Verbal comprehension	60	0.4
Perceptual organisation	94	34
Freedom from distraction	68	2
Perceptual speed	66	1

Case conceptualisation and formulation

Ashley's presentation was unusual. There was no clear reason for his actions on that Sunday night when he went missing from home. It was evident that he had wanted to get away from a stressful situation (sitting for the GCSE mock examination) and it was his way of coping with a difficult situation. The underlying problem, however, was one of intellectual or learning disability as shown by his educational, social and cognitive difficulties. Although his educational difficulties had been recognised by school, its impact on other spheres of activity had not been appreciated. Consequently his problems had gone unrecognised and had become known only following a crisis situation. Examination showed that he had considerable intellectual disability and social and educational impairment.

His difficulties in understanding concepts, abstract thinking and impaired general knowledge found on examination were a reflection of his poor cognitive abilities relative to his age. Although he was 15 years and 9 months his cognitive abilities were that of a much younger child. His level of abstract and analytic thinking, general knowledge and social competence showed significantly below that which would be expected of someone for his age. This was confirmed by his scores on WISC. Additionally, he was impaired educationally and socially. On the basis of these findings he was considered to have global intellectual (learning) disability. The degree of intellectual impairment was mild/moderate but significant. His difficulties in dealing with stressful situations were thought to be related to poor abilities in problem solving. The cause of the intellectual disability was not clear; no particular medical cause was found.

The other possible explanations for the clinical picture included

1 autism spectrum disorder (ASD)
2 specific learning disability (sLD) and
3 a major psychiatric disorder.

ASD is characterised by the triad of social impairment, communication difficulties and stereotyped behaviours (*see* Chapter 7). Ashley did show considerable difficulties in relating to peers and maintaining relationships and did not have many friends. But his social difficulties arose from being excluded by peers because of his naivety rather than from self-imposed social isolation. He did not show preoccupations, rigid routines or stereotyped behaviours. His social difficulties were a reflection of the overall impairment of general cognitive level rather than a specific deficit.

Specific learning disability (sLD) refers to impairments in one (or more) dimension of performance such as reading in the context of normal intelligence and IQ. Specific reading retardation (sometimes known as dyslexia or specific language impairment) is an example of sLD. Ashley's difficulties were spread across most domains of cognitive, social and emotional functioning. The possibility of a mental illness was raised by the GP possibly because of his seemingly irrational behaviour on the Sunday night. On mental state examination, however, there was no indication of delusions, hallucinations or thought disorder to indicate that he had a psychiatric illness such as schizophrenia (*see* Chapter 16). The possibility of undisclosed drug misuse was left open. It was possible that Ashley may have gone out on that Sunday and been involved in drug misuse. This was explored with him in later sessions. Ashley admitted that he had experimented with cannabis previously, but he had not liked the experience. He denied using any drugs thereafter.

Based on the above findings the following formulation was made: Ashley is a 15-year-old boy with mild intellectual disability; his disabilities were global and generalised and involved cognitive, social and emotional domains; he showed significant functional impairments in the social, educational and emotional spheres. In short, his mental age and functioning appeared to be equivalent to that of a much younger (8- or 9-year-old) child. Given these limitations Ashley's adaptive behaviour to the stress caused by demands of the school and friendships has been unusual and dramatic. This was considered to be an example of abnormal behaviour (absconding) to a normal situation (school examination and demands of peers) in a person with limited cognitive and emotional resources.

Theoretical perspectives

A number of different terms have been used to describe the entity of intellectual disability. Both DSM-IV and ICD-10 use the term 'mental retardation' in their classificatory systems. In the UK the term 'learning disability' (LD) is preferred because of the pejorative connotations of the term 'mental retardation'. (In the US the term 'learning disability' refers to specific learning disability such as reading disorder.) Others have used the term 'generalised or global learning disability' (gLD) to distinguish it from specific learning disabilities (sLD). Recently the term 'intellectual disability' has been gaining currency and may replace the terms 'mental retardation' and 'learning disability' in the near future. The name 'intellectual disability' has the added advantage of emphasising the global nature of the cognitive impairment. Often parents and teachers believe, or are led to believe, that only learning is deficient in the child with LD and that the rest of the functioning is adequate, while it is clearly not the case as the definition implies (see below). This is a major error of description and judgment because it is a misrepresentation of the difficulties the child has and tends to minimise the breadth and extent of impairments in the child. This inevitably results in inadequate educational support to, and inappropriately high expectations from, this vulnerable group of children.

Intellectual disability is lifelong and reduces the chances of employment and independent living. Two criteria have to be met for a diagnosis of intellectual or learning disability to be made:

1 significant impairment of intellectual functioning (below 70 IQ) *and*
2 concurrent deficits or impairments in adaptive functioning.

These dual criteria feature in all definitions of the condition. The American Academy of Mental Retardation, for example, defines it as 'a disability characterised by significant limitations in both intellectual functioning and in adaptive behaviour as expressed in conceptual, social and practical adaptive skills that originates before the age of 18' (AMA, 1992).

Intelligence or intellect refers to general mental capability. It involves the ability to reason, plan, solve problems, think abstractly, comprehend complex ideas, learn quickly, and learn from experience. Although not perfect, intelligence is represented by Intelligent Quotient (IQ) scores obtained from standardised tests. In regard to the intellectual criterion for the diagnosis of intellectual disability it is generally thought to be present if an individual has an IQ test score of approximately 70 or below. The theory that underlies IQ (called the psychometric theory of intelligence) is based on the assumption that most human abilities are underpinned and anchored on a basic and fundamental cognitive ability or general intelligence or g and that in the population intelligence scores are distributed in a bell-shaped normal distribution curve. A total of 68% (two-thirds) of the population falls within one standard deviation of the mean (85–115), while 95% of the population have IQs within two standard deviations of the mean (70–130).

The severity of intellectual disability is graded from mild to profound depending on the IQ:

- Mild Intellectual Disability: IQ between 50 and 70
- Moderate Intellectual Disability: IQ between 35 and 50
- Severe Intellectual Disability: IQ between 20 and 35.

Within the group of intellectual disability (using a cut-off of 70 IQ) two subgroups with distinct correlates may be identified: an 'organic' group and a non-organic ('subcultural') group. The organic group comprises of people with known prenatal, postnatal and chromosomal causes. Invariably they have moderate to severe intellectual disability (IQ below 50). Down's syndrome is the commonest disorder in this group. The non-organic or subcultural group is considered to be the normal variant representing those at the lower end of the normal Gaussian distribution of intelligence. They have no organic conditions, neurological or otherwise, tend to have mild intellectual disability and are more likely to belong to a low socio-economic group.

Psychometric testing using the Wechsler Intelligence Scale for Children, fourth edition (WISC-IV) or British Ability Scale, second edition (BAS-II) are useful in providing a profile of the child's cognitive strengths and weaknesses, but is not necessary in all cases. These are specialised tests that are carried out by trained clinical or educational psychologists. It is important that CAMHS practitioners are conversant with the criteria for referral and interpretation of such tests as well as the psychometric theory behind their use.

Adaptive behaviour refers to a collection of conceptual, social and practical skills that are necessary for functioning that are expected for the person's age in one's everyday life. Significant limitations in adaptive behaviour may affect the ability to respond to particular situations in the environment. The American Association of Mental Retardation (AMA, 1992) lists 10 areas of functioning: communication, self-care, home living, social skills, community use, self-direction, health and safety, functional academics, work and leisure. Limitations in two or more of these domains existing concurrently with subaverage intellectual functioning is necessary for a diagnosis of mental retardation to be made. Most workers agree that adaptive skills help shape the ultimate life success of people with intellectual retardation. The Vineland Adaptive Behaviour Scale is one of the most popular scales for the assessment of adaptive functioning. It also provides extensive population norms against which the subject's scores can be compared.

Mild intellectual disability: Of those with intellectual disability, 85% have IQs falling within this range. Although IQ <70 occur in about 2% of the population, when the impairment criterion is included the rates are around 1%. This is because many children and adults whose intelligence fall within this range manage life reasonably well educationally and socially. Many children with mild intellectual disability function reasonably well and go undetected at school and may not come to the attention of CAMHS, but a significant proportion requires special services including special educational help. Nevertheless, mild intellectual disability is over-represented in the population of children seen in CAMHS. This is especially so when they have other coexisting developmental problems such as autism or other developmental problems. Even when such problems are mild or do not meet all the criteria for a diagnosis of another developmental disorder (subclinical), the resulting disability tends to be cumulative and may cause significant problems for the child which may manifest as behavioural emotional or educational problems. The main features of mild intellectual disability are summarised in Box 4.1.

Box 4.1 Key features of mild intellectual (learning) disability

- An IQ between 50 to 70 *and* significant impairments in social, educational and personal domains.
- Cognitive impairment involves all, if not most, areas of cognitive functioning.
- Comorbidity with other developmental disorders such as autistic spectrum disorder, dyspraxia or hyperkinetic disorder are common.
- They are vulnerable and prone to decompensate under stress more easily than their well endowed counterparts.
- Mental health problems are twice as common.

Another important reason for the increased frequency of intellectual disability in clinic populations is increased prevalence of psychiatric disorders in this group (Deker and Koot, 2003). While as a group all psychiatric disorders are over-represented in children with intellectual disability, externalising behaviour disorders such conduct disorder and hyperkinetic disorder are particularly increased. The third reason for children with mild intellectual disability to be referred to CAMHS is when their adaptive behaviour may sometimes break down under the stress of life's demands. Children with low intellect are a vulnerable population and their abilities to respond to stressful situations in the environment are often compromised. This was particularly the case with Ashley.

In any generic assessment of a child presenting with possible intellectual disability, a clinical evaluation of the level of intellectual functioning is obligatory. This should include an assessment of the following:

- conceptual skills: money concepts, abstract thinking, concept of time
- scholastic skills: reading and writing
- speech and communication: receptive and expressive language
- social skills: gullibility, interpersonal skills, naivety, avoiding victimisation
- practical skills: personal activities of daily living; dressing, preparing meals, route finding, using the telephone, shopping, ensuring personal safety.

Conceptually mild intellectual impairment is considered to be a normal variant made up of those at the lower end of the normal distribution of intelligence. Many first-degree relatives have borderline IQs (around 85). In most cases of mild intellectual disability no medical cause is found. Both environmental and genetic factors are thought to contribute to their low intellectual abilities.

Moderate and severe intellectual disability: Most accounts on intellectual disability in the literature and textbooks are mainly about moderate and severe intellectual disability (IQ <50). Organic causes including chromosomal abnormalities account for the majority of this group, e.g. Down's syndrome, fragile X syndrome; other medical conditions such as epilepsy are common.

Treatment choice and management

Intellectual disability is managed rather treated unless there are accompanying mental disorders or complications. Experience over the last few decades in managing those with intellectual disability indicates a multidisciplinary approach is essential for managing the many difficulties in such children and adolescents.

Education: In the UK, children with uncomplicated mild learning disabilities are educated in mainstream schools. Children with more severe learning disabilities may attend special schools; frequently they have associated medical disorders, and sensory impairments, as either a cause or a correlate of the learning disabilities. By law, local educational authorities are required to provide the necessary provisions for the education of children with learning difficulties. Under the Education Act 1993 local education authorities have a duty for ensuring that special educational provision is made for pupils with special educational needs. The Act contains duties to identify, assess and provide for such children in need. The Education Act 1993 has established a Code of Practice which sets out detailed guidance. It identifies a continuum of need to be dealt with in five stages:

- Stage 1 – Class teacher or form/year tutor has overall responsibility.
- Stage 2 – Special Educational Needs Co-ordinator (SENCO) takes the lead in co-ordinating and drawing up individual educational plans.
- Stage 3 – External educational, usually from an education psychologist, support enlisted.
- Stage 4 – Statutory assessment by Local Education Authority (LEA).
- Stage 5 – Statement of Special Educational Needs issued by LEA.

In practice, the process of getting a 'statement' can be lengthy and laborious. Sadly, financial considerations tend to prevail. The education of children with mild and moderate intellectual disability is now governed by the principle of inclusion. Although the definitions of inclusion vary, in general it refers to the right of the child to be educated in the mainsteam educational environment while acknowledging the need for special schools. The advantages of inclusion are said to be lack of stigma, enabling children to learn from peers, increasing opportunities for educational, social and personal advancement. It is thought to enhance self-esteem, academic achievement and personal functioning. While proponents of inclusion have provided evidence for this view, others have pointed out that many children with intellectual disabilities continue to be stigmatised and tend to underachieve in mainstream schools.

Support for family and young person: Many families with children who have mild intellectual disability need support and help, but currently there are no special provisions for this group. At a minimum, parents need to be made to understand the various limitations in the child's functioning as well as his or her strengths. Career advice, mentoring and 'buddy' systems may be necessary. This group of children are particularly vulnerable to abuse and exploitation.

Child mental health services: The role of CAMHS with this group of children and adolescents is primarily in the treatment of coexisting mental health difficulties. As mentioned before they are more at risk of mental health problems. Although rates of most mental disorders are increased, behaviour problems are the most common complications. For clinicians, identification of major mental disorders in children with intellectual disability may be challenging because the presentations are often different from those with normal intellectual functioning.

Clinicians working with children with special needs have a responsibility to liaise with educational professionals to ensure the provision of appropriate educational input and services. Although the ultimate responsibility for such decisions lies with the local education authorities, CAMHS clinicians have an important role in presenting the child's difficulties in such a manner as to optimise the chances of getting the appropriate educational provision for the child.

Progress and outcome

Following assessment Mr and Mrs Clerk were given feedback on Ashley's difficulties and the findings of the clinical and psychological assessment. Intellectual disability was described to them as a general and widespread impairment of development affecting cognitive, social and educational/vocational functioning. However, in the case of Ashley, the impairment was mild and with support and help a good outcome could be expected. It took some time for them to alter their previous belief that learning disability affected only scholastic learning. Initially they were in denial and hoped that Ashley would 'catch up' with his peers.

Ashley refused to go back to school saying that the place 'did his head in'. He was enrolled in the local college for a learning skills course when he turned 16. Initially he was enthusiastic and attended college regularly. But soon he said he found the course difficult. More worryingly, he could not get on with the others in the class. He claimed that they had got him to smoke cannabis and use drugs. He got into conflicts with another boy and got into a fight. Following this he was afraid of attending college and kept away from going to the town centre for fear of retaliation from the boy and his friends. He spent most of his time at home and became frustrated and irritable. He started a part-time job in a supermarket but could not carry on with it because he was not happy with the pay. Most of his anger was turned against his parents for not helping him enough.

He and his family were seen on a number of occasions to get them to work better as a family. The aim was to get his parents to understand Ashley's difficulties and to have realistic expectations of him. Individual sessions were offered to Ashley to get a perspective on his difficulties. In the sessions Ashley came across as an unhappy boy who was acutely conscious of his limitations. He had little confidence in himself and felt that he was getting left behind. He kept contact with a few friends and went out with them, but he described himself as a 'loser'. Although aware of his difficulties, he was unrealistic in his expectations. He wanted his mother to give up her work and be at home with him. He said he hated to be on his own, it was boring. He called it child abuse for him to be left all alone at home. On other occasions he had invited other young people home without his parents' permission. On one occasion some electronic items were stolen by some of them. This made his parents bar him from inviting friends home.

When seen together their problems were framed by the therapist as problems that most families with teenagers face. Ashley was described as being rebellious and, owing to his intellectual difficulties, was less inclined to understand the problems, let alone solve them. The main needs for Ashley were outlets for socialisation, guidance from a mentor and recreational activities until he was ready to undertake some form of vocational training of his choice. The family was helped to access a number of community resources for young people with leaning disabilities in the locality.

Three months after Ashley was discharged from the service, he took an overdose of paracetamol following an argument with his father over doing paper rounds and was admitted to hospital. When seen in the ward he said his father would be arrested because he had made him take the overdose. It was December and he refused to go back home, saying that he wanted to live on his own without any interference from his parents. When seen in the ward with his mother, he said, 'Give me my Christmas presents; I want to leave home. I am 16 and old enough to be on my own.' At this point social services were asked to get involved. After one more day in the ward, he decided to go home.

There have been a number of crises in the family since the overdose. On a number of occasions he has tried to leave home. Fortunately, his uncle has been able to keep Ashley with him each time for a few days to defuse the situation. Eighteen months after the referral to CAMHS, Ashley continues to live at home and attend college. His place at college has been under threat because of his behaviour. For example, he has been seen masturbating in class and using sexualised language with female teachers and students. There has been no input from social services. When he turned 17 he was referred to adult learning disability services. He was said not to meet their criteria. At the time of writing the CAMHS takes referrals up the 17th birthday but he is being followed up in clinic. The long-term future for Ashley would depend on finding a suitable supportive environment such as supported living or a group home.

Comments

Ashley represents that group of children whose intellectual disabilities go unrecognised in school and are left to sink quietly without real help. While officially he had been statemented and had an IEP, in reality this meant very little apart from 'some help in literacy'. In spite of an IEP he was made to do subjects well beyond his abilities. His difficulties had mounted as he got older and the demands on him increased. Of everyone, Ashley appears to be the only one who had been aware of the increasing discrepancy between his chronological age and his abilities. Unable to verbalise his difficulties, his very insight into his difficulties had made him very unhappy and had even made him feel suicidal. In one of the individual sessions he said, 'I feel like a seven-year-old'. This was a remarkably accurate description of himself. Without help from the mainstream school and with the provision of a special school denied because he was 'too good' for a special school, children like Ashley are victims of the principle of normalisation. In Ashley's case it was nothing less than a disaster.

It has to be recognised that mainstream education is not suitable for a small minority of children and they need a 'special school'. There are no agreed criteria for placement in special schools and there is vast variation across the local educational authorities. In recent years there has been a consistent decline in the number of special schools in the UK. At present only those with severe learning disabilities or severe behaviour problems get places in special schools.

This has no doubt been due to financial considerations, although inclusion is upheld as the justification. This is an injustice to the principle of inclusion and the children involved.

Would Ashley's problems have been prevented if he had received appropriate help while at school? Early recognition of his problems and proper educational provision would no doubt have been helpful, but would have been unlikely to have addressed the other difficulties that occurred in later teenage years. These require integrated services involving social services, education and community support services to provide support, mentorship, leisure activities, vocational training and career advice. Currently services are weak and poorly coordinated. There are few dedicated learning disability services for children and adolescents (and probably none for the mildly disabled group) in the country and those that exist are selective in what they provide. For example, services for major psychiatric disorders, challenging behaviours and forensic populations are available for those with intellectual disabilities in some parts of the country. Very few CAMHS are resourced sufficiently to provide a service for this group of children whose needs are different and the support services necessary are very different to that of the population seen by specialist CAMHS. Children with mild to moderate intellectual disability require a service that is firmly based on their educational, social and mental health needs. A psychosocial model of service delivery rather than rather a mental health model is likely to meet these needs better. Despite the laudable ambition of The National Service Framework for Children to include learning disability within generic CAMHS, the requirements for a service to this group of children are somewhat different from what a traditional CAMHS could provide. Properly resourced services based on validated models that target this vulnerable group are needed rather than depending on an already overburdened specialist CAMHS.

An important message that Ashley's case conveys is that the impairments in mild intellectual (learning) disabilities may not be mild at all. His parents had great difficulty understanding how his so called 'mild' disabilities resulted in such great problems. What about the future for Ashley? One alternative is for him to be referred to adult learning disability services when he is old enough for the services. Given the current climate, one can foresee a long debate among various potential service providers about taking up Ashley's case. The learning disability services in the area do not take those with mild to moderate degree of disability and it is highly unlikely that he will be offered a service. Another possibility is that he might 'act out' his distress and his behaviour might become disruptive or he may take further overdoses. In such situations, due to lack of any other provision, by default he might be considered a suitable candidate for psychiatric services. Involvement of adult psychiatric services in the absence of an identifiable mental disorder would be most inappropriate and damaging to Ashley. There is also the possibility that he might wittingly or unwittingly break the law and enter the criminal justice system.

> **Box 4.2 Research on mild intellectual disability says that . . .**
>
> - Mild intellectual disabilities occur in at least 1% of the population.
> - Mental disorders are two to four times more common in children with intellectual disabilities; 30% have a diagnosable mental disorder.
> - About a third of children referred to CAMHS have some degree of intellectual disability.
> - Children with mild intellectual disability often need extra provisions such as educational input and family and social support.
> - Parents and teachers should be aware of the impact of intellectual disability in areas of the child's functioning other than learning; a range of provisions are necessary for this group.

References

American Association on Mental Retardation. *Mental Retardation: definition, classification and systems support.* 9th edn. Washington, DC: American Association on Mental Retardation; 1992.

Deker MC, Koot HM. DSM-IV disorders in children with borderline to moderate intellectual disability I: Prevalence and impact. *Journal of the American Academy of Child and Adolescent Psychiatry.* 2003; **42**: 915–22.

Chapter 5

Parental divorce and separation

Dear Team

Many thanks for seeing Tim, a 10½-year-old boy. His mother complains that he is shutting himself away in his bedroom and refusing to communicate with other members of the family. She says that he paces his room up and down, talking to himself and muttering to himself in anger. He agrees that he is angry all the time, has tantrums and gets angry very easily. On one occasion he had left the house and been missing for some three hours. His mother had to inform the police and he was found roaming in the neighbourhood. He is said to be aggressive towards his sister. He does not like the word 'no' and challenges his mother whenever possible. He complains of not having any freedom. There have been problems at school too. He has been falling behind in his work and takes a 'don't care' attitude towards schoolwork. I understand he had been subject to some low grade bullying at school. He has few friends and is unhappy both at home and at school.

His parents are separated and went through an acrimonious divorce. At one stage, Tim's father took Tim and his sister away. They were returned to their mother following a Court Order. The children now reside with his mother and his stepfather. I feel that Tim has been adversely affected by the divorce, separation and the events that followed. Surprisingly, his 8-year-old sister, Susan, is well adjusted and is doing well at school. I would be most grateful for your advice and intervention.

Yours sincerely

Dr Smith

GP

The referral letter, although short, provided sufficient details about the case and viewed the problem as a response to the messy parental separation and divorce. It was not clear when the separation was or what the contact arrangements with the father were. There was no indication as to whether there had been difficulties that predated the divorce. At the time of referral the legal process of the divorce had been completed and the mother had custody of the children. In short, there was no ongoing custody or legal issues. It was therefore decided to see the mother, children and the stepfather as a family initially. It was recognised that various members of the family may have to be seen separately or in various combinations to make a full assessment. Meeting the father of the children, or inviting him for one or more sessions, was considered necessary at some point in the course of assessment and treatment.

Clinical presentation and background

A family session was arranged to which all members of the current household were invited. The session was attended by Tim (10½ years), his sister Susan (8 years), Wendy, his mother, and Simon, the stepfather. Tim's mother described Tim as a polite boy who sometimes put on a front but his mother felt that he was sad, lonely and angry. She said he was different from day to day. He was snappy and abrupt towards her and had little respect for her. He called her names and was quite aggressive towards his sister. She found it difficult to discipline him. Whenever he was asked not to do something or was refused something he went into a temper or he would go to his room, pace the floor, talking to himself, saying things like, 'I am always wrong, I am always at fault'. She was most worried about the way Tim excluded himself from the family. He would not join in with family activities and spent most of the time in his room.

Of late, he had started having his meals in his room and refused to join the family during mealtimes. She was very upset and concerned when, following an angry argument, he left the house and was missing for 3 hours. She had to call the police and Tim was angry that she had called the police. She also felt that he knew just how to upset her. Tim would often explode into angry outbursts but these had decreased over the last few months. When angry he would kick doors and talk to himself. He also had lots of physical complaints, such as headaches, sore throats, and aching muscles. They had made several visits to the GP over the last 2–3 years but no physical illness had been found. His behaviour had been reasonably good until he was 6 or 7 years old. Her view was that the change in him was the result of the breakdown of the marital relationship or the consequence of witnessing his father's violence towards her before and after the separation. He had also seen her very distressed during her 'struggle with her depression'.

The interview was a tense one. While his mother talked about her concerns, Tim looked out of the window and, at times, his eyes were filled with tears. His sister moved close to her mother and held her hand. Simon said little until he was addressed directly and asked what he thought the problems were. Simon said that he agreed with Wendy's account of Tim's behaviour. He felt that Tim was angry, sad and confused. His behaviour was worse following visits to his father. Simon had tried his best to develop a relationship with Tim. Simon was a PE instructor and Tim was interested in sports. Although Tim liked football he refuses to go to football matches with Simon. He described Tim as a boy who could be polite and fun to be with. But he was so full of anger that he resisted relating to the family in a normal way. Simon was most concerned about Tim's lack of respect for his mother. He was rude to her and took every opportunity to put her down. At this point, Wendy intervened to say that Tim blamed her for 'sending his dad away'. Simon felt that Tim deliberately kept himself away from the family and all attempts by Simon to get involved with Tim have not been successful so far. Simon was unsure as to how much he should get involved in disciplining Tim and left most of it to his mother. However, there were times when he had felt that he should intervene, especially when Tim was rude to his mother.

During the family interview, Tim did not say very much. When questioned about his feeling towards his mother and Simon, Tim said that he thought he got on quite well with Simon but he said that he found his mother to be too interfering and that he wanted to be left alone. On direct questioning he said he could not think of an instance where they had a good time as a family and he added, 'We hardly talk.' He said he was supposed to visit his dad once a week at weekends but in practice visits have become infrequent. Dad's girlfriend had her family living with him and there was not enough room for all of them. Asked about school, he said he was reasonably good at his schoolwork but he had only one friend, whom he had known from Year 2. They visited each other. He felt that the other boys in his class were rather mean and on a number of occasions there had been some bullying. He had fallen behind in his schoolwork because he felt he was not paying enough attention to what was going on in class, not done his homework in time and, in general, been out of step with classwork. He said he got on well with his teachers but he was not enjoying school as much as he did before. He said he liked his nan (paternal grandmother); when he went to his nan's he met his cousins, some of whom were around his age and they got on well. More recently he had been visiting nan instead of his father.

His sister, Susan, said that she agreed with her mother that Tim had a bad temper and he would blow hot and cold. She did not know whether to speak to him or to avoid him. She said that he was 'horrible' to her mother. She felt sorry for her mother that she has had to put up with Tim's outbursts. At this point Tim snapped back at her and said that she (Susan) was horrible to him and that she was not keen to visit their dad and that she was being 'ungrateful'.

Developmental history: Tim was a planned pregnancy and delivery was normal. His mother described him as quite hard work when he was a baby. He did not sleep much and was a voracious feeder. She breastfed him until the age of one, and she described it as one of the happiest times of her life. Her relationship with her husband was good at this time and they had just moved into a flat of their own. Tim's developmental milestones were within normal range. His medical history was unremarkable except for recurrent ear infections as a toddler. He got on well with kids in his class and there were no problems in school.

His mother said that Tim used to be a lovely boy but recently his good qualities had been overshadowed by other problems. He liked football and she had enrolled him in football training and he had been going once a week over the last 4 months. Unfortunately he was not selected for the football team but she felt that Tim had dealt with the disappointment quite well. He was good at maths and science and when asked what he wanted to be when he grew up, he said he wanted to be a scientist or an inventor. Following the family interview, an individual session was arranged with Mrs Pickering with the aim of collecting more information about the family break-up and the events preceding it.

Individual session with Mrs Pickering

Tim's mother had been married to her former husband for 8 years and been living with him for the previous 11 years. Initially they had been happy. After getting married they had moved to a flat and her relationship with her husband was good. But soon he became very controlling towards her. She felt stifled and increasingly oppressed by him. He restricted her from socialising with friends. She said things changed after Tim was born. She was living in a high rise flat with the baby and had little support from her husband. He was rude and threatening towards her initially and later started hitting and punching her. She had had postnatal depression but had not realised it at that time. Her husband was sexually very demanding. She had very little help from the extended family and found it difficult to cope with the baby.

The main problem was the deteriorating relationship between her and her husband. He took every opportunity to put her down. The violence became increasingly more severe. Things got worse after the second baby was born. Her husband spent more time away from home on the pretext of work. He was away from home for most of the month and when he came home he behaved like a visitor. He took little notice of her or the children and the slightest disagreement deteriorated into arguments and resulted in physical violence. She had been punched, kicked and pushed down the stairs.

When Tim was about 7 years her husband had told her that he had formed another relationship. Mrs Pickering was devastated by it. Within a month of breaking the news to her he left home. But he would come back home regularly on the pretext of seeing the children and demand sex from her. There were lots of arguments and he would be violent towards her. On one occasion following a row he had pushed her down the stairs. She informed the police this time and he was arrested and warned to keep out of the house. She had hurt her back and had to have an operation on her spine. Tim had been a witness to the incident but had never talked about it. A month later her husband had tried to run her and the children down with a car. At this point she contacted lawyers and a Court Order was made, preventing him from having any contact with her or the children. However, one day he had taken the two children to his house without her permission and kept them with him for 2 weeks. She reported this to the police and got the children back. Currently there was a prohibition order preventing him from visiting her or the children at home.

The children were supposed to visit him every week and stay over Friday and Saturday nights but, in effect, their visits were occasional and when they did visit him they came back the same day. Her husband had said that the living arrangements at home were not satisfactory, that there was not enough room for the children. Tim had started visiting his paternal grandmother instead of going to his father's house. His father visited him at these times. Susan was not keen to visit her father and had not been to see him for quite some time.

Wendy said that she found the separation very difficult, especially because of the power he held over her. During this period she had become quite depressed and she had been treated by the GP with antidepressants. On one occasion she had taken an overdose and had been admitted to the hospital. She had known Simon for some time. They started a relationship 2 years ago. He had moved into the family home 18 months ago and they got married soon after. She had been cautious in introducing Simon to Tim and wondered how the two would get on. But she felt that Simon had not imposed himself on the family and his introduction into the family had gone well. Simon would usually keep out of the way when Wendy and Tim got into arguments or disagreements. She felt that Simon and Tim got on reasonably well. Next, Tim was seen individually.

Individual examination of Tim

Tim was an articulate boy and expressed his views quite well. He was chatty and wanted to tell his side of the story. He said that he and his mother were not getting on at all; they got into arguments over small things and not a day passed without an argument. When asked what he thought the main problems were, he identified the following:

1 the relationship with his family, which included mum, Simon, and Dan (11-year-old son of his father's girlfriend) and
2 his anger; he said he found it difficult to control his anger; he was snappy and had a bad temper.

He said he was quite unhappy with the situation as it was. He was not happy when he was at 'mum's house' nor was he happy when he was at his 'dad's house'. He felt his dad paid more attention to Dan, the 11-year-old, than to Tim. He said his dad was in a difficult position because he had Tracy, his girlfriend, and her children living with them. His mother blamed his dad for not seeing him regularly and often said that his dad was not interested in him or his sister. He said this was not true. His father was a long-distance lorry driver and he loved to go in dad's truck in the past but more recently there had been no opportunity for such trips. He said that when he was at school he kept thinking about dad and sometimes mum. This made him quite unhappy and when other children teased him, he cried easily. The happiest time at the moment for him was when he went to his grandmother's and met his cousins. But the grandmother and his mother did not get on well and, in fact, did not speak to each other. He felt that his mother was not happy with his visits to his grandma.

Tim was close to tears when talking about his father. He said his father was 6 feet tall and very strong. He was a good driver and they used to enjoy it when he took Tim in his vehicle. He remembered that during holidays his father would take him in the truck. They would drive hundreds of miles and go on long journeys. He worked in different places and it was fun going with dad in the truck. He could not remember when he had had a good time with his dad recently. He blamed his mother for not taking his dad back. He was aware that his dad had come back several times and wanted his mother to take him back. He was angry with her for turning him down. 'I am without a dad because my mother sent him away,' he said. He felt they could be one family together if only his mother would have his dad back. During the session Tim's mood fluctuated between one of anger and sadness. He talked about his dad with fondness but there was also a feeling of sadness and loss associated with it. He appeared quite angry when discussing his current predicament and often said, 'Why can't we be a normal family?' His appetite and sleep were normal and, apart from the misery he exhibited, there were no features of depression.

Case conceptualisation and formulation

Tim was a 10 years 6 month old boy who presented with a mixed picture of emotional and behaviour problems. He was sad, upset and unhappy following the separation and divorce of his parents. He had been isolating himself from the family, preferring to spend time in his room, usually ruminating over past events. He was also an angry young lad. He held his mother responsible for the break-up of the family and for depriving him of his dad and, therefore, directed all his aggression and anger against her. Although he had not been very close to his father in the past, since the separation he had felt the loss of his father acutely and now idealised him and yearned to be with him. Obviously the fact that he could not maintain contact with his father because of his father's current commitments and living situation only made Tim feel the loss more acutely. In addition he idealised his father. In psychoanalytic literature this has been called 'defensive idealisation of the absent father'.

He was torn by loyalty conflicts. In his mind a normal, loving relationship with his mother meant that he was being disloyal to his father. The continuing conflict between the parents was a major factor in maintaining Tim's difficulties. He felt lonely and powerless as most children who go through the separation and divorce of their parents do. It was easy for him to see one parent as good and the other as bad (splitting). He had had to cope with a number of changes: change of school, friends and home. A positive factor in the family for him was that he was quite accepting of Simon and had a reasonably good relationship with him. Obviously he was grieving the loss of his father, which he had not even begun to acknowledge and hence was full of blame and anger. It was highly likely that he did not see the separation of parents as final and probably fantasised that his father could come back and rejoin the family. Although the separation and divorce had been the major factor in causing Tim's difficulties, another factor that maintained the problem was the reconstitution of the family by Simon's entry into the family. Simon felt unsure of his position as stepdad and was ambivalent about his attitude towards Tim. His son's visits to the family created minor perturbations in Tim, resulting in Tim feeling pushed out by Simon's family.

In spite of the difficulties that the family encountered, there were a number of features that were encouraging and positive: a definitive decision had been made (including a Court Order) that the children stay with their mother, thereby eliminating custody battles; Simon was accepted within the family by Tim although the relationship was not very close; the mother had recovered from her depression and was functioning reasonably well. The main destabilising factors were the unsatisfactory contact arrangements with the father, his overt and covert undermining and demeaning of the mother and her role, and Tim's idealisation of his father.

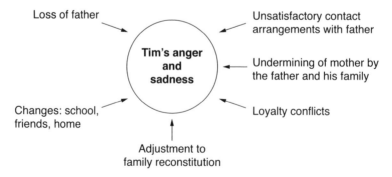

Figure 5.1 Factors associated with Tim's difficulties in adjusting to parental separation.

In psychiatric terminology, the emotional and behavioural features exhibited by Tim following the separation and divorce of his parents would be termed 'adjustment disorders'. Adjustment disorders are defined as the development of emotional or behavioural symptoms in response to identifiable stressor/stressors that produce marked distress and significant impairment in functioning. The various factors leading to and maintaining Tim's adjustment problems are shown in Figure 5.1.

Theoretical perspectives

Separation and divorce are classed as the second most stressful life events in an adult's life, second only to death of a spouse. For children, parental separation is equally stressful but this is little acknowledged by parents. Family life is changing all over the world and parental separation and divorce are becoming common. Currently the divorce rates are around 150 000 a year in the UK. It is now estimated that one in three first marriages in the UK and one in two second marriages end in separation or divorce. Two-thirds of those divorcing have children under the age of 16. At least one in three children will experience parental separation before the age of 16. It is estimated that about 2.5 million children will grow up in stepfamilies.

Recent approaches to divorce, separation and stepfamily formation have moved away from considering them aberrations of 'normal' family life that were deficient and pathogenic, to thinking about them as normative life transitions that give rise to new challenges. It has been postulated that within the next decade the stepfamily will be the most prevalent type of family in Western countries.

For the child, parental separation and divorce is primarily a loss: the loss of the non-resident parent. This produces bereavement reactions and they go through the usual stages: an acute phase during which there is rage, aggression and depression; and a transition phase when they disengage from the parents. Bereavement affects not only the child but also the parents. Furthermore, the children and the parent go through each step of the bereavement process at different rates; often the grieving process of the children is not compatible with that of the parents, especially when the parent remarries.

Current research consistently indicates that parental separation is best viewed as a process rather than a single event. The extent and significance of the chain of events and a sequence of experiences that begin before divorce itself and continuing long after has been emphasised by most authorities (Wallerstein *et al.*, 2000). For children, these transitions involve exposure to marital conflict and, in many cases, intra-familial violence, followed by the experience of disruption in the parental relationship and living arrangements. Loss or partial loss of a parent, loss of contact with grandparents, change of peer group and change of school are common. Additionally, for most children, within the next few years of divorce there is also another change – the entry of a stepparent into the family which necessitates further alteration in family organisation and functioning.

Effect of parental separation and divorce on children

Research into the effects of parental divorce and separation on children over the past three decades has produced two consistent findings (e.g. Hetherington, 1993):

- the vast majority of children who experience parental separation and divorce do not exhibit severe or enduring behaviour problems and most develop into reasonably competent, well adjusted adults, and
- a significant minority of children show emotional, behavioural, educational and social problems. For example, about 10% of children in non-divorced families score above a clinical cut-off on total emotional and behaviour problems on the child behaviour checklist versus 20–30% in divorced families (Hetherington, 1993).

Following an extensive review of the literature of over 200 studies linking parental separation and outcomes for children, Rodgers and Pryor (1998) concluded that children of separated families compared with intact families:

1   are at risk of behavioural problems, withdrawn behaviour, aggression and other antisocial behaviour
2   tend to perform less well at school and gain fewer educational qualifications
3   are more likely to report health problems, visit their doctor or be admitted to hospital
4   are more likely to leave school without qualifications; leave home prematurely and form cohabiting partnerships
5   tend to report higher levels of depression and drug misuse in adolescence and adulthood.

Other studies have found that children of separated families tend to grow up in households with lower incomes, poorer housing and greater financial hardships than intact families. They are more likely to leave school and home when young and more likely at an early age to become sexually active, form cohabiting partnerships, become pregnant, become a parent and give birth outside marriage. Although the differences in outcome are clear, it cannot be assumed that parental separation is the underlying cause. The multiplicity of factors that impinge on families before, during and after separation indicates a process, rather than a single event, that merits careful examination.

What about the long-term effects of divorce? The Virginia longitudinal study of divorce and remarriage carried out by Mavis Hetherington (1993) attempted to answer this question. The study began in the early 1970s and followed up a cohort of children who experienced divorce for more than thirty years. Her findings confirm that about 25% of children of divorce show serious social emotional or psychological problems compared to 10% of children living with two parent families. But 20 years later the children from divorced and never divorced families were more similar than different. She concludes thus: 'Divorce is usually brutally painful for the child, . . . but the negative long-term effects [of divorce] have been exaggerated to the point where we now have created a self-fulfilling prophecy' (Hetherington and Kelly, 2002).

Factors affecting outcome

Adverse outcomes are more likely under certain circumstances. Parental conflict before, during and after the separation is, by far, the most damaging to children's psychological well being. Children exposed to hostilities, mutual denigration and recrimination between parents are subject to loyalty conflicts and feel pressurised to forge alliance with one parent and reject the other. Most children are simply not prepared to make such a choice and would prefer to maintain relations with both parents.

The ability of parents to recover from the psychological distress associated with their separation is important for children's own ability to adjust. Two lessons are clear from research. First, in the first year after divorce parents are often preoccupied with their own anger and emotional upheaval that they are unable to respond sensitively to children's needs. Second, in most divorcing families there is a period in the first year after divorce when mothers become depressed and function poorly. During this period divorced parents tend to become ineffectual in dealing with children and tend to lose control of them. Their ability to parent children authoritatively is impaired.

Continuing contact with the non-resident parent may benefit children's adjustment following separation but there is no simple relationship with frequency of contact. It is the quality of contact, rather than the quantity, that appears important. Under ideal circumstances, the custodial and non-custodial parents work together to avoid conflict with each other, share resources, rights and responsibilities and support each other's parenting for the benefit of their children. When contact does not work, it is mainly for two reasons: lack of parents' commitment to contact and parental conflict. Contact is a significant source of stress for children when contact arrangements do not work. Children report difficulties with new partners of non-resident parents, in establishing a meaningful relationship with the contact parent and with not being consulted about contact. Resident parents find the continuing emotional engagement with the former partner difficult.

In some studies marital conflict *before* the separation has been found to be a more important predictor of child adjustment than divorce itself or post-divorce conflict. Many large-scale longitudinal studies have found that as many as half of the behavioural and academic problems of children in marriages whose parents are later divorced were observed 4–12 years *before* the separation. This research shows that regardless of parents' marital status, a high level of marital conflict experienced during childhood could be linked to a number of psychological problems and disorders in children and adolescents. Violence is more likely to occur in high conflict marriages and has an independent effect on children's adjustment. Repeated exposure to violence leads to children's adjustment difficulties and has a more significant effect than marital conflict. Often intrafamilial violence is accompanied by child abuse.

Wider kin networks, especially grandparents, can play an important part in supporting children and grandchildren around the time of separation. They are an additional resource when one parent is absent and other parent is upset, and can communicate with their grandchildren while supporting their own child. Clinicians need to be aware that grandparents and friends are key figures for children.

Treatment choice and management

In contrast to the voluminous literature on the effects of and outcomes in family divorce and separation, there is a marked lack of systematic studies on interventions that work with children and families. Controlled trials of therapeutic interventions with post-divorce families are limited. A recent review of research on interventions for separated and divorced families notes that adequate research on this topic is meagre (Kelly, 2000). Three types of interventions have been studied:

1 School-based interventions, which typically involve groups of children from divorced families. Most involve educational and therapeutic activities and are of short duration.
2 Parent-focused interventions using group therapy to help parents deal with the stresses of divorce to improve their coping skills and to promote their adjustment and usually only secondarily to improve parenting and family relationships.
3 Divorce mediation has been shown to reduce conflict and re-litigation and also increase father involvement in child rearing. It has not been found to promote the mental health of either children or parents.

A number of parent-based projects have been conducted in the US and evaluated (Emery, 1999). These group therapy based programmes consistently report high levels of parent satisfaction but parental gains have do not show beneficial impact on children. School-based divorce intervention programmes have shown modest improvement in children's feelings about self and the family, coping abilities and perceived self-competence. But the effect sizes were small and it is doubtful whether they were successful in alleviating more severe problems such as conduct problems and depression. Divorce mediation offers parents a forum to resolve their disputes about financial settlements, custody disputes and contact issues. Although mediation has been shown to be more effective than litigation in settling disputes between ex-spouses, its effect on child and adult mental health measures has been very little indeed.

   In CAMHS settings most frequently used interventions are individual therapy for the child (including play therapy), individual therapy for the parents, couple therapy and family therapy, each of these alone or in various combinations. When providing help to children, professionals need to focus on the child's view of the world rather than being preoccupied by the breakdown in the parents' relationship as partners. Research into children's wishes and feelings has shown that (Cockett and Tripp 1994):

1 Children need an explanation. They need to understand that their parents can no longer live together but they will remain interested in and responsible for them. It also helps to free the children from the idea that they have been responsible for the break-up.
2 Maintaining good relationships with both parents minimises the chances of adverse effects on children.
3 Continuing conflict between parents is by far the most damaging for children.
4 How well the parent, especially the resident parent, adapts to the divorce and its consequences has a significant impact on the adjustment of children.
5 Major psychological or psychiatric problems that antedate the divorce or are precipitated by the divorce have an adverse influence on children's adjustment to divorce and separation.

Management plan for the Pickering family

The aims of therapy for various members of the Pickering family were as follows:

- For Tim:
  1 Help recognise and come to terms with the loss of his father.
  2 Develop a realistic understanding of the reasons for the family break-up, especially the violence his mother had suffered at the hands of his father.
  3 Assist him in re-establishing a good relationship with his mother.
- For Mrs Pickering (mother):
  1 Avoid blaming or denigrating her ex-husband.
  2 Support contact for Tim with his father.
  3 Strengthen her relationship with Tim.
  4 Overcome her bitterness and anger with her former spouse and avoid conflict.
- For Simon (the stepfather):
  1 Develop a positive relationship with Tim and avoid taking a disciplinary role until a close relationship has formed.
- For Neil (the father):
  1 Come to terms with the divorce.
  2 Maintain parental boundaries and avoid using Tim to 'get at' his ex-wife.
  3 Avoid denigrating and blaming his ex-wife.
  4 To be honest with Tim as to how much contact is feasible and keep to the promises he makes.

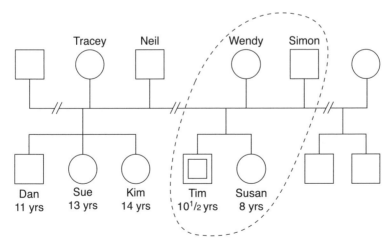

Figure 5.2 Genogram of the Pickering family (the current household is indicated by the oval).

Family sessions: The first few therapy session involved Mrs Pickering, Simon, Tim and his sister, Susan. Together with the family, the therapist spent some time drawing the family genogram, emphasising the changes that had taken place in the family (*see* Figure 5.2). A number of issues surfaced during the family sessions: the mother's lack of understanding of the changes for children that the divorce had involved, Tim's strong loyalty to his father, his perception that his father was the victim and the unacknowledged sense of loss for all family members especially Tim. The various changes that the family had gone through and the difficulties in coping with them were discussed with each member of the family. Excerpts from the family session are given below:

Clinician (to the mother): How have things changed for you since the divorce?

Mother: You mean . . . after I pulled myself together? I have become more confident. I manage the finances, something I could not do before. I am more settled, happier (glances at Tim) and, begun to enjoy life after a long time.

Clinician: What about the finances?

Mother: Neil's earnings are no more and Simon does not earn as much. The family income has suffered and I am unable to afford things I have been used to. I try my best to prevent the children noticing the difference. But I have to budget for everything.

Tim (surprised): You mean we are poor?

Mother: Yes, I suppose so.

Tim: You never said this before. Are you sure?

Mum: I have managed without you children noticing it. I don't want you to think, 'Oh now that dad is not there we can't afford this or the other . . .'

Clinician (to Tim): I wonder what differences you have noticed in mum since the divorce?

Tim: She does more . . . She goes out more . . . I suppose, suppose she is a lot happier.

Clinician: A lot happier? How do you know?

Tim: I can see it. She laughs more (smiles). She talks more (smiles). She does more things for me and Susan.

Clinician: Such as . . .

Tim: You mean . . . What she does for us? Well . . . she got me to join the football club and takes me there every Friday and she takes Susan for music lessons, don't you mom?

Clinician (addressing Tim): Things have not been as they used to be for you. How have things been different for you since your parents separated, Tim?

Tim (thinks for a while): Not much . . . (appears unsure). Well, I have had to go to a different school.

Clinician: That's a big change.

Tim: It has all been different . . . difficult. I did not have any friends here.

Clinician: You mean you have lost all your friends? That would have been hard.

Tim: I don't like the new school. I have no one there who I know. The kids are mean and horrible . . . I am getting used to it now . . .

Clinician: What else has changed?

Tim: I can't see my (paternal) grandma as before. I miss her and Tiger (the dog). I don't see Kevin, my best friend.

Mother (surprised): You never mentioned Kevin before. You can call him home over a weekend. He is a nice boy, you know . . .

The discussion moved on to how life was different for Tim in his daily life after the divorce. His mother was surprised to hear how different life had become for Tim and was moved by the sacrifices he had had to make. The clinician encouraged the mother and son to talk about their experiences of life before and after the separation. The conversation about 'differences before and after' the divorce was extended to encompass his mother's experiences before the separation. Mrs Pickering described how she had been depressed after Tim's birth although at that time she did not realise it was postnatal depression. To witness each step in Tim's development appeared to have been a wonderful experience. But there were times when she felt so drained of all energy that she could not manage to get up from bed and when he cried for feeds she had to literally drag herself from bed and crawl on the floor to get to make his milk (when he was a toddler). Tim listened intently to her account of postnatal depression and how it affected her. At one point his eyes filled with tears and he looked up at the ceiling to hide his tears.

One of the main tasks was to think about the losses the family had faced and how each of them was coping with them. Mrs Pickering described the main loss as a fall in family income and the adjustments it entailed. Things had improved for her after Simon came into the family. Although Simon did not earn much, he was caring and has been supportive to her. Tim said that things had been miserable for him since his dad left, he missed him a lot and wished he was 'there with them'. He said it did not feel the same now that his father was not there. He was observed to fight his tears as he spoke of his dad. When his mother tried to comfort him he pulled himself away from her and shouted, 'Don't touch me. You sent him away.' Mrs Pickering felt helpless and said, 'He gets very upset when talking about his dad.'

It was clear that Tim blamed his mother for the break-up of the marriage and subsequent departure of his father. His perception of the reason for the break-up of the marriage was his mother 'sent his father way,' depriving him of his father. Consequently (this was not said) he was punishing his mother by isolating himself from the family and especially by avoiding interacting with her. He appeared to be ignoring the violence and ill-treatment she had suffered at his father's hands. When asked about how the divorce had been explained to him, he said that he remembered his mother telling him that she was breaking up with his father. As for the reasons for the break-up, no one had told him why she broke up with his father. His father has always wanted to come back and told him several times that his mother was not taking him back; when his father had come home his mother had called the police to get him out. 'She sent him away,' he said repeatedly, staring at his mother.

In contrast to Tim, Susan's loyalties were with her mother. She considered her father to be horrible and sympathised with her mother. The alliances within the family were clear. Susan was totally and completely aligned with her mother and although Tim's loyalties were divided he appeared to be aligned with his father. The therapist remarked that Tim's behaviour at home was one way of keeping his father's memories alive lest the family members would forget his father. This led to a discussion about how the family could preserve memories of the good times they had had with Neil. Tim suggested hanging family photographs in the living room and he wanted Neil's possessions like trophies displayed in the living room. It was left to the family (including Simon) to discuss the issue at home and come to a decision about how they wanted to remember the past.

In family sessions the mother was encouraged to talk of the happy times that she had had with Neil. She described the time before the children came as full of happiness. With encouragement from the therapist she went into examples of their 'happy days'. She was also asked to describe the qualities she found in Neil that were positive (she had been primed for this in previous couple sessions). She described Neil as a good provider and a protective husband. Tim was seen to pay careful attention to her as she described incidents from the past that showed his father in a good light.

Individual sessions with Tim: In one of the individual sessions with Tim the issue of violence towards his mother was brought up. He remembered seeing his mother beaten and kicked on a number of occasions. This was explored in the session:

> *Clinician*: How did seeing your parents quarrel affect you at that time?
>
> *Tim*: We were sort of scared. When I heard them arguing in their bedroom I thought to myself 'Here we go again, next he is going to throw things at my mom, he is going to hurt her pretty bad.' We used to put our ears to the wall to see if we could hear anything.
>
> *Clinician*: At that time why do you think dad hurt your mom?
>
> *Tim*: You mean when we were in the old house? (Reluctantly) I used to think that mom must have done some bad things.
>
> *Clinician*: You don't seem to be very sure. What do you think now?
>
> *Tim*: I think dad was pretty horrible to mom. He is screwed up, badly screwed up.
>
> *Clinician*: It needs of a lot of courage to say things like that about your father.
>
> *Tim*: Umm..
>
> *Clinician*: How has seeing dad's violence towards your mum affected you?
>
> *Tim*: (Long pause) I am not sure. I think I sort of feel sorry for mom . . .
>
> *Clinician*: How else?
>
> *Tim*: (Long pause) I lose my temper quickly . . . with mum.

In later sessions he stated seeing his mother as a strong and determined person to have stood up to his father. Drawing from his own experience, he said it needed a lot of courage to stand up against bullies and his mother had been brave to stand up against his father. He admitted that it caused him a lot of pain to be talking 'bad' about his father. He loved his father and missed him. The therapist pointed out the difference between not liking a person and not liking a person's actions. He was helped to make a list of things he liked and disliked about his father; he was relieved to see that the list of things he liked about his father was longer than the list of things he disliked about him. He did a similar exercise about his mother. The therapist introduced the idea of the sort of a man he would like to be when he grew up, especially with regard to his attitude towards women. Tim was initially not forthcoming about it, but later said that he did not want to be like his father.

One of Tim's more important grievances was the loss of the 'normal family'. On numerous occasions he had said, 'Why can't we be a normal family?' The implication was that he considered his family not to be the norm and, to him, it appeared abnormal. In discussing these issues, he was asked about those of his classmates, neighbours and extended family who did not fit his description of normal (two parent) families. Initially he denied knowing any. Later he remembered a classmate whose mother was a single parent. He was asked to act as an investigator and discreetly find out about his friends and family members who had experienced divorce or separation. Over the next few sessions Tim had made a long list of friends and acquaintances who had experienced divorce and separation. He was surprised to discover that there were so many of them. More importantly, some of his classmates whose parents had divorced appeared to be 'normal'.

Loss of his father as he knew him as part of the family in the past was a major issue for Tim. Although he was sure that there was no possibility of them getting back together, dealing with the permanence of the divorce and the losses it entailed was painful for Tim. He was not sure of his father's love and was worried that, over time, he may forget him. He desperately wanted to have a good relationship with him and contact visits were, in his mind, one way of measuring it. He felt that his mother was not in favour of his visits to dad because she was angry with his father. She made insulting comments about his father and asked too many questions after each visit. It was remarkable that he remembered the contact visits vividly although there had been no visits to his father over the previous four months or so. He received birthday cards and presents. He was free to telephone his father whenever he wanted. He did not like it if his father's girlfriend answered the phone.

In a later session he said that he was angry with his father too. His father was not good at keeping his promises. For example, he would cancel Tim's visits to him at the last moment. Tim used to look forward to the visit to his father all week. This made him angry and sad. He would punch the door and kick furniture. On one occasion he had put his hand through the glass window. The anger lasted for days and he could not pay attention to class work or bother to talk to his classmates. The therapist framed it as disappointment leading to frustration. He also wondered if Tim was probably directing the anger he had against his father towards his mother. The more important issue for him was to think about how he could deal with disappointment without necessarily getting angry.

Couple sessions and sessions with the mother: In the couple sessions Mrs Pickering and Simon were seen together several times. Some of the sessions were attended by Mrs Pickering alone. In these sessions she admitted that she was very angry with her former husband for all the pain and suffering he had caused her. She could not forgive him for the abuse that she had suffered and wished that she had been stronger and put an end to it early in the marriage. Mrs Pickering had difficulty in believing that contact with the father was a good thing and seemed to rationalise this by pointing to the problems in contact arrangements. A number of hypotheses were put forward as possible explanations for her lack of motivation to promote contact. Could it be possible that the lack of commitment to contact was her way of showing her anger against her husband, or even seeking revenge? Did she want to do all the caring for the children herself and deprive him of taking part in the children's lives? Was she envious of his girlfriend? What part did Simon play in all this?

During these conversations the importance of separating her (mostly angry) feelings for husband from the needs of the children was emphasised. It was pointed out that Tim was 50% his dad's and the latter had as much right as her. Whatever the flaws of the parents, children like to carry a positive image of their parents in their mind. The more useful position for her to take would be to encourage contact so that the children could come to their own opinions and conclusions without imposing her view of their father on them. It was not only necessary to support contact but she should be seen to be doing so. Mrs Pickering said it was hard for her to take a detached position regarding the contact visits, but was prepared to give it a try.

By the end of the couple sessions it was agreed that Mrs Pickering would try her best to support contact visits and not be disparaging towards her former husband. After contact visits she was not to ask Tim questions about the happenings at dad's place unless Tim volunteered to do so. Rather she would talk about how she and the rest of the family spent their time during Tim's absence.

In individual sessions with Mrs Pickering, she described to the therapist the violence she had been subjected to. Tim had witnessed some of the attacks but they had never talked about it. The therapist felt it would be helpful if the abuse were to be discussed in family sessions so that the children understood her experience of it. It was important that she talked about how she experienced it at that time without seeming to launch into an attack on her ex-husband (she had had the opportunity of doing this in the individual sessions). So, when during one of the family sessions, she was asked to say why she decided to break up with her ex-husband, Mrs Pickering described the abuse she had suffered in some detail. The children listened in silence and Susan held her mother's hand as if she felt her mother's pain. Tim looked at the floor and said nothing. When she had finished telling about the abuse, she turned to Tim and said, 'It is now all over. I don't want to talk of it again, but I felt that you children should know what I went through.'

Sessions with the father: The therapist wrote to Mr Pickering about Tim's referral and invited him to a meeting with himself. He failed to attend the first appointment. This was not unexpected. Next the therapist spoke to him on the telephone and explained that it would be helpful if the therapist and he could discuss issues related to Tim. He explained that Tim was a bright boy, but was somewhat confused about things after the family break-up. The therapist described some of Tim's problems including loyalty conflicts and said that the purpose of the session with him would be to think about the best way to parent the children *after* the divorce. He reluctantly agreed to attend one session.

Mr Pickering was a well built man with an aggressive manner. He was keen to counteract his ex-wife's version of events and tell his side of the story. After listening to him for some time, the therapist told him that the main purpose of the interview was to think about how best he could help Tim. Tim missed him a great deal and was angry with everyone, him included, for the current state of affairs. The therapist drew his attention to the unsatisfactory contact arrangements that prevailed. Mr Pickering went on the defensive and said that his girlfriend had a family and that it was not physically possible to have the children for overnight visits. He was angry about the prohibition order on him to visit the children at their (mother's) home. The therapist stressed that it was not so much the physical arrangements that mattered but the message that he gave Tim and his sister. Within the constraints of his family situation, how could he let the children know that cared for them and had not relinquished his role as their father? What would he need to do to set aside his anger and ill feeling with his ex-wife and make some time for the children?

Contrary to expectations, the session went well and Mr Pickering agreed to think about the various issues discussed in the meeting. He also agreed to come for a second session. At the next meeting he was more relaxed and talked freely about his difficulties in arranging contact visits for the children. He said his girlfriend was not keen on seeing them and made every excuse to stop them visiting him. He agreed that the children had a right to see him. Following further discussion he thought it might be a good idea if he could see them at his mother's house. The important point though was to make a realistic plan for contact visits and adhere by them so that the children were not disappointed. He agreed that he should be honest with the children and promise them only that which he could deliver. The issue of contact settled, the therapist discussed the need to maintain boundaries between the parents and children. The importance of keeping adult affairs and problems such as the ones between him and his ex-wife to themselves and not burdening the children with them was stressed. Divorce and separation provoke strong emotions that take time to settle, he agreed, it was difficult to be objective and think about what was best for the children. He was glad that he had come for the sessions.

In later sessions with the family Tim joyfully reported that he had started seeing his father at his grandmother's house.

Progress and outcome

In total, treatment took nine months. A follow-up was arranged three months after the conclusion of therapy. Tim's angry outbursts were reported to be less though not completely abolished. He was taking part in family activities; Simon and he were spending more time together. The contact visits at the grandmother's house initially worked well but Neil started reneging on his promises. The contact was irregular and when Neil did meet Tim at his grandmother's house he spent very little time with him. But Tim regularly went to his grandmother and felt content as if, for him, she and her house represented his father. Perhaps, he was protecting his father by appearing to be happy with visits to his grandmother. Mrs Pickering learned to come to terms with her ex-mother in law and allow the visits to occur, although she realised that her ex-husband hardly kept to his side of the bargain. Susan refused to go on contact visits. In general, within the household relationships were improving and a new family unit was emerging.

Comments

The Pickering family made good use of therapy. Although Tim was seen as the 'symptom bearer', the whole family was going through a phase of reorganisation and change. Tim's grievances and complaints were preventing the family moving forward. All three – Tim, his mother and father – felt they were the victims in the divorce and separation. Mr Pickering's participation in the sessions proved to be crucial. It helped to reduce hostilities in the family and made him take responsibility for post-divorce parenting. That he did not carry it out well is another matter. For Tim, his father was making efforts, however feeble, to see him.

Divorced and separated families are best served by taking a family therapy/ systemic approach. Typically they are seen in family therapy clinics. In this instance therapy was carried out by a single clinician for want of family therapy facilities. There was no family therapy clinic at the time the Pickering family were seen. The pressure on the service was so high no co-therapist was available either. It could be argued that use of a CAMHS was, in this instance, inappropriate and it was not good use of the clinician's time. This may be true. Unfortunately, there is no single service other than CAMHS that addresses these issues or a clear pathway for dealing with them once the main problems are identified.

Separated and divorced families are over-represented in the population of children referred to CAMHS. Therapists need to be aware that:

1   Families may seek help from CAMHS at any point in the course of the divorce – parental conflict before the decision to divorce, during the upheavals caused by the divorce itself, in the post-divorce single parent stage and during the stepfamily phase, and the therapeutic aims may be different for each stage
2   Many families seek help through their children by presenting them as the ones in need of help. It is a well recognised phenomenon that some children 'bring' their parents for therapy by taking on the role of symptom bearers for the family.
3   Various adult members of the family may have different agendas when getting referred to mental health services. Custody disputes (e.g. who should the child live with?), legal issues surrounding the divorce (e.g. who should get the family home?) and the inability of one or the other parent to make a decision (e.g. should I seek divorce?) sometimes masquerade as concerns for the child (e.g. 'he is upset and I want the best for the child'). Unwary clinicians can find themselves caught in the crossfire, with one or the other parent seeking the support of the clinician against the other or when asked for court reports as to what is in the best interest of the child.

Apart from these potential hurdles, clinicians working with separated, divorced and reconstituted families need to be aware of their own prejudices and how their world views might affect the work with these families. It may be fitting here to quote Forma Walch (2003), a well known scholar in this field: 'We need to be aware of the implicit assumptions of normality that we bring to our work with families from our own world views, including cultural standards, clinical/research paradigms, and personal/family experiences.'

Box 5.1 Research into the effects of parental separation and divorce on children shows that . . .

- The majority of the children from divorced families eventually weather the stresses and strains of parental divorce and emerge as competent individuals.
- However, a significant minority (about 20%) are two to three times more likely to show psychological problems than children in intact families.
- Divorce is best viewed as a process than an event.
- Children from divorced families are over-represented in treatment populations.
- There is paucity of methodologically sound studies of divorce interventions.

References

Cockett M, Tripp J. *The Exeter Family Study: family breakdown and its impact on children*. Exeter: Joseph Rowntree Foundation/University of Exeter Press; 1994.

Emery RE. *Marriage, Divorce and Children's Adjustment*. New York: Sage Publications; 1999.

* Hetherington EM, Kelly J. *For Better or For Worse*. New York: Norton; 2002.

Hetherington EM. An overview of the Virginia Longitudinal Study of Divorce and Remarriage with a focus on early adolescents. *Journal of Family Psychology*. 1993; 7(1): 39–56.

Kelly JB. Children's adjustment in conflicted marriage and divorce: a decade of research. *Journal of the American Academy of Child and Adolescent Psychiatry*. 2000; **39**: 963–73.

Rodgers B, Pryor J. *Divorce & Separation: the outcome for children*. York: The Joseph Rowntree Foundation; 1998.

* Wallerstein JS, Lewis J, Bakeslee S. *The Unexpected Legacy of Divorce: report of a 25-year landmark study*. New York: Hyperion; 2000.

Walch F. *Normal Family Process*. 3rd edn. New York: Guilford Press; 2003.

Chapter 6

Looked after child

The initial referral from the GP was brief. He was referring two children, Brandon aged 6 years and Amy aged 10, for behaviour problems. They were living with their grandparents, who were long-standing patients of his. The main reason for their visit to the GP was the difficulties that school was experiencing with both children, especially Brandon. His behaviour at school had been extremely disruptive and he was considered a danger to other children. The school was finding it difficult to manage him and he was attending school only in the mornings. His grandparents, both in their late sixties, had been finding it difficult to manage him, and after the school's decision to send him home after morning lessons, they found managing the two of them onerous. The GP mentioned that the grandfather had heart problems and the grandmother had arthritis of the hip and was awaiting hip replacement. He was aware that a social worker was involved. He indicated that the situation was reaching crisis point and the grandfather's health was being put at risk. The GP had also attached a copy of a report from school that had been sent to the LEA, presumably requesting extra help for him at school. It read as follows:

> Brandon exhibits unacceptable behaviour at school that has not improved despite a range of behaviour strategies as suggested by support services. He is also a danger to himself and other children in class. Brandon disrupts other children's learning and deliberately tries to provoke other children by poking, pushing and pulling them. His behaviour is erratic and unpredictable. I have noticed there seems to be no catalyst which stimulates his disruptive behaviour. This concerns me because he can become violent towards other children and staff. Brandon concentrates for very short periods of time (5 to 10 minutes), even if he is doing an activity of his own choice. This term he has had one-to-one support and this appears to have had no impact on his concentration.
>
> He puts very little effort into learning. Most of his energy and time is spent disrupting the learning of others. Brandon appears to want to be friendly with his peers but he has no idea how to form a friendship. In the end other children have become scared of him because of the violent behaviour he exhibits. Quite often children in the class have been hurt by him. Also parents instruct their children to keep away from him.
>
> I found it very difficult to identify an area of strength. His main problems may be summarised as follows: attitude towards adults and peers, violent and aggressive behaviour, poor concentration and following instructions, not following through and completing a set

tasks and inability to form relationships with children. Brandon has had IEPs and reviews as appropriate at 'school action' and has been given work to help him achieve his targets. The consultation with the educational psychologist gave us strategies that had been tried out. Brandon, however, has made very little progress in terms of behaviour and learning. The strategies suggested have not been appropriate for Brandon. As a result of intense discussion between the school, carers and social services, we have requested an urgent formal assessment.

The referral was discussed in the CAMHS team meeting. Admittedly, the report from school described how desperate things were. But the referral raised more questions than it answered: Why were they in the care of grandparents? What about the parents? What was the role of the social worker and social services? What was the legal status of the children, for example were they being accommodated with the grandparents or did they have a residence order? More importantly, why was the referral coming from the GP/school rather than from the social worker? Team members were somewhat puzzled that the request had not come from social services because the CAMHS held weekly consultations with social workers where referrals and potential referrals from social services where were discussed. It was decided to contact the social worker to find out more about the case. A member of the CAMHS team telephoned social services and was directed to the social worker dealing with the case. When told about the referral by the GP she was totally apologetic and said that she was, in fact, in the process of making a referral to CAMHS. She had just taken over the case. A date for consultation with the social worker was arranged.

The consultation

Two members of the CAMHS team met with the social worker. The consultation that took place is described below under different headings to aid conceptualising the process but, in reality, it took the form a discussion that systematically focused on various aspects as the consultation progressed.

Exploring the history of social services' involvement and their current role

Finding out what happened for social services to be involved, and tracking the passage of the case through the social services system, is an essential part of the consultation and provides a longitudinal view of the child's history. It also clarifies the current role of social services and their short- and long-term plans. In the case of Brandon and Amy, they came to the attention of social services two years ago when the primary school that they were attending reported their concerns to social services. Brandon had started school in September of that year and had settled well in his new class. He was described as a delightful boy who made friends quickly. At the beginning of the next year the class teacher had noticed a dramatic change in his behaviour. In a letter to the social services she had set out her major concerns:

1   Brandon's attendance had become erratic and there were frequent unex-
    plained absences.

2 His appearance became unkempt and there were occasions when he was teased by his classmates because he was smelly.

3 The children had head lice that had remained untreated despite several letters home drawing attention to the problem. On one occasion, the class teacher actually washed their hair with Malathion shampoo because Brandon was in obvious discomfort.

4 On several occasions during PE lessons (for which Brandon had to change clothes) he was noticed to have scratch marks on his arms and greenish-brown bruising on his lower left buttock. Brandon said that the family dog had jumped up at him causing the scratch marks. As for the bruises, he said he had fallen off his bicycle onto his bottom, thereby sustaining the bruise marks. The teacher was not entirely convinced by these explanations.

5 On six different occasions Brandon had arrived at school with no packed lunch. He explained that his mother had forgotten to set the alarm clock and they had overslept; staff provided him with sandwiches and drink at lunch-time.

The headmistress had attempted to make contact with their mother Juliet on several occasions and later by letter to discuss her concerns. Appointments offered were not kept and messages left on the mother's mobile phone went unanswered.

Social services became involved at this stage. During the home visit the investigating social worker described the home as dirty and unhygienic with rubbish everywhere. She found a large collection of soiled nappies behind an armchair and two beds with no blankets or duvet. The stairs and landing were littered with rubbish and the kitchen floor was piled up with dirty clothing and bags of rubbish. There was no food in the house; there was a very strong smell of excrement. The social worker was unable to find clean clothes for the two children after an extensive search. Their hair was full of nits and lice.

The children had no contact with their father. Juliet lived with a 30-year-old man called Tony Curry. He had numerous convictions for offences of drink-related violent behaviour. She denied drinking excessively. She told social services that her liaison with Mr Curry was a disastrous mistake and that she was trying to get her life sorted. During this time, in an entirely unrelated incident, Mr Curry was involved in a violent attack on a man and was imprisoned for 2 years. The children were placed for a brief period with their grandparents. On the way to the grandparent's house, the children described their 'parents' as violent and drunk; Amy described being hit by Mr Curry with a shower pipe. Amy and Brandon described a family friend who came to the house, drank cider and pulled up their drawers and touched their private parts. A child protection case conference was held and the children's names were placed on the Child Protection Register under the category of neglect. Social services records showed that the children were returned to the mother after a brief stay with their grandparents.

Matters came to a head when the police received an anonymous telephone call one morning the same week from a neighbour reporting a domestic disturbance in Juliet's address. The report stated that two young children could be heard screaming in the background amidst the sound of furniture being thrown around the room and the breaking of glass. The police arrived at 10.30 am and found Juliet with a black eye, smelling strongly of drink and with slurred speech. The room was littered with empty beer cans and bottles and broken furniture. The children were quickly located in the bedroom hiding in a cupboard. There was no one else in the house. Juliet was taken to hospital and the children underwent a medical examination. Juliet admitted that her care of the children had become neglectful and that she was drinking excessively. The row, she explained, came about after a prolonged drinking session the night before and her refusal to part with benefit monies the following morning to permit her boyfriend to purchase more alcohol. The social services emergency duty team was contacted by the police and an application for an emergency protection order (EPO) was made and obtained that evening while the situation was investigated. The children were placed with their grandparents.

Care proceedings were initiated in the Family Proceedings Court. A risk assessment carried out by the then social worker on Juliet's parenting reported that her lifestyle was not conducive to the care of the children. More specifically, her drinking and chaotic relationships were thought to put the children at risk of neglect. Both children had remained with the grandparents, Mr and Mrs Myatt, under a succession of interim care orders for a period of 13 months. The social worker had visited them on several occasions and found that their home was not particularly child-oriented. The arrival of the children had severely disrupted the pattern of their day-to-day lives. Mr Myatt took early retirement on grounds of ill health after the arrival of the children. He suffered from angina although this now appeared to be under control. He drove the children to school, a full half an hour drive, because the children had remained in their former school. They would prefer them to attend a local school. Mrs Myatt gave up her part-time job as care assistant in a retirement home in order to devote more time to the children. Their finances were strained and they had been seeking financial assistance from the local authority.

Juliet visited the children three times a week. On Wednesdays she met with them after school from 5.00 pm to 7.00 pm and on Saturdays and Sundays between 10.00 am and 3.00 pm. All contact had taken place at her parent's house and had not been formally supervised. Over the previous six months Juliet's contact visits had been sporadic. Visits had been cancelled at short notice and on at least three occasions her parents had refused to allow her into their house because she was reportedly unsteady on her feet and smelling strongly of alcohol. She denied turning up at visits drunk but she admitted that there had been occasions when she had to cancel contact visits because she had been short of money. She felt that her parents wanted to assume the role of parents and wanted her out of the picture.

Exploring the reason for the referral to CAMHS

Next the current concerns were explored, taking care to get a behavioural description of the problems. When Brandon came to the grandparents, he would overeat and it was many months before he could stop when he was full. Initially he would only agree to stop if his grandmother saved what was left of his meal or his snack. The grandparents felt he seemed like a child who never knew where the next full meal would be coming from, so he had to stock up. They described him as having terrible nightmares, from which he would wake terrified; some of these were about someone hurting him. Sometimes he would get up in the night and be very destructive. There was one occasion when he flooded the bathroom. Over the months his behaviour had been getting better and his grandparents felt it was a great achievement. But over the recent few months his behaviour had deteriorated. Although Brandon had lived with them for 13 months, they felt they still did not know what to expect from him. At times he seemed to be loving and wanting cuddles, at other times he kicked and screamed.

The social worker's immediate concern was the partial exclusion of Brandon from school. This had placed an extra burden on Mr and Mrs Myatt. They had not expected to look after him during school time. His grandfather had claimed that, if anyone could control Brandon, it was he who could do it. Currently Brandon attended school three mornings a week and was at home the rest of the time. Now Mr Myatt too found it difficult to control Brandon's behaviour. Brandon used 'foul' language and destroyed his toys in temper. His behaviour was becoming more extreme, arguments at bedtime were common; he had also started biting, kicking and spitting. On the way to school he had turned and run across the road in front of a car. He was defiant when told off. He was said to be very restless after contact visits and cried a lot. He had soiled and smeared twice just after visits from his mother. He had been repeatedly saying that no one loved him. The social worker was concerned about the escalation in his bad behaviour.

Amy too was showing problems but in a different way. She was reported to be well behaved and compliant in a superficial way. She talked about the 'wonderful' times she had with her mother and Tony. She spoke of her mother with great admiration and denied any problems when she was living with her, something that infuriated the Myatts. The grandparents felt that she made up the stories. She was known to tell lies and steal things from school. They had found several items such as ribbons and pens that did not belong to her. She had claimed that her friends gave them to her. She was known to openly 'flirt' with male visitors who come to the house. Mrs Myatt had spoken to her teacher who was also concerned about Amy's dishonest and deceitful behaviour.

Mapping the family and other system(s) involved

Building up a picture of the family *and* the professional network was the next task at this stage of the consultation. What did the social worker know about the family – the grandparents, Juliet and her partners? Who else was involved with the children and the families?

The social worker, having just taken over the case, was not fully acquainted with the various family issues. She was aware that there were several volumes of notes and reports about the family in social services records but was not completely in possession of all the facts. She had visited Mr and Mrs Myatt on a number of occasions. They lived in a comfortable semi-detached house in an upmarket area. They were somewhat embarrassed by the behaviour of the children, especially when Brandon threw tantrums or ran out screaming. Mrs Myatt, the social worker felt, was full of energy and in no way an older woman. In spite of her arthritis she was active and full of life. Mr Myatt was the sort of person who complained about health all the time; he considered himself an invalid and was anxious about his health. Both of them seemed 'old fashioned' and very conservative in their lifestyle. They were frequent churchgoers and wanted the children to come with them to the church and were annoyed that contact visits interfered with their attendance at church. The social worker felt that both of them were committed to looking after the children. They had worked hard with them and were proud of what they had achieved. They had given endless examples of how badly the children had been neglected by their mother. They felt the children were happy with them, they were well fed and looked after, whatever the difficulties they presented. They felt that the children were better off with them. They were critical of their daughter's lifestyle and considered her irresponsible. Their main social support was from their friends in the church.

The social worker was not clear about the family history apart from the fact that Juliet was adopted by Mr and Mrs Myatt when she was 4 years old. Amy and Brandon were by different fathers. The social worker had found Juliet to be pleasant and cooperative. Apart from one occasion, she had not found Juliet under the influence of alcohol. She was concerned that the previous social worker had recorded in the notes that, on an unannounced home visit, Juliet was with a man whom she introduced as David, her new boyfriend. There was reference in the notes to the two of them drinking at 10.00 am. They had refused access to the kitchen stating that it was untidy. The notes indicated that David was her former boyfriend Tom's brother. Juliet had vehemently denied having a drink problem. The social worker was not sure of Juliet's current living arrangement and wondered what the Myatt's meant by her 'chaotic lifestyle'.

The other 'systems' involved with the family were the school and the school health services. The school was managing Brandon by mostly excluding him from school. The headteacher was frustrated with her efforts to get more help from the education department. She wanted formal assessment of his educational needs as soon as possible so that more help would be available to the school in managing him. She had attended a number of meetings with social services and was urging them to support her in her request. Brandon had also been seen by a community paediatrician. His opinion was that Brandon had mild learning difficulties and showed massive behaviour problems probably because of the neglect and possible abuse he had suffered. Apart from the regular 'medicals' there was no further involvement from the community paediatrician.

Social services plan and their future role

In any consultation with social services, the future role of social services needs to be verified, including their short-term and long-term plans. In the case of Brandon and Amy, the current social services plan was to keep the children with Mr and Mrs Myatt in the foreseeable future. Social services were hoping to get a full care order and secure the children's future with their grandparents. But the problems that the school was encountering had thrown the plan into disarray and doubt. This unexpected turn of events had complicated matters and the social worker and her team manager were not sure what the way forward was.

Exploring referrer's expectations

By now a clear picture was emerging. The consultant summarised the social worker's dilemma as, 'This seems a complicated case. While the involvement of the grandparents at the time of crisis had been helpful and was seen as the solution for the problem and the situation eased for some time, a number of problems had surfaced recently throwing some doubt into the social services plan for the children.' The social worker agreed that when she took up the case it appeared that the problems had eased and the children were happy with the grandparents and the child protection issues were a thing of the past. She felt that Brandon's disruptive and difficult behaviour was rooted in his early experience: witnessing violence in the family, lack of attachment and possibly abuse and trauma. She was hoping that CAMHS could help by treating Brandon's behaviour problems by individual psychotherapy and the grandparents be helped to manage him better, possibly through family therapy. And, incidentally, she wanted to know if CAMHS could attend a meeting with education to stress the need for securing a formal statement of educational needs so that the school got more help with managing him.

The consultants observed that it was most unlikely that there was a simple solution or a 'quick fix'. It was understandable that the social worker was overwhelmed with the problems thrown at her. Like the grandparents she had not bargained for an eventuality where the social services plan had been thrown into doubt and disarray. Now that things had not worked out as was expected, it appeared that (like most families seen in CAMHS) the social worker's expectations were vague and unclear apart hoping for a magical solution ('the fix it approach'). In order to get clarification, at this stage the consultants posed the question, 'What is the question we should be looking to answer in this case?' This led to further exploration of the issues leading to greater shared understanding of the problem. It was very clear the social worker was very anxious about the current situation and the consultants wondered what caused her and her team manager the greatest concern, i.e. the 'mega worry'. Reluctantly, the social worker said that her main worry was that the Myatts may give up on the children and the children may end up with foster parents. As an afterthought she added that Juliet might mount a legal battle for custody of the children. And get them back!

Formulation of the main issues

Following some discussion the consultants and the social worker were able to come to a mutual understanding of the problem. On balance the chances of breakdown of the placement were considered to be high. There were problems in all three domains that affect placement (see later): Brandon showed considerable behaviour problems, the grandparents were not managing the situation well and social services plans were not working.

Together with the social worker the problem was conceptualised as follows. The children had two set of carers but neither of them was considered problem-free nor even 'good enough'. The mother had been found unfit to be a parent but she had not given up on the children. Then there were the grandparents; they had gone to rescue the children from their daughter at a time of crisis. They were well intentioned and committed to the children; they had been happy looking after the children as long as there were no problems but once problems arose they had found it difficult to manage the children's behaviour. They were experiencing heath problems themselves and the long-term viability of the placement was uncertain. Incidentally, the consultants observed that they had sought help from the GP rather than from the social worker. What did this say about their relationship with the social worker? Although there were two sets of parents none of them had been assessed as regards their current capacity to parent the children. It appeared that Juliet had been written off although she was the mother. Admittedly she had been neglectful and put the children at risk. But her current situation was far from clear. Her parenting behaviour including contact visits appeared to depend on her level of functioning and the partner she was with at the time. Her drinking too was an issue. What was her relationship to the parenting role? Was she committed enough to parenting the children to be able to submit herself to surveillance by social services regarding her drinking (e.g. blood tests)?

It was noted that Juliet was 26 years old. This meant that she would have been 16 years when she had Amy. Little was known about her life with her parents apart from the fact she was adopted at 4 years. Although Mr And Mrs Myatt were critical of Juliet's ability to parent the children, they had not done a good job themselves either!

The consultant wondered what sense the social worker made of the children's behaviour. In short, what the meaning of their behaviour was? This led on to a discussion about the burden on the children and their feelings about the move to their grandparents, and their sense of belonging. After all, they too appeared to be in a predicament, having to justify living with and be loyal to their grandparents, while having a mother who in their eyes was a perfectly capable loving parent. As the consultants and the consultee discussed this further, they started wondering whether the children's behaviour was a normal reaction to an abnormal situation. The question then was, 'When would their current behaviour be considered normal?' If the children considered their situation to be unusual or abnormal (living away from their mother), then rebelling against it by behaving badly would be 'normal'. A question raised by their behaviour was: what was it intended to achieve? As the consultation proceeded it started making sense to think of the meaning of their behaviour and the function it was serving. Was it possible that they wanted to go back to their mother, who, in their perception, had done nothing wrong? Could it be that their actions were a form of attachment-seeking behaviour rather than rejection of the grandparents? What better way was there than to show up their conservative grandparents through bad behaviour at school? If they made it too hard for the grandparents would they give up so that they could go back to their mother?

The social worker remembered that Amy had said to her teacher that she would be going back to her mother soon. 'Mom will come and fetch us when she has a new house; we are with granny for a short time,' she had said. She had told the social worker how her mother visited her regularly although 'she does not get on with granny, but she comes for our sake'. When asked about the wishes of the children (as to with whom they wanted to live), the social worker was unsure but said, 'it would be with their mother, obviously'. It had been taken for granted that the children would live with the grandparents because it was the social services plan and everyone appeared to have forgotten to ask or think about with whom the children *wanted* to live!

Another way of approaching the problem was to ask the question: what was destabilising the placement with the grandparents? Was it the frequent contact with the mother and what went on during contact visits? Who was destabilising it, Juliet, or possibly Amy? It had been noted that Amy was a strong character and there was a strong sibling bond. As the older of the two is it possible she was instigating the drive towards disrupting the placement and Brandon was doing the 'acting out' on behalf of her? An alternative hypothesis was that the children were not sure of their place with the Myatts and were testing their grandparents' commitment by their misbehaviour and testing of boundaries.

Agreeing on future plans and documentation

At the end of the consultation through reflection and discussion the social worker and the consultants were able to arrive at a common understanding and a shared formulation of the case. It was summarised as follows: Amy and Brandon showed considerable behaviour problems that were severe enough to put their placement with their grandparents at risk. Although children's wishes had not been ascertained, it was highly likely that they would want to go back to their mother. While Brandon's behaviour was the main cause for concern, the role that Amy, the older of the two children, played was considered to be crucial. The level of attachment to their mother and grandparents or the loyalty conflicts they were experiencing were unclear. It was suggested that the social worker under-take a piece of work with the children to find out through play, drawing and conversation their views and feelings about where and with whom they wanted to live. It felt that an assessment of Juliet's current parenting capacity should be undertaken as well as an assessment of the grandparent's. Social services and CAMHS would support the school's request for statutory assessment of Brandon's educational needs. It was agreed that the social worker and her team manager would think about some of the issues raised. Assessment of the children by the CAMHS was considered not necessary. The social worker would request another consultation with CAMHS in the future if necessary.

A letter summarising the consultation was sent to the social worker. It read as follows:

Dear Ms . . .

    Regarding: Amy – (date of birth) Age: 10 years
    Brandon – (date of birth) Age: 6 years.

Thank you for coming for the consultation meeting on (date) regarding the above children. In the meeting we discussed your current concerns regarding the children. Brandon in particular shows severe behaviour difficulties at school and is close to exclusion. His behaviour with the grandparents has been difficult as well. They had been placed with them following a child protection investigation on the basis of neglect (actual) and had been with them for the last 13 months. You were concerned about the possibility of breakdown of the placement if problems continued.

    We discussed the likely reasons for the destabilisation of the placement with Mr and Mrs Myatt. A number of ideas were considered:

- The children, especially Amy, might want to go back to her mother. The children might believe that they were with their grandparents for a temporary period and saw no need to make attachments to them.
- On the other hand, Juliet too may be working under the assumption that

---

she would be getting the children back and hence undermining the current placement in subtle ways. We understand that the contact visits are frequent and are unsupervised.

- We wondered about the possibility that the children's behaviour might be designed to secure better attachment with their grandparents and test the grandparent's commitment to them.
- There was little information about Juliet's adolescence and current life style. We agreed that an assessment of her parenting capacity including her relationship to the role of parenting, her alcohol use and current relationships may be necessary.
- Lastly we felt that building a working relationship between you and the children was important and could be a prelude to doing some work with the children including finding out about their perception of where they want to live. This work would be especially significant for Amy who is now 10 years and appears to be the stronger of the two. We felt that this work may need another worker in addition to your self.
- CAMHS was not planning to offer an appointment for the children but would be pleased to have another consultation with you in the future, if necessary.

We discussed the complexity of the case and how the difficulties it presented might seem overwhelming particularly because you had come into it recently. We hope that you found the consultation exercise useful. We would appreciate if you could keep us informed of the progress of the case. Please do not hesitate to contact us if necessary.

Yours sincerely

(Signature 1 and signature 2)

Theoretical perspectives

The process of consultation: The seven-step process of consultation employed in the case of Brandon and Amy was based on the case-centred consultation as described elsewhere (Thambirajah and Rai, 2004). The knowledge base that informs the thinking behind case centred consultation comes from two sources. The first is from the classical work of Caplan (1970) (elaborated upon later by Sternberg, 1989). They defined consultation as 'any activity undertaken by one professional (the consultant) to help another (the consultee) with a problem or issue in the consultee's work'. They stress three aspects of the consultation:

1 The emphasis is on helping the consultee make the most effective use of his or her own skills.
2 The consultee remains autonomous in deciding whether to use or not to use what has been discussed in the consultation.
3 The consultant has no formal authority over the consultee.

Based on their research they identified three forms of consultation:

1 client-centred (where the case is the focus)
2 consultee-centred (helping the consultee deal with the case) and
3 organisation-centred (addressing organisational issues).

Consultation to other services requires an additional set of attitudes, knowledge and skills to that required for working with a child and/or family independently. It calls for the practitioners to understand the roles and responsibilities of professionals working in contexts different from their own. Having an understanding of the perspectives, language and culture of other professionals can inform how consultation is conducted. The main attitudes underpinning such consultations are:

- **Respect for each other's expertise**: Each one is an acknowledged expert in their own field and has independent decision-making abilities and powers. It also means that each has the right to assert his/her view without being dominated by the other or being coerced into accepting the other's view.
- **Adopting a professional and honest approach**: The consultation is the meeting of two professional minds and it is considered important that they are open and honest and express their views, however unpalatable, clearly during the consultation.
- **Working collaboratively**: A consultation is seen as a collaborative effort in which both parties strive to share views and arrive at a common understanding of the problem as much as possible.

Many authors have written extensively about how to conduct a consultation, especially in the case of low income, crisis-ridden, multiple problem families. The main aims of the consultation may be summarised as follows (Reder, 1986):

1 Clarify the reasons for the referral ('what is the question that needs to be answered?').
2 Clarify expectations ('what is the social worker expecting as the main outcome of the consultation and what can realistically be offered?').
3 Arrive at a shared formulation or view of the case, bringing together the 'bottom up' information provided by the social worker and the 'top down' process from the consultant.
4 Agree on a future plan of management, including the roles of each agency, and document what has been agreed.

The second source of knowledge that underpins consultations is derived from the work of family therapists. During the consultation, timely and well-placed questions are used as a way of eliciting appropriate information and promoting thinking. One has to be particularly mindful of the nature of the questions and the intent embodied in them. A number of family therapists have drawn attention to creating certain contexts when working with agencies and families that aid responses to certain questions. This requires both the framing of such questions to be carefully considered as well as the timing of them. This has been referred to as 'warming the context' in an attempt to nurture the best possible outcome for the child being referred.

It is essential that each system understands the 'other'. For CAMHS professionals this involves getting to know the structure and organisation of social services, the way social services functions and the processes involved in the passage of the case through the social services system. Inevitably this involves a good grasp of legislation and statutory requirements, including The Children Act (1989) and the *Framework for the Assessment of Children in Need and their Families* (Department of Health, 2000) and child protection procedures. In addition, it is important to have a good grasp of how the *local* social services teams are organised and how they work. Typically children's services within social services departments are now divided under two or three main areas, each of which may respond to children in need of protection. A brief account of the procedures is given here. The reader is advised to consult the original documents and the local policy documents for details.

Local authority social services departments have a duty to safeguard and promote the welfare of the children in their area. Upon referral to social services on child protection issues, the initial assessment is to be completed within 7 days of the children being referred. The referral information and the results of the initial assessment will determine what action is required. This should result in one of the following outcomes:

1 Initial assessment only (and no further action).
2 Child protection (Section 47) investigation: Section 47 of The Children Act 1989 states that the local authority has a duty to investigate when they suspect that a child who lives, or is found, in their area is suffering or likely to suffer significant harm. If the child is felt to be at risk, an initial child protection conference may be held, the purpose of which is to decide if the child's name should be placed on the Child Protection Register.
3 'Core assessment': The core assessment is a more detailed assessment within the three domains detailed in Assessment Framework and should be completed within 35 days from when it is commenced. It is carried out when the eligibility criteria have been met for a child in need. The Assessment Framework consists broadly of three domains:
    1 child's developmental needs
    2 the capacity of the parents or caregivers to respond appropriately to those needs and
    3 the impact of the wider family and environmental factors on parenting capacity and child development.
   From such an assessment carried out by the social services it is hoped that clear professional judgements can be made. These judgements include whether the child is in need, whether a child is suffering or is likely to suffer significant harm and what actions must be taken.

Many family therapists view the process of case-oriented consultations as analogous to that of meeting a family in the first family therapy session. Undoubtedly there are similarities between the two: both involve the process of understanding how the other system (family/social services) works, its rules, beliefs, power structure and boundaries; their respective expectations from the referral; and the beliefs and hypotheses each hold about the presenting problems. Working with professional systems differs from working with families in that the organisation and culture of the 'other' system can be incredibly difficult to unravel and that, in case-oriented consultations, the meeting may be limited to one, or at best to two, consultations, unless it is agreed to have regular ongoing consultations. There is, therefore, a need to plan and prepare for the consultation in some detail.

There are thus three parts to the process of consultation – preparation, the consultation and conclusion – all of which are equally important. It is not uncommon for only the second part, the consultation, to be seen as the main task and, therefore, the other two parts to be carried out usually in haste, by professionals who are overworked and under-resourced.

In most CAMHS the usual practice is for two persons (preferably from different disciplines) from the CAMHS to be available to do the consultation. There are at least two valid reasons for this practice. First, having two people from the consultant's organisation mirrors the perceived hierarchy within the organisation. Second, it is useful to have two people with differing expertise so that the second person can confirm or reinforce the views of the first, or offer a different view. Also the second worker may want to adopt a 'meta' position vis-à-vis the first consultant and the consultee.

Preparation for the consultation necessarily involves reading the referral letter, talking to any clinicians who may previously have been involved and reading the old notes, if any. At times the referral letter may be accompanied by lengthy legal reports, case conference minutes and other reports. It is useful to identify areas or aspects of the case that are more significant than others. Reading the above material would often lead to formation of rudimentary hypotheses or, in the least, raise further questions for which answers have to be sought in the consultation process.

At times it may be more helpful for the social worker (or another member of the CAMH team) to telephone the referring social worker, on a colleague-to-colleague basis and invite the referrer to elaborate on the background to the case. Often such preparatory work is more revealing than an impersonal letter or a checklist. It also helps keep abreast of changes when cases get passed on from one worker or team to another, and identify the person with whom it is best to have the consultation.

There are several possible outcomes to the consultation process:

- **Consultation only:** When it is felt that there is no role for CAMHS involvement, this should be spelt out clearly, together with the reason for it. A clear statement has to be made that there is no role for CAMHS in direct work but it may be useful to try to offer new ideas or a different perspective of the problem to the social worker. Social workers may find such reframing useful, especially when it fits with their understanding of the case.
- **Further consultations:** If the consultation exercise has been found to be helpful for both parties in thinking about the problem, the participants may want to continue to consult each other to think about how best to manage the case. Since many cases tend to have long-standing and intractable problems with no immediate and satisfactory conclusion, regular consultations may prove to be the best way to help manage them.
- **CAMH assessment:** Here the CAMH team offers an initial generic assessment of the child and the family. We emphasise the need for a general assessment in all cases because we believe that proper and all-rounded assessment is a prerequisite for formulating a management plan and, in this, cases referred through Social Services are no different to those coming from General Practitioners or others. The tendency for more specialised workers within the CAMH team to bypass the stage of generic assessment and begin family

therapy, individual child psychotherapy or drug treatment is fraught with dangers.

At the end of the consultation, the discussion, formulation and the conclusions are summarised, documented and copied to the social worker to avoid confusion as to what was agreed.

'Looked after' children

Children may not be able to live with their parents for a variety of reasons including parental physical or mental ill health, child neglect or abuse. Substitute or alternative care for children is provided through adoption or fostering. The term 'looked after' was introduced by the Children Act (1989) to refer to children who are subjected to care orders and those who are accommodated. In March 2004 there were 61 000 children looked after by English local authorities, a rate of 55 per 10 000 or 1 in 250 children under the age of 18. Of these, 68% were in foster care. Looked after children may be placed with relatives (kinship foster care), foster families or in group residential care (children's homes).

Looked after children are faced with a vast array of psychological challenges and trials. These include the following: several losses (loss of parents, school, pets, extended family, friends); uncertainty and lack of stability or sense of permanence; sudden and unpredictable changes; difficulty forming attachments; loyalty conflicts; lack of a coherent narrative including why they came into care; memories of past abuse, violence, neglect or rejection and confused identity about themselves and belongingness.

The specific problems seen in maltreated children depend on the intensity, duration, timing and nature and type of the neglect and abuse. The common manifestations of abuse and neglect are:

- **Aggression:** Typically abused and neglected children lack empathy. This combined with lack of impulse control leads to aggression and cruelty. Aggression accompanied by a callous and uncaring attitude is one of the most disturbing features of abused and neglected children.
- **Developmental delays:** Delay in language, motor and cognitive and social domains.
- **Eating:** Hoarding food, overeating and hiding food.
- **Soothing behaviour:** Immature and bizarre behaviours like rocking, head banging, biting themselves and self-injury, especially at times of distress or perceived threat.
- **Indiscriminate show of affection:** Overfamiliarity with strangers and 'indiscriminate attachment'.
- **Repetition compulsion:** Abused children tend to abuse other children or adults (and their children when they are parents); sexually abused children often show sexualised behaviour.

There is now considerable evidence that the rates of emotional, behavioural, social and educational problems found in looked after children is substantially higher than that in the general population. A recent Department of Health survey (Meltzer *et al.*, 2003) of the mental health of over a thousand young people (11–15 years) in public care in England using ICD-10 criteria found that 45% had a disorder compared to 10% in controls, i.e. the overall prevalence of mental disorders were five times higher than those children living with their families. The rates of mental disorders varied between different types of placement. Children in foster care showed lower rates (about 40%) compared to those in residential placements (60%). All psychiatric disorders were common: 40% had conduct disorder (6% in controls), 12% emotional disorder (6% in controls) and 7% had hyperkinetic disorder (1% in controls). Other studies confirm these findings. Unfortunately, the study did not examine post-traumatic symptoms or attachment difficulties. This study also highlighted educational difficulties experienced by this group: 60% had some difficulty with reading, spelling and maths; over 62% were at least one year behind in their intellectual development; about two thirds of the children had special educational needs. Where children had a mental disorder, the educational problems were even higher. For example, those children with mental health disorder were three or more years behind in learning and intellectual development. Another important finding from research is that educational under attainment in fostered children is particularly marked even after they are settled in long-term placements. In those children with severe abuse or neglect a normal family environment appears to be insufficient to compensate for early deprivation (Viner and Taylor, 2005). The implication of this finding is that these children require additional and continuing educational input from schools.

Figures provided by the government Social Exclusion Unit (SEU, 2003) presents a depressing picture of short- and long-term outcomes for children who have been in public care. In the period 2001/2, only 8% of children in care achieved five or more pass grades in GCSEs compared to the national average of 60%; only 1% of care leavers aged 18–21 gained access to higher education, compared to around 40% of their peers. The social cost of this failure was evident in other spheres too. For example, in 2001/2 only 46% of care leavers were in employment, education or training compared to 86% of all 19-year-olds. Over a quarter of rough sleepers had been in care; around a quarter of adults in prison had spent time in care; care leavers were two and a half times more likely to be teenage parents (SEU, 2003). A long-term follow-up study of children in public care in the UK over a 30-year period (Viner and Taylor, 2005) confirms the all-round poor outcome for the group as a whole. This study involved the follow-up of a 1970 British birth cohort at 5, 10, 16 and 30 years. A total of 343 (3.6%) had been looked after before the age of 17 years. Controlling for socioeconomic status, men with a history of public care were less likely to attain high social class and more likely to have been homeless; they had more convictions, higher psychological morbidity and had poor general health. The authors conclude that 'public care in childhood is associated with adverse adult socioeconomic, educational, legal, and health outcomes in excess of that associated with childhood or adult disadvantage'.

Factors affecting placement: There is widespread concern regarding the stability of placements in foster care. Breakdown of foster care placements is common and carries adverse outcomes for the children. A number of studies have tried to identify the factors associated with placement breakdown and stability. One such study was carried out across seven local authorities and involved 400 children placed in foster care during a 14-month period (Wilson *et al.*, 2003). Successful placement and lack of disruption was dependant on three aspects:

- **Child's characteristics:** The personal qualities of the child were important to the foster carers. Children perceived as attractive, responsive, loving, good-natured and able to give something back were more likely to have successful placements despite the difficulties encountered. The 'chemistry' between the child and the carer was an unpredictable element that led to both sides not knowing whether the placement would work.
- **Qualities of the foster carer:** Successful placements had foster carers who showed 'responsive parenting' such as warmth, firmness and ability to recognise and interpret behaviour as 'emotional communication'. Avoidance of power struggles and reinforcing negatives cycles of interaction leading to rejection was considered an important skill. Handling behaviour, setting predictable limits and clear boundaries, communicating love and providing a secure base by demonstrating sensitivity, availability and consistency were found to be essential. Foster carers who were able to tolerate challenging behaviours and use such testing situations to build intimacy, self-esteem and promote attachment had better outcomes. The success of the placement was predicated on the development of compatibility between the foster parents and the child where both ultimately felt rewarded.
- **Conditions or the context:** For placements to succeed a shared agency view of how to support the placement and meet the needs of the child was found to be important. The other ingredients to a successful outcome included a proper care plan for the child, supportive social worker involvement and management of contact with the birth family.

In the case of Brandon and Amy there were problems in all three of the above domains. First, it was clear that Bandon showed severe behaviour problems, second, the grandparents were either unwilling or unable to manage his behaviour and third, the medium-term plans for the children were unclear. A number of studies have examined the risk factors for breakdown of long-term foster placement and the following factors have been repeatedly shown to be the common causes (Minty, 1999):

- Conduct problems in the child such as aggressiveness and sexualised behaviour.
- Older age of the child at the time of placement; in children over 11 years one third of the placements break down in 1–2 years.
- Presence in the family of children under 5 years or a child of similar age to the one fostered.
- If foster carers believe that the wellbeing of their own child is threatened.

Support for foster carers is important if the placements are to succeed. Triseliotis *et al.* (1998) asked a group of long-term foster carers what they found most useful. Foster carers valued the following:

1   meeting with the social worker regularly and discussing child management
2   opportunities for respite care for the child if and when necessary
3   the provision of specialist standby services
4   support when false allegations are made against them and
5   being paid in time.

   Management in foster care: For this group of children traditionally three main forms of interventions have been available:

1 use of existing services, including CAMHS, to mange the child's behaviour and support the parents or foster parents
2 placement with 'specialised' foster parents and
3 therapeutic foster care.

In most CAMHS the 'looked after teams' provide training for foster carers on management of child behaviour problems. But the efficacy of such well-intentioned methods has been called into question by the findings of a recent study. This study was a randomised controlled trial involving 182 children in which the treatment group received specific training for foster carers on a protocol based on communication and attachment. Despite being well received by foster carers, the training was found to be not sufficient to make an impact on the levels of child behaviour problems (Minnis *et al.*, 2001). A more recent study, however, provides more hope. Using existing services, Pallett *et al.* (2002) provided a manualised 10 session programme for groups of foster carers in local communities. This involved a programme of training for foster parents to manage behaviour of the children in this notoriously difficult population. It has been evaluated and proved to be effective in improving care, confidence and child outcomes. It has now been published as a manual (Pallett *et al.*, 2005). Taken together these studies emphasise the need to exercise care in choosing the method of training foster carers in managing this population of children.

'Specialised foster care' refers to the provision of foster carers who have been especially chosen and trained to a high level of competence; usually they receive enhanced payments. The type of training and the quality of such carers vary across the country. Although a number of therapeutic foster care programmes have been adopted in various parts of the Western world, most notably in the US, the best known and researched model is the Multidimensional Treatment Foster Care (MTFC) programme devised by Chamberlain in Oregon (Chamberlain, 2003). MTFC is a community-based treatment programme that is based on longitudinal research over 30 years on the development and treatment of antisocial behaviour. It was initially developed as an alternative to institutional, residential and group care placements for youths with severe and chronic delinquent behaviour and has been extended to work with children and adolescents referred from both mental health and child welfare systems. In MTFC the foster parents are the primary intervention agents. The main components of the programme that contribute to its success are: a proactive approach to reducing behaviour problems; a consistent, reinforcing environment for youth; and separation and stratification of staff roles. MFTC is a well structured 'wrap around' service with the following features:

- Carefully selected foster carers trained in social learning-based behavioural principles; a behaviour management programme based on behavioural principles consisting of a three-level point system in which the child earns points by meeting clear behavioural expectations throughout the day.
- A foster carer takes only one young person at a time, and advice is available to them 24 hours a day.
- Family therapy for the family of origin along similar lines; individual therapy for the young person as required; close school liaison.
- Active case management by a senior member of staff to coordinate the various services.

- Staff consisting of a programme manager, behaviour support specialist, youth therapist, family therapist, consulting psychiatrist, parent daily caller and a case manage/clinical team supervisor.

Research into MTFC has produced some impressive results. Chamberlain has provided follow-up data on groups of hard-to-place youth, including those showing delinquent behaviour and those discharged from mental hospitals, in which the MTFC programme has been effective. Cost analysis for delinquents treated has shown that for every dollar spent on the programme 14 dollars were saved. A modified form of MFTC called MFTCE is being piloted in 20 local authorities in England. The TFC model in England (TFCE) attempts to replicate MFTC for children aged 10–16 years with some modifications. Each TFCE team is designed to undertake work with 8–10 youths. It is likely the service would be targeted mainly at youth placed out of the Local Authority and other specialised foster care and other services would be required for those with less severe problems.

Progress and outcome

Following the consultation the social worker kept CAMHS informed of the progress of the case through letters and informal discussions. Additionally, two more consultations were held at the request of the social worker. She had discussed with her team manager the outcome of the consultation with CAMHS. They had decided to assess the wishes and feelings of the children first before undertaking any other work. Unfortunately, no additional social worker was allocated to the case. After meeting with the children on a few occasions the social worker had become convinced that the children wanted to go back to their mother. Amy had been found to be intensely loyal to her mother and was keen to get back to her. She considered the grandparents to be too old and had made derogatory comments about them. Her view was that it was her mother's boyfriend that caused all the problems and her mother had told her that she would never take him back. The social worker felt that Amy had taken over the role of mothering Brandon. Brandon took the lead from her and the two of them had developed a strong sibling bond.

Next the social worker had visited Juliet. Juliet had been hostile towards the social worker and blamed the social services for taking the children away. It had taken the social worker some time to forge a good working relationship with her. Juliet was functioning reasonably well and had no partner at the time. However, it was not clear whether she was drinking excessively or using drugs. In her discussions with Juliet the social worker had been able to find out more about Juliet's childhood and adolescence. She had pieced together Juliet's early history by talking to Mr and Mrs Myatt. She had also read social services records of Juliet when she had been in local authority care.

Juliet's biological mother had suffered with severe bouts of depression following Juliet's birth and Juliet spent much of her early life in and out of various foster placements. She had been placed in long-term foster care with Mr and Mrs Myatt. Initially her mother had been in contact with her but later decided to move to Scotland to make a new life for herself. Juliet was freed for adoption and adopted by the Myatts at the age of 4. Juliet had been a difficult child all along. Her adoptive parents found it hard to manage her. She had been excluded from school on numerous occasions. She went to a special school because of her behaviour difficulties. As a teenager she had truanted from school and associated with older teenagers. On more than one occasion she had been returned home by police in a drunken state. She was permanently excluded from school just before her 15th birthday. The same year Mrs Myatt had become concerned about Juliet's health and taken her to the GP. She was found to be 4 months pregnant. She gave birth to Brandon when she was 16. Two years later she left home to live in a hostel for young mothers with small children. Since then she had lived in a variety of locations in and around the area. She and her parents did not get along well at all and had not seen each other until the children were placed with them.

Given her chaotic childhood history, the social worker was concerned about Juliet's ability to look after the children. She was also anxious about how well the grandparents could care for them, especially when faced with Brendan's behaviour. The grandparents were particularly worried that his behaviour at school would be seen as a reflection of the level of care they provided for the children. Social services decided to undertake an assessment of Juliet's parenting abilities. The social worker felt that Juliet was very keen to get the children back and be in the role of a parent. The social worker had observed a number of the contact visits and found that the children related to their mother quite well and were looking forward to the visits. She had found Juliet to be quite responsive and caring. The social worker wanted to test out Juliet's motivation to have the children back, and if possible, engage her in some work regarding parenting. She had approached Juliet with the question: what help would she need if she were to have the children? While social services were prepared to offer her practical help, it was important for Juliet to demonstrate that she could provide a stable and healthy home environment for the children. In particular, it was important to show that she was not drinking excessively or using drugs. The social worker felt that Juliet was an intelligent and competent person but her ability to look after the children depended to a large measure on the male partner she had at the time. Moreover, there were concerns about her abilities to parent (as distinct from her desire to parent) because of her childhood history. The social worker was impressed by the efforts that Juliet was prepared make to change her lifestyle in order to get the children back. For example, she had agreed to be tested regularly by the GP for alcohol misuse.

Following an assessment of Juliet's parenting capacity, social services decided to return the children to her on condition that the children would remain on an interim care order until the placement was found to be stable. Juliet was agreeable to this. She also agreed to attend the family centre run by social services and eventually enrolled herself in a parenting group. The family was allocated a sessional worker to help with practical day-to-day issues. The children were formally assessed by the educational psychologist and received statements of special education and extra support at school. Brandon continued to show difficult behaviour at school and was receiving help there. Juliet decided to move from the housing estate in which she had been residing.

Over the next six months regular reviews were held. A core group consisting of the social worker, the children's teachers and the sessional workers met regularly to review the case. Juliet made good progress in caring for the children. Brandon's school problems continued but at a lower level of intensity. In due course, the children's names were removed from the child protection register and the interim care order was not renewed.

Comments

There is much confusion in the literature as to what constitutes consultation to other agencies and services. The consultation approach described above refers to case-centred consultations where one practitioner seeks consultation from another. A variety of working relationships (other than simple referrals) may exist between agencies, services and practitioners, ranging from liaison to consultation to supervision. Unfortunately, there has been a tendency to view all types of working together as consultation. Many consultations with social services described in some textbooks (e.g. Southall, 2005) are supervision exercises rather than proper consultations. This begs the question about how social workers are supervised and what professional support is available to them. In spite of the non-hierarchical attitudes advocated by many authorities and the playing down of the 'expert' role, in practice, many practitioners seek consultations from those who are more experienced, knowledgeable and more skilled. For consultation to be effective and useful it is crucial to observe boundaries between services and professions. Often supervision carried out under the name of consultation has the effect of making the consultee feel deskilled and ultimately dependent of the consultant.

CAMHS practitioners working in looked after teams frequently feel overwhelmed by the demands made by social workers and the over-reliance of social workers on them. Rather than using their expertise and assessment tools, social workers could come to depend on CAMHS workers to make decisions about their cases. Consultation skills are all the more critical in such situations to enable the CAMHS workers to help demarcate and delineate their respective roles. The type and quality of supervision that social workers get within their service is very variable and sometimes not sufficient for the arduous tasks that they perform. By definition, the cases that social workers deal with are complex and complicated. They affect the lives of the children and families concerned in a profound way. Yet they get very little recognition for the work they do. Any improvement to the working conditions of social workers should begin with increased status and respect for the work they do. For example, it is a travesty that reports from social workers who have known the families and children for long periods are not considered worthy enough by courts, resulting in the commissioning of expensive reports from 'experts' who see the child and the family a few times just for the purpose of reports.

Note

I am grateful to my colleague Kamesh Rai for permission to use part of the material from a previously published article in which she was the co-author. I am also grateful to her for her comments on the first draft of this chapter.

References

Caplan G. *The Theory and Practice of Mental Health Consultations*. London: Tavistock; 1970.

Chamberlain P. *Treating Chronic Juvenile Offenders: advances made through the Oregon Multi-dimensional Foster Care Model*. New York: American Psychological Association; 2003.

Children Act. London: The Stationery Office; 1989.

Department of Health, Department of Education and Employment and the Home Office. *Framework for the Assessment of Children in Need and their Families*. London: The Stationery Office; 2000.

Meltzer H, Gatward R, Corbin T *et al*. The Mental Health of Young People Looked After by Local Authorities in England: Office of National Statistics/The Stationery Office; 2003.

Minnis H, Pelosi AJ, Knapp M *et al*. Mental health and foster carer training. *Archives of Diseases of Childhood*. 2001; **84**: 302–6.

Minty B. Outcome in long term foster family care. *Journal of Child Psychology and Psychiatry*. 1999; **40**: 991–9.

* Pallett C, Blackly K, Yule W *et al. Fostering Changes: a manual for foster carers*. London: British Association for Adoption and Fostering; 2005

Pallett C, Scott S, Blackly K *et al*. Fostering changes: a cognitive behavioural approach to help foster carers mange children. *Adoption and Fostering*. 2002; **26**: 39–48.

Reder P. Multi-agency family systems. *Journal of Family Therapy*. 1986; **8**: 139–52.

Social Exclusion Unit (SEU). *A Better Education for Children in Care*. London: SEU, Office of the Deputy Prime Minster; 2003. Available at www.dfes.gov.uk/educationprotects/index.cfm.

* Southall A, editor. *Consultation in Child and Adolescent Mental Health Services*. Oxford: Radcliffe Publishing; 2005.

Sternberg D. *Interprofessional Consultation*. London: Blackwell Scientific; 1989.

* Thambirajah MS, Rai K. Deconstructing the referral question: a framework for case centred consultation with social services. *Child and Adolescent Mental Health in Primary Care*. 2004; 1(4): 106–14.

Triseliotis J, Borland M, Hill M. Foster carers who cease to foster. *Adoption and Fostering*. 1998; **22**: 54–61.

Viner RM, Taylor B. Adult health and social outcomes of children who have been in public care: population-based study. *Pediatrics*. 2005; **115**: 894–99.

Wilson K, Petrie S, Sinclair I. A kind of loving: a model of effective foster care. *British Journal of Social Work*. 2003; **33**: 991–1003.

Chapter 7

Asperger's syndrome

'In what follows, I will describe a particularly interesting and highly recognisable type of child. The children I will present all have in common a fundamental disturbance which manifests itself in their physical appearance, expressive functions, and, indeed, their whole behaviour. This disturbance results in severe and characteristic difficulties in social integration. In many cases the social problems are so profound that they overshadow everything else' (Asperger, 1944, translated by Frith, 1991). So begins Hans Asperger's original paper published in 1944, in which he described the syndrome that bears his name now. The following case report departs from the chapter format in the rest of the book in that it tells the case of Christopher, now 21 years, in narrative form as it follows his journey from the time the first difficulties were noticed to the present day. He came into CAMHS when he was 8 years of age.

Christopher, now 21 years, is the firstborn child of Mr and Mrs Brookes. They had been married for 5 years and were overjoyed when Christopher was born. It was a planned pregnancy and the delivery was normal. Christopher was a delightful baby. He slept and fed well and everyone who saw him remarked how handsome he was. His developmental milestones were normal; he spoke his first word at 12 months and was able to put two words together by 18 months. He sat up at 6 months and was walking by 13 months. He greeted his parents with a charming smile and could wave goodbye in his second year. As he moved into toddlerhood, he was becoming stubborn and wilful. He displayed temper tantrums and insisted on doing things his way. He had boundless energy and 'was on the go' all the time. He would run rather than walk and was into everything in the house. His mother found that she was getting exhausted trying to keep pace with him. None of these were perceived as problems at this stage. His parents felt that he would 'slow down' once he went to a nursery and mingled with other children.

Preschool and primary school: He started nursery school when he was four years and it was then that he ran into problems. Although Christopher went to school willingly and had no separation difficulties, his behaviour at the nursery caused a great deal of concern. He refused to co-operate at the nursery and shouted 'no, no, no' and ran around the nursery. He became overexcited easily, jumping up and down and shouting out. In group activities he lost attention and would fidget and touch other children. He was reported to 'pounce' on other children for no apparent reason and be surprised by their response to his actions. He would go up to other children, and without warning, push them or grab them or put his hands around their neck. This was happening about three times a day. Teachers reported that he interacted with other children on his own terms. For example, when playing at the dough table, he took dough from another child without saying a word. He preferred to play on his own or side by side with other children. He found it difficult to share toys and equipment with other children and, if asked to, he ran around the room shouting, 'I can't, I won't.' When upset his reactions were extreme and out of the ordinary; he would try to bang his head on the floor or wall or he would hit the fist against the temple.

Teachers had noticed that at times he seemed to be in a 'world of his own' and tended to ignore the rest of the children. School reports at the time indicated that Christopher 'showed good verbal ability for his age although his had a detached manner and did not always respond appropriately to questions'. At times he used words and phrases that children of his age did not understand. Instead of saying 'I like' he would say 'I prefer' and use the word 'however' to mean 'but'. In a report to educational authorities requesting additional resources to support Christopher, teachers reported that 'He will initiate conversation with other children by calling their name but cannot sustain a conversation because he cannot give relevant sensible answers to their questions or requests.'

At this time parents and teachers noticed that he liked routine. If anything happened to disrupt the routine he resorted to temper tantrums. He liked to eat from a particular plate and insisted that the food be placed on the plate in a particular order. For example, he always wanted the vegetables to be served last. Any deviation from this routine produced massive outbursts in Christopher. The school had not realised his preference for routine until one day when the police had come to school to talk to the children. The music lesson was cancelled as a result. Christopher went berserk and completely lost control of his emotions and had to be firmly held by a teacher to stop him hurting himself. The teachers had not realised what caused his outburst at that time. There were other times too when the teachers found it difficult to understand his behaviour. A visiting theatre had come to school and Christopher had enjoyed taking part in the activities, but within a short time he had started shouting out and rocking himself forwards until his head touched the floor.

Another piece of behaviour that was puzzling was his tendency to spin around and flap his hands. This happened especially when he got very excited during activities. He jumped up and down shouting out loudly and flapping his hands about. The hand flapping and running around was not a problem at home but the school found it hard to manage and the other children were shocked by his behaviour. Teachers described his hand flapping and running around in circles as 'Christopher's bird dance'.

At the age of 5½ years his physical development was considered to be good. However, he found it difficult to jump with feet together, hop on one foot, walk along a plank and jump off; and he could not catch a ball. He held the pencil in the pincer grip and had little control over scissors, paint brushes and crayons. Using a fork and knife had been a challenge to Christopher all along. He says that he mastered their use only when he was a teenager. As early as 4 years of age, his parents had noticed that Christopher enjoyed dance, interpreted the music well and was creative in his movements. He had a lovely tuneful singing voice. The teachers commented that he enjoyed 'conducting' the children during percussion and singing. He had an extraordinary memory for music and songs. He could repeat a song or tune he had heard once or twice with incredible accuracy. In general he had an astonishing memory and was able to repeat conversations and remember incidents that others had long forgotten. His parents felt that he gave the impression that he was not listening or paying attention but would repeat the conversation almost word for word much later. Their overall impression was that he was a bright child who became frustrated and distracted easily.

The teachers in the nursery were concerned about his behaviour, especially in view of the impending transfer to primary school. They felt that he may have special educational needs and requested help from the LEA. He was also referred to the community paediatrician. The education psychologist who saw him reported: 'Christopher is an attractive, interesting little boy who functioned in most of the areas of development at the level expected for his age. His main area of difficulty seems to be social behaviour. He has made good progress in the nursery with hard work and thoughtful support given by his teachers.' He concluded that his educational needs included:

1 access to the full mainstream curriculum
2 early interventions to avoid him becoming overexcited
3 a structured approach to improve his co-operation and attention and
4 encouragement and managed opportunities to help him develop social skills and relationships within his peer group.

He was provided with 15 hours of extra help a week at school.

His parents too were becoming aware of other problems apart from his overactive and boisterous behaviour. Quite often when spoken to Christopher looked at them apparently not understanding what was being said to him. He would just walk away without saying a word. Then an hour or two later he would suddenly respond in a relevant and sensible way to the earlier conversation. He played with his trains, cars and building blocks for hours and would create his own play world where he acted out stories. He loved books and would have stories read out to him or read them himself, having memorised the stories. The parents found it difficult to understand his behaviour. On the one hand he was stubborn, strong-willed and determined and wore down anyone who was looking after him, but on the other hand he was a 'charmer' who won the hearts of the adults he came in contact with. They were inclined to feel that his difficulties stemmed from lack of contact with other children of his age and that, over time and with help from school, they hoped he would improve and be integrated with his peers.

One of the other concerns for his parents was Christopher's eating habits. He was picky in what he ate and wanted the same items of food for every meal. For example his school dinner consisted of jam sandwiches and he refused to have any other items of food. (This lasted till he was 10 years of age and was replaced by cheese sandwiches for the next 4 years.) He avoided any food that was mushy or soggy. For example, he refused to eat mashed potatoes, ice cream or cooked vegetables. The items of food had to be separate and not touch one another; they had to be set in a particular order. He did not like tea or coffee. His persistent refusal to try new items of food became a problem when they visited friends or went on holidays.

Christopher was noted to have unusual interests from an early age. This was first noticed when he started at the primary school. He became interested in taps, water and sewers. He asked the teacher where the water came from and where it went. On a number of occasions the teacher took him to the toilet and explained how the flushing system worked. His interest in sewers and drains was initially considered to be part of childhood curiosity and the teachers took extra interest in explaining about sewage disposal and the environment. One of the teachers even organised a trip to the sewers to show him how sewers worked. Soon the teachers found that he was wearing them out with questions about sewers, drains, cesspits and gutters. In conversations in class and outside, he was found to steer the talk to discussing sewers and drains. He did the same with the other children in class and they started avoiding talking to him. The conversations at home too were about sewers. He wanted his father to take him to see the sewers and, when he refused, Christopher started drawing toilets, sewers and drains. Whenever friends or relatives visited the family Christopher's conversation was about sewers. The parents were so embarrassed by some of his questions that his father forbade him to talk about sewers when visitors came or when the family went out.

One of the behaviours that annoyed his mother was his tendency to argue over minor things. For example, if he was asked to get the trousers from the drawer, to get ready in the mornings, Christopher would bring the trousers but not the shirt and socks. If he was made to go again to fetch them he would get annoyed and argue that he did what he was told and it was unfair to get him to do it again. Similarly, if asked to empty the bin he would empty it but not the basket. These minor disagreements led to arguments and Christopher would end up in a temper. According to him it was wrong to expect him to do things he was not asked to do. His parents felt that he acted silly in order to deliberately annoy them. It was not until they met with the CAMHS clinician that they realised that Christopher was not being silly or naughty, rather he interpreted things literally. They had taken for granted that he understood what they meant, while he only understood what was said.

The other annoying behaviour was his tendency to 'switch off'. It had been noted that from his toddlerhood Christopher had a tendency to 'ignore' what was said and not pay attention. There were periods lasting up to five minutes when Christopher appeared to be 'not there' and was preoccupied with his own thoughts during which he did not respond to requests or questions. Initially his mother had felt that he was hard of hearing. A hearing test was done and it proved to be normal. The family believed that he was deliberately ignoring what he was being told. They were convinced that he was using it as a ploy not to do things requested of him. Often this led to arguments.

Both teachers and parents had noticed that from an early age Christopher had the habit of not looking at the person who was speaking to him. This had been identified as a problem at the nursery and later at the primary school. The teachers had made it a point to get him to maintain eye contact every time they spoke to him during conversations, by saying 'Christopher, look at me'. The parents had been told to do the same. Although there had been some improvement in eye contact, family members had to sometimes remind him to look at them when spoken to.

His educational needs were reviewed after transfer to primary school. The teachers and the education psychologists were pleased with his progress both socially and educationally. It was decided that he 'no longer needed the protection of a Statement of Special Educational Needs'. In view of his progress at school the extra help he received was withdrawn when Christopher was 7 years old. But things at home were getting worse. He was particularly difficult on return from school; he 'had a mad half an hour' during which he became defiant, ran around the house and was completely out of control.

The education psychologist referred him to the community paediatrician during this time. The community paediatrician who saw Chrisotopher was puzzled. His developmental milestones including those of speech had been normal and everyone agreed that he was an intelligent boy. Apart from mild dyspraxia, there were no positive features of developmental delay. However, some of the behaviours were certainly odd and did not make sense. The paediatrician referred him on to CAMHS.

Clinical presentation: Christopher was 8 years of age when seen at the CAMHS. The parents' descriptions of Christopher's behaviour were rather vague. They found it difficult to be precise about the difficulties, at times they could not give examples of the behaviour they were complaining about. Mrs Brookes said, 'He acts silly, but he is not stupid.' The family was concerned about his 'annoying' behaviours and 'immaturity'. They had come to realise that his sister Susan who was three years younger than him had more common sense than him. His behaviours did not make sense to them because on the one hand he was reasonably good at reading and writing and was quite intelligent, but on the other hand he was irrational, argumentative and often acted like a younger child. The other complaints were that he was preoccupied with certain topics and talked only about the subjects he was interested in. He was outgoing and talkative but his conversation was odd and he had no friends and was finding maths difficult. He lacked social graces.

When seen in the clinic Christopher seemed like any other 8-year-old, so much so that a trainee who sat with the clinician during the interview said that during the first half an hour of the session she felt that he was just an active little boy who appeared quite normal. During the session Christopher played with the toys in the room but was seen to keenly follow what his parents were telling the clinician. He answered questions readily and appropriately. Unless asked to look at the clinician he preferred to answer without facing the clinician and continued with his play. His drawings were colourful and well executed. He said he liked drawing, but the drawings consisted mainly of patterns, designs and geometric shapes.

During later sessions, when Christopher had come to know the therapist well and he was more talkative and spontaneous, some of his difficulties were more apparent. For example, the avoidance of eye contact was more noticeable. He would look out of the window while answering questions. At other times he fell silent during conversations and had to be reminded about the question. Although he was articulate and chatty and keen to talk about his current subject of interest, at times he used long and unusual words. For example, when asked about whether he had been to school that day, Christopher looked out of the window in his usual fashion and replied: 'Affirmative.' On another occasion he said his dress was an anachronism. When asked for the meaning of these words, he was not sure. No one was sure from where he got the word 'anachronism'. When asked about his use of long words, his mother said that he was known to use big words from the time he was in primary school. For instance, he had used the word 'telecommunication tower' one day at the primary school and his teachers had been surprised that he did not say 'TV tower' like other children. He was known to surprise visitors to the family with his use of long words. When asked about his age when they were on holidays by a relative stranger he had said 'I am approximately eight'. Asked about his experiences in the theme park he had said, 'It is captivating.'

Parents found it difficult to remember all his difficulties in the first few sessions and were asked to make a note of behaviours (with examples) they wanted to discuss. One example that they had recorded was about an instance in school when he was said to have dabbed paint over a boy. Christopher had been punished for it and his mother was called to school to talk about a complaint about his behaviour. When the incident was discussed in the clinic Christopher said that they were working in pairs and the class was asked to draw a boy on a particular sheet of paper. (It appeared that they had been given scenes from the class and asked to draw them.) Next they were asked to paint the boy (meaning draw the boy with paint). Christopher had literally painted the boy who was his partner!

When the family was asked to give examples of such 'misunderstandings' by Christopher, they came up with a long list of them. On one occasion, his father had postponed a trip to the garden centre. He had said, 'I have changed my mind.' Upon hearing this, Christopher who was not involved in the conversation had retorted, 'You can't change your mind.' Surprised by the interruption, his father had asked him why he could not change his mind on a matter such as going to the garden centre. Christopher had said, 'You can't change your mind; you will have to have a brain operation.' Similarly, one day while in the car with Christopher his mother had said, 'It is raining cats and dogs.' Christopher had looked up at the sky and said, 'It's not. There are no cats or dogs there.' His mother said he had difficulties understanding expressions such as 'catch you later', 'over the moon' and 'spill the beans'. The family had come to understand that Christopher took things literally and had learned to avoid the use of metaphors.

Christopher liked certainty and wanted to know exactly what was going to happen next. For example, if they were going out he would want to know at what time they were going out and what time they would be back, what route they would take and where they were going. Any deviation from the plan resulted in protests and arguments from Christopher. On one occasion they had been to a friend in Manchester and Christopher had been told that it would take 2 hours to get there. But they had difficulties finding their way in Manchester. Christopher had become angry and agitated and started a massive argument. He had shouted, 'It is not fair. You said two hours.' His wailing had gone on for a long time, so much so that his father had threatened to get him out of the car and leave him on the road. His mother had come up with a solution. She had suggested playing his favourite music tape and when it was finished they would be at the friend's house. As it happened, they found the friend's house before the tape ran out and were pleased to be there sooner than expected. But Christopher had shouted at them that the tape was not yet finished and his mother was breaking her promise. He had yelled 'You said we will be there only when the tape is finished, you liar,' and refused to get out of the car.

Over the years his parents had learned to tell him things only when they were very sure of their plans and to give him just enough information so that he would not hold them to it. This meant that most of the time they had to keep things away from him. This strategy produced its own problems, as Christopher blamed them for not telling him things. The family had also learned to tell him things in simple clear language so that it could not be misinterpreted.

Another of Christopher's difficulties was that he had hardly any friends. His parents had not considered this a particular problem when he was young. They described themselves as rather reserved and short of friends. As he had got older Christopher had started complaining that nobody liked him and he was not getting invited to birthday parties. He found himself alone during break times. The parents had made an effort to 'engineer' friendships by inviting his friends home. But after playing with them for a few minutes Christopher lost interest in them and was back in his room playing on his own and his friends ended up playing with his sister, whom they considered 'wonderful'. Christopher then blamed his sister for stealing his friends.

His parents attributed his difficulties in making friends to his selfishness and lack of interest in their activities. They felt he had few interests in common with them. His teacher reports had consistently mentioned his isolation from friends and his difficulties in adapting to friendships. Christopher said he longed to have friends and the other kids were not interested in him. He found it difficult to talk to them about football and take part in their games. He felt excluded by them and blamed them for not taking him into their groups.

He said he found it difficult to understand what they expected of him and when he butted into their conversations they laughed at him. On the other hand he did not understand some of their conversations. For example, he did not understand some of their jokes and had to pretend to laugh at them. Sometimes he had asked them to explain the jokes and they had called him 'tube light'. For sometime he did not know why they called him tube light and asked his mother what it meant. She had explained that fluorescent bulbs took some time to light up after they were switched on. It had taken him some time to understand what it meant. When he did realise what it meant he was heartbroken.

His parents had always felt that 'he was out of sync' with how other people thought about things. When they watched television programmes as a family he frequently asked them questions about the jokes in them and wanted to know what they meant. His sister found it annoying and used to shout at him. This was true of other people's actions as well. He repeatedly asked them why they did/said one thing or the other.

At the time he was seen by the CAMHS his main preoccupation was capitals of the world. Following a period of extreme interest in sewers, he had become interested in the sea (where the sewers ended) and later it was oceans of the world. His interest in capitals of the world included finding out the names from atlases and books, writing down the names in a book and collecting information about each capital, including their population. He had a remarkable memory for their names and other details and had an encyclopaedic knowledge of most countries in the world. He started researching the flags of various countries and spent hours drawing them out in great detail. He had a vast collection of various paper cuttings, maps and drawing of flags and made it a point of showing them to everyone who visited them. The family was most embarrassed when while travelling by plane on a holiday to Spain he had asked a lady 'Do you know the capital of Iceland?' As he became familiar with the CAMHS clinician, the first question he asked on entering the clinic room was 'Do you know the capital of . . .?' He then proceeded to tell him all he knew of the country.

As he got older his interests changed. From interest in capitals of the world, it shifted to a preoccupation with football clubs. He knew the names of *all* the players in the various football clubs. Unlike other children of his age, he went round collecting a vast quantity of information about each of the players and knew them by heart. He knew details of each of the players including where they came from, their ages and birthdays and other personal details and often used his superior knowledge to outwit (or so he thought) his peers.

Following assessment in the clinic a diagnosis of Asperger's syndrome was made. The various difficulties that Christopher was showing were explained in terms of features of Asperger's syndrome. One of the difficulties the parents had encountered was that he had a variety of problems that, in their view, were incomprehensible. Although they were not keen to 'label' Christopher, when the features of Asperger's syndrome were explained to them his behaviours started making sense to them. The parents were given a booklet on Asperger's syndrome and asked to underline the features that applied to him. When it was discussed in the next session his mother said that it appeared to describe him accurately. Admittedly he did not show some features like hypersensitivity to noise, light or touch, but he showed the main features – difficulties in communication, impairment in social relationships and the presence of preoccupations.

It took Mr and Mrs Brookes more than two years to fully realise Christopher's difficulties and how handicapping they were for him. One of their main difficulties was that they were never sure whether what they witnessed was ordinary laziness, misbehaviour and unwillingness to learn things or deficits resulting from Asperger's syndrome. As his mother put it, 'We can never be sure whether it is Asperger's or simply Christopher.' Because of the unusual nature of his difficulties and their subtleness, it was also difficult for them to explain to others what his difficulties were. Years later, in one of the sessions, Mrs Brookes said, 'He sees the world in a very different way. It took me a long time to realise this. Yet, I do get annoyed and frustrated with him. I know I should not.'

The parents made contact with the National Autistic Society and found attendance at the meetings helpful. He was re-referred for speech therapy but he was considered to be 'too good' to need therapy. His mother who was a civil servant gave up her job to become a voluntary helper at school. The school was welcoming of this because they had number of children with various special needs and were short-staffed. During this time Mrs Brookes had realised that her husband too showed some Asperger-like features. She described him as a loner and one who liked to spend time on his own. In the early part of their marriage this had led to a number of marital problems. She resented him for not spending his time with her but over the years she had come to understand that he 'liked his own space'. But it had taken her a long time to come to terms with it. His particular preoccupation was DIY and he spent long periods of time working in the garage. He did not like to join parties or family gatherings. She remembered one occasion when they had gone to a neighbour's party and in the middle of the party he was nowhere to be seen. Later she discovered that he had left the party without telling anyone and gone into his garage to do his jobs, which he found more interesting than the party.

Secondary school: The time of moving to secondary school was an anxious one for both the clinician and the parents. They were not sure whether Christopher would adjust to the new school and if the school would be flexible enough to accommodate his difficulties. Before Christopher transferred to the secondary school the clinician met with the headteacher and the SENCO of the new school to get them to understand what his difficulties were. Since he had no Statement of Special Educational Needs they could not give him the extra help. It was explained to them that Christopher was an intelligent boy but he was socially naïve. This meeting proved to be enormously important. The clinician gave them a profile of his difficulties and strengths.

The first year in secondary school was challenging for Christopher. The introduction to school was gradual. The SENCO took him around the school to familiarise him with the layout and show him where the various classes were. He had a student mentor with whom he could spend time. In later years Christopher was to say that he found the help and support that he received in the first term in secondary school made a big difference to him. To this day he remembers how the SENCO got him to give a speech to the class about capitals of the world. His classmates were impressed with his depth of knowledge. It also proved to Christopher that he could give a performance to an audience.

In year 7 (at 12 years) he took part in the school play, 'Lady Jane'. He was assigned to the chorus, but, fortunately for Christopher, the boy who was to play the character 'Rattlesnake' was taken ill and Christopher was asked to do his part. He was overjoyed to take on the part and even happier when he drew applause for his performance. Christopher remembers this incident and the sudden realisation that he was good at drama as a turning point in his life.

Christopher's academic performance had always been good. He passed his GCSE examinations and obtained Cs in six subjects and 2 AS level passes. He went on to do his A levels and passed them. At the age of 18 for a short period of time he worked part-time in a bar. The till at the bar was old and did not indicate the change. He got worried whether he could deal with the money. His sister had several days of practice sessions with him so that he could learn to give the correct change to the customer. To his surprise he managed well in the job but it was a temporary arrangement and Christopher had to look for other jobs. He had been asked to help in the local theatre company to assist with props. He says that he was later given the high-sounding title of assistant stage manager but the work involved little more than helping with 'following the spots'. However, he liked the job because he liked theatre.

University: At the time of writing this chapter Christopher is 21 and attends university and is doing a degree course in drama. He likes the atmosphere at the university and says that people are more tolerant of diversity and 'they take you for what you are'. He has a support helper at the university who helps to organise his work and with time management. His parents feel that he lacks motivation and easily settles down to a life of a recluse, avoiding responsibilities and becoming dependent on them. He has no close friends but has a girlfriend. He lives with his parents and goes out very little. He is dependent on his parents to take him to friends and places. For example, he had to go for a performance in a nearby town and was expecting them to take him there at night and bring him back, irrespective of the inconvenience to them. His social development has been quite delayed. He started travelling by bus on his own at the age of 16 and it took him one more year before he could go out with friends. Frequently he comes across to his parents as uncaring and selfish. He is not known to enquire about their day or offer to make them a cup of tea. He comes across as unmotivated and lacking in enthusiasm about his career or looking for part-time jobs. They complain that he needs prodding. The parents feel that he has no social niceties and that he is irresponsible. Christopher claims that these are features of Asperger's syndrome and the parents feel that it is Christopher syndrome.

It was noticeable that his interests and activities had become more 'normal' in terms of their content, although he remains preoccupied with them and prefers to talk about them than other subjects. He also spends a great deal of time collecting, arranging, filing and hoarding things that he finds interesting. His current preoccupation is his hair and his music. He spends hours doing his hair until he gets it right; he does this several times a day. He has to do things in a particular order. He plays the guitar for long periods of time and can forget himself in it. He has to read the papers first thing in the morning and takes a long time over it. Consequently everybody at home gets delayed in the mornings. His mother has been given a regular paid job in the school and helps with children with special needs.

He admits that he has no friends. He describes his mates as acquaintances rather than friends. With a group of peers he tends to remain in the background and not say much. He is not sure what others think of him. 'I feel I am left out a lot; often I feel like an outsider. But now I get on with people. But talking to adults seems much easier,' he says. At the age of 21 he has not spent a night away from home. He admits that he finds it difficult to initiate and maintain conversations. He says he is good at disguising his difficulties and pretending to join in conversations. His diet continues to be restricted and he avoids foods he considers mushy; he is averse to trying new items of food and prefers to eat the same food. But he eats a reasonably varied diet. Christopher admits that he is not good at talking about emotions and says, 'I don't understand why people keep talking all the time about how they feel.' He says that when he is with his friends his greatest difficulty is to 'read between the lines'. ('A few years ago I would not have understood what this meant', he quips.)

His case was presented at the local postgraduate training centre. Contrary to expectations, he readily agreed to be available in person at the presentation and answered questions without much hesitation or anxiety. When asked about the experience he said, 'It is easy if you think of it as a great big show.'

Theoretical perspectives

The first person to describe autism was Leo Kanner (1894–1981). He was an Austrian-American physician known for his work related to autism. Kanner was born in Austria but he immigrated to the United States in 1924. He was the first physician in the United States to be identified as a child psychiatrist and his first book, *Child Psychiatry*, published in 1935, was the first English language textbook to focus on psychiatric problems in children. His seminal 1943 paper 'Autistic disturbances of affective contact' formed the basis of the modern study of autism. Kanner's original study consisted of 11 children and introduced the concept called 'early infantile autism'.

Asperger's syndrome is named after Hans Asperger (1906–1980), who was an Austrian paediatrician. Born in Vienna, Asperger published the first definition of Asperger's syndrome (AS) in 1944. In four boys he identified a pattern of behaviour and abilities that he called 'autistic psychopathy', meaning autism (self) and psychopathy (personality disease). The pattern included 'a lack of empathy, little ability to form friendships, one-sided conversation, intense absorption in a special interest and clumsy movements'. Asperger called children with AS 'little professors' because of their ability to talk about their favourite subject in great detail. He was convinced that many would use their special skills in adulthood. He followed up one child, Fritz Vee, into adulthood. Vee later became a professor of astronomy. Asperger died before his identification of the pattern of behaviour became widely recognised because his work was mostly in German and was little translated. The first person to use the term Asperger's syndrome in a paper was a British researcher, Lorna Wing, in her paper, 'Asperger's syndrome: A clinical account', published in 1981.

Autism spectrum disorders (ASD)

It is now believed that autistic traits are widely distributed in the normal population and many 'normal people' show isolated autistic traits. Current evidence indicates that autism could represent the extreme of a quantitative distribution of autistic traits that are present in the normal population. Increasing evidence supports the hypothesis that autism is a quantitative or dimensional spectrum, with no clear distinction between traits found among individuals with the disorder and the general population. Thus it is now common to talk of an autistic spectrum of disorders (ASD). Figure 7.1 shows the various disorders in the autistic spectrum as is currently understood. When the traits are marked, prominent and involve multiple domains, they are likely to cause social and personal impairments. Recent surveys of the prevalence of autism in the community indicate not only the number of cases meeting conventional criteria, but a disproportionate increase in the number of milder cases that fail to meet full ICD/DSM criteria.

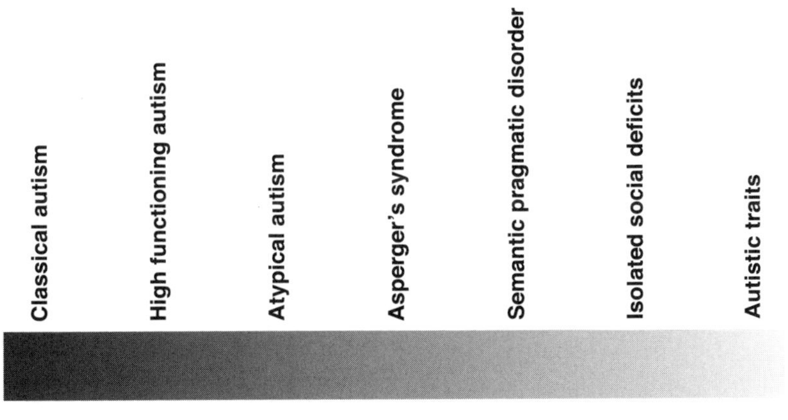

Figure 7.1 The autism spectrum.

The autistic spectrum disorders consists of a group of disorders of development with lifelong effects and that have in common a triad of impairments (known as Wing's triad), consisting of impairments in:

1 social interaction,
2 communication and
3 imagination and behaviour (narrow repetitive pattern of behaviour).

ASD includes 'classical' autism originally described by Kanner and Asperger's syndrome, but is not limited to the two conditions. The triad of impairments occur in children with all levels of intelligence, from the most learning disabled to those with average and superior cognitive abilities. The following are thought to come under the umbrella of ASDs:

'Classical' (or Kanner) autism: Autism is a neurodevelopmental disorder with a strong genetic basis. Features of autism are thought to manifest before 36 months although in 70% of cases the problems in development had been evident from infancy. In 'classical autism' most children have low IQs (in 70% the IQ is below 70 and in 50% below 50). About half of those with Kanner autism never develop useful speech. Although classical patterns vary depending on severity, all children with autism demonstrate some degree of qualitative impairment in reciprocal social interaction, qualitative impairment of communication and repetitive and stereotypic behaviour patterns of behaviours, interests and activities. Children with the classical clinical picture are usually identified during preschool years by community paediatric services and child development clinics and rarely get to be referred to CAMHS.

'High functioning' autism: This refers to a group of children with autism who are usually of normal intelligence and function reasonably well socially and educationally. They usually attend mainstream schools and many of their difficulties are often mild. However, they show deficits and impairments in all three domains described above. Notably, language development is impaired and many show difficulties in language comprehension and pragmatics (see later). Frequently, children in this group are not identified by services until middle childhood and often present to CAMHS with other problems such as behaviour difficulties, anxiety or inappropriate behaviour.

Atypical autism: Autism is now known to be a very heterogeneous disorder, with milder forms being more common than the classical form. Partial syndromes of autism are more common than classical autism and Asperger's syndrome put together. Those with atypical autism (also known as autism not otherwise specified, NOS) show one or more features of Wing's triad of impairments but do not meet all the criteria for a diagnosis of autism or Asperger's syndrome. Those presenting to CAMHS have significant impairments in the social and communication sphere and many professionals and parents find it difficult to understand the problems faced by the child because of lack of a diagnostic label.

Asperger's syndrome: Distinguishing between autism and Asperger's syndrome can be difficult and some have argued that such distinctions to be of little more than academic interest. At the present time, the main differences between the two conditions rest mainly on the relatively normal development of language and cognitive functions in Asperger's syndrome. DSM-IV stipulates that there be no clinically significant delay in language development in Asperger's syndrome (as indexed by single word use by age 2 and communicative phrases by age 3). The hallmark of children with Asperger's syndrome is that they are verbally articulate individuals of average or normal intelligence. The main features of Asperger's syndrome are shown in Table 7.1.

Apart from language and intelligence, other subtle differences have been demonstrated in a number of studies. Children with Asperger's syndrome are responsive to their parents and show normal greeting, comfort-seeking and attachment behaviour. Their social impairment really manifests itself when they begin to interact with other children in nursery or playgroups at primary school, where they are aloof, isolated and interact with their peers in inappropriate ways.

Table 7.1 Key features of Asperger's syndrome

1 Qualitative impairment in social interactions	2 Restricted repetitive and stereotyped pattern of behaviour, interests, and activities	3 Subtle impairments in language and communication
• Marked impairment in the use of nonverbal behaviours (e.g. eye-to-eye gaze, facial expression) • Failure to develop peer relationships appropriate to developmental level • Lack of spontaneous seeking to share enjoyment, interest or achievements • Lack of social or emotional reciprocity	• Intense preoccupation with stereotyped and restricted pattern of interest • Inflexible adherence to specific, non-functional routines or rituals • Stereotyped and repetitive motor mannerisms (e.g. twisting, twirling) • Persistent preoccupation with parts of objects	• Pragmatic language difficulties (concrete interpretation, difficulties understanding sarcasm, metaphor, jokes) • Difficulties in understanding emotional cues

There are also clear differences in imaginative play. While the autistic child rarely shows imaginative play and uses toys in a symbolic way, the child with Asperger's syndrome displays symbolic play albeit somewhat later than normal children. But the play in the child with Asperger's syndrome is repetitive, lacks creativity and is rarely used to promote social interaction. They insist on playing the game 'their way' or the play will end. Motor clumsiness has been observed to be more common in children with Asperger's syndrome.

Although language development is almost normal and gross defects in speech such as neologisms, echolalia and pronoun reversal are uncommon, subtle difficulties in the use of language are evident in most children with Asperger's syndrome. Their superficially normal speech often conceals other language difficulties such as literal interpretation of other people's speech, pedantic use of language and pragmatic language difficulties

The skills that we use to interact effectively, share meaning and communicate with each other are known as *pragmatics*. The word refers to the social use of language. Communicating is not just about using appropriate words and sentence structure because it goes beyond these skills. As a listener, to interact effectively means interpreting what the speaker is meaning to say and reading between the lines. As a speaker, it means that we imply more than what we say and as listeners we infer more meaning than is actually said. We use language for a purpose (function) and in context. Some purposes are: forms of politeness, jokes and humour, sarcasm, wit and irony. For the child with Asperger's syndrome, implied rules of language and behaviour are difficult to decode. Literal reading of other people's statements and concrete interpretation of speech are common.

The main failing of the child with Asperger's syndrome is in the social sphere. In spite of their desire to have friends, they find that they have difficulties in understanding social cues and responding appropriately. Hence children with Asperger's syndrome find themselves friendless and on the periphery when in a group. The main differences between classical autism and Asperger's syndrome are shown in Table 7.2.

Table 7.2 The main differences between autism and Asperger's syndrome

Classical autism	Asperger's syndrome
70% have an IQ below 70	Normal intelligence
Delay in speech development	Normal speech development but subtle difficulties, e.g. in pragmatics
Social impairments pronounced	Social impairments prominent
Preoccupations and routines present	Preoccupations and routines present

The difficulties of the Asperger child continue into adulthood. Although the contents of preoccupations and interests may take a less idiosyncratic form and be less visible, the social impairments may be more handicapping. A study by the National Autistic Society of adults with Asperger's syndrome showed that 3% were living independently, 12% had a full-time job and one third had no outside social contact.

Semantic pragmatic disorder (SPD): This term has been used to describe a group of children who show difficulties primarily in the use of language (pragmatics) and semantics (meaning conveyed by words and sentences). In the past it was considered as exclusively a language and communication problem (and hence dealt with by speech therapists), recent research findings indicate that it does belong within the autism spectrum and has the same underlying triad of socio-cognitive deficits as those found in high functioning autism. Current consensus among authorities is that there is no value in separating it from the autistic spectrum (Bishop, 1989). Although in children showing the SPD picture, speech and language difficulties appear to be the more prominent problem, they show variable but not insignificant difficulties in the other two domains of functioning.

Prevalence of ASD: In the past autism was considered a rare disorder and earlier studies estimated the prevalence of autism to be 4–5 in 10 000 persons. Recently, a major increase in the diagnosis of ASD has been observed in the UK, US and Denmark. Analysis of figures show that the apparent increase in ASD is due primarily to change in diagnostic practices, such as improved identification and availability of services. An important recent study of a population of almost 57 000 children aged between 9–10 years has confirmed the view that the prevalence of autism and related ASDs is substantially greater than previously recognised (Baird *et al.*, 2006). In this study the prevalence of classical childhood autism was found to be 38.9 per 10 000 and that of other ASDs was 77.2 per 10 000. Taken together, the prevalence of ASD was shown to be 1% of the child population and the authors consider it to be an underestimate! The study concluded that 'Services in health, education, and social care will need to recognise the needs of children with some form of ASD, who constitute 1% of the child population' (Baird *et al.*, 2006).

Aetiology: Between 10–15% of those with classical autism have a medical disorder and 5% have a chromosomal disorder such as fragile X syndrome. Genetic factors have been shown to be strongly implicated in the aetiology of autism. Multiple genes are thought to be involved. In clinical situations it is not unusual for a family with one autistic child to have a number of members in the extended and nuclear family to have ASD of varying severities.

Psychological deficits: A number of theories have been put forward to explain the core deficits in ASD. Unfortunately, none of the theories adequately explain all different aspects of the disorder. The best known is the 'theory of mind' (also called mentalising) hypothesis proposed by Baron-Cohen *et al.* (1985). Theory of mind is a somewhat misleading term that has been used to describe the cognitive abilities concerned with understanding other people's mental states – beliefs, desires, intentions – and use this knowledge to predict the behaviour of others. A number of studies have shown that children with ASD have a significant deficit in theory of mind tasks. The difficulties of children with ASD to understand how other people's minds work and modulate their behaviour accordingly may be considered to be the result of lack of theory of mind. This may explain the social difficulties that children with ASD exhibit. Another popular theory is that they have 'executive function' deficits. Executive functions refer to the cognitive activities involved in planning, problem solving, behaviour shifting and inhibition. Many studies have demonstrated that children with ASD have executive function deficits. Although these theories do explain some of the features of ASD, they do not adequately account for others, most notably the preoccupations and repetitive behaviours.

Comments

Since CAMHS practitioners are now seeing more children with ASD in their day-to-day clinical practice, they need to increase their font of knowledge and expertise in identifying and caring for these children. Families expect the clinician to guide them through the plethora of behavioural, educational and alternative treatment options available for them. Early diagnosis of ASD is challenging in the context of CAMHS, because there is no pathognomonic sign or laboratory test to detect it. Thus, the practitioner must make the diagnosis on the basis of the presence or absence of a constellation of symptoms. ASD is a phenomenological rather than an aetiological disorder (such as Down's syndrome), making the diagnosis more challenging. Clinicians must rely on parent report, clinical judgement and the ability to recognise criteria-based behaviours that define ASD.

The generic assessment of children seen in CAMHS should include screening for ASD whatever the presenting problem. Practitioners need to be proficient in identifying ASD because it may present in a variety of ways: behaviour problems, inappropriate behaviour or social isolation, to name a few. Moreover, the presentation changes with age and those coming into CAMHS during middle childhood or adolescence may not show the typical presentations. Keeping a watchful eye for ASD is particularly important in light of the recent findings that about two thirds of primary school children excluded from school have social and communication problems (Gilmour *et al.*, 2004) and that many adolescents who commit offences and are seen by Youth Offending Services show features of the full or partial syndrome.

Early diagnosis is dependent on listening carefully to parents' concerns about their child's development and behaviour. Current research has revealed that parents are usually correct in their concerns about a child's development. Any concern by the parents should be valued and should lead to additional investigation by the practitioner.

The burgeoning recognition of autistic disorders is putting a great strain on local CAMH services.

References

Baird G, Simonoff E, Pickles A *et al.* Prevalence of disorders of the autism spectrum in a population cohort of children in South Thames: the Special Needs and Autism Project (SNAP). *Lancet.* 2006; **368**: 210–15.

Baron-Cohen S, Leslie AM, Frith U. Does the autistic child have a 'theory of mind?' *Cognition.* 1985; **21**: 37–46.

Bishop DVM. Autism, Asperger's syndrome and semantic-pragmatic disorder: Where are the boundaries? *British Journal of Disorders of Communication.* 1989; **24**: 107–21.

Frith U, editor. *Autism and Asperger's Syndrome.* Cambridge: Cambridge University Press; 1991.

Gilmour J, Hill B, Place M *et al.* Social and communication deficits in conduct disorder: A clinical and community survey. *Journal of Child Psychology and Psychiatry.* 2004; **45**: 967–78.

* Wing L. Asperger's syndrome: a clinical account. *Psychological Medicine.* 1981; **11**: 115–30.

Chapter 8

Anorexia nervosa

Rachel was referred by her GP who, in addition to making a faxed referral, made a telephone call to CAMHS to express her concerns regarding Rachel Parkinson, a 15½-year-old girl, whom she had seen in her surgery that morning. The GP had been shocked by the appearance of Rachel, who seemed to have lost a vast amount of weight. She looked extremely thin, with a bossy forehead and drawn face. The GP remembered having seen Rachel a year ago when she seemed quite healthy and had attended surgery for a respiratory infection. Over the past year Rachel had been cutting down on her food, so much so that at the time of referral she was eating very little. She missed lunch and breakfast and had a small meal in the evening. Her current weight was 83.5 lbs and her height was 5 feet 2 inches. She had not had her periods for the past six months. The school had been very concerned about Rachel for some time. In the previous week she had fainted whilst at school and had been sent home with a note from the teachers asking her parents to seek help from their GP. The GP had taken blood samples to run some tests, but she did not think there was a physical disorder that could account for the illness. During the interview Rachel had been glum and resistant and uncooperative, giving single word answers to most questions that the GP asked. When the GP had seen Rachel on her own, Rachel had mentioned that she looked too fat and wanted to be thin. She wanted Rachel to be seen as soon as possible.

Clinical presentation and background

The first appointment was attended by Rachel, 15 years, her parents, Christopher and Ann Parkinson, and her younger sister, Tanya, aged 14 years. No one in the family was sure when Rachel started losing weight. She had tried various 'diets' over the past couple of years, but about a year ago she had started to cut down on her food drastically, saying that she had no appetite. She had started avoiding certain foods which she thought were fattening. Initially she stopped eating chips, fried food and fast food, claiming that these were unhealthy. She had been trying to restrict her calorie intake and had become an expert at the calorie content of various items of food. She kept a close check on the number of calories in the food that she ate. The parents had found out she had not been eating school meals. She usually took a packed lunch to school and they had discovered that on a number of occasions the lunch was still there in her schoolbag in the evening. When questioned about it, Rachel had said she had no appetite or that she had forgotten to eat it. At home she did not sit with the rest of the family for meals, preferring to eat on her own. Usually she served the meals herself and at times cooked her own meals. She was said to be a good cook and read a number of cookery books and was a good in making Chinese dishes, although she did not eat them. She had always been a girl interested in physical exercise, sports and other activities. After coming back from school she went jogging. They had also heard her jog in her room at night. They said they had been aware that Rachel had been losing weight but had not realised that she had lost quite a lot. They felt she had lost about 10 lbs in the previous 3 months, although they had not weighed her regularly or known her accurate weight. Rachel began having her periods at the age of 12, soon after she began secondary school, but her periods had stopped 9 months ago.

Mr and Mrs Parkinson described Rachel as a somewhat shy girl, unlike her sister who was extroverted and outgoing. She was good in her schoolwork and had a few friends with whom she got on well. She liked PE and physical activities and wanted to be a gymnast. There had been no previous problems, she had been well behaved and they had nothing to complain about. Her early development had been normal, and apart from the usual childhood illnesses, Rachel had been a healthy girl and there was no significant past medical history.

Rachel was born at 41 weeks gestation following an uncomplicated pregnancy. Her mother was due to be admitted to hospital to be induced but went into labour naturally. Labour was prolonged and, as is quite common with epidural anaesthesia, Rachel was eventually delivered by ventouse. There were no complications, and she was a healthy baby. Her development was uneventful and she was always a happy and confident child. There were no separations between Rachel and her mother during infancy and her mother worked in the nursery that Rachel attended. Academically Rachel was said to be bright and she was expected to obtain good grades in her GCSEs next summer. There had been no major problems of conduct at school, though Rachel had suffered some bullying over the years and her mother had gone to school on a couple of occasions to sort this out. There had been instances of arguments between Rachel and her parents over her choice of friends but her parents believed that this was normal for her age. She had a few good friends with whom she shared an interest in music and fashion. Rachel did not smoke or drink. She had no allergies or sensitivities and she was not on any medication at the time of examination.

Rachel was the elder of the two children in the family. The parents had been married for 17 years. Mr Parkinson was a management consultant and often worked away from home, spending up to a week away when he had to go to outstations on work. Her mother worked part-time as a supply teacher. The family was somewhat isolated and the grandparents lived far away. There was no history of any psychiatric disorders in the family or in the extended family. Mrs Parkinson had had concerns about her own weight for a long time and had been on diets off and on. She was keen on healthy eating and preferred to cook at home and avoid 'junk food' and preprepared meals.

Examination: When seen on her own, it was clear that Rachel had lost a vast amount of weight recently. Her face was thin, with prominent cheekbones; her forehead appeared protuberant and her fingers were quite thin and long. She was pale with drawn-in cheeks. She was wearing two jumpers and a baggy coat over it, presumably to camouflage her emaciated appearance. She denied having any problems and said she had come only because her parents wanted her to. When asked what her parents concerns were, she said they felt she had lost weight and were worried about her getting ill. However, she did not consider herself to be ill and, in fact, thought that she should lose some more weight. She said her ideal weight would be 65 lbs. In the past she had been quite plump and there had been some name-calling at school on account of it. Her highest weight that she had ever reached was about 100 lbs. She admitted that she had been cutting down on her food to reduce weight. She did this by avoiding 'fatty food' and not eating her school lunch. A typical meal consisted of some cornflakes in the morning with milk, no lunch and a small meal in the evenings consisting of boiled vegetables, one slice of bread and some white meat or fish. She claimed that she did not feel hungry and, in fact, she was repelled by the sight of food. On closer enquiry about what she ate, it became clear that she measured the amount of milk carefully before pouring it into the bowl of cornflakes or rice crispies. She also weighed the rice crispies to make sure that she was not eating too much. She said she kept a close count of the calories that she took because she was worried that she would put on weight. There were a number of food items that she avoided such as bananas, ice creams, cakes, crisps, chips and fried foods. She said she had been on a diet on and off as long as she could remember but had never felt in control of what she ate. She felt that her parents were unduly interfering and dictated what she should eat. Even if she were to eat half the amount of what her parents wanted her to, she said she would put on weight and become fat. She made a drawing of how she felt she looked and how she wanted to be (*see* Figure 8.1).

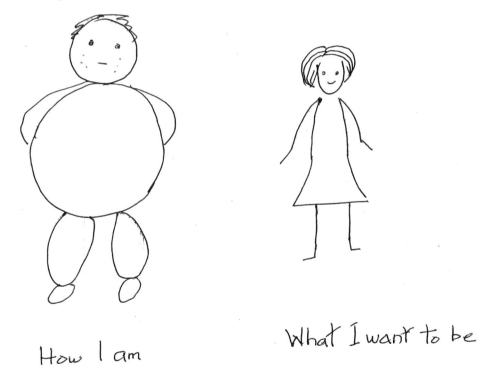

How I am

What I want to be

Figure 8.1 Drawing of self.

When questioned directly about what she felt about her appearance and body shape, she said she hated the way her body looked. She felt that she was fat, obese and ugly. More specifically she felt that her thighs were too fat and her abdomen was protuberant because of the 'fat inside'; she felt her face was too big and her cheeks were too full. She said she did not like to look at herself in the mirror because it reminded her of how fat she was. As for her mood, she did not feel particularly depressed but was unhappy about her looks and the shape of her body.

She reluctantly agreed that, of late, she had been feeling very tired and had, in fact, had several fainting attacks. She also felt cold and lethargic. She admitted to doing excessive exercising. She used to go jogging around the house and also jogged in her room whenever she had thoughts about feeling too fat. She denied inducing vomiting or taking laxatives to lose weight. She felt that her parents ate too much, especially her father, and she hated to sit at the table to eat with them because it was so repugnant to her to see them 'gobble up so much food'. She was convinced that she was overweight and needed to lose some more weight. She said she was envious of models on TV advertisements and fashion shows. It made her realise how fat she was. To her being thin mattered a lot and she felt driven to take measures to reduce weight. She 'was worried sick' that she would put on weight. 'I dare not weigh myself because it might be bad news,' she said. Her parents did not understand how she felt and had become rather critical of her after the visit to the GP. This had lead to a number of arguments over food.

She wanted to be a gymnast or a PE teacher. Rachel claimed that she had an active social life but would not eat with her friends. She liked swimming and dancing. She granted that she had been unable to take part in them recently, but it was because she was losing interest in sporting activities rather than because she felt tired. She was a perfectionist and if she could not do something well she would rather give up. Her schoolwork was tidy and well presented, she hated disorder and her room was always clean and well kept.

A physical examination was carried out by another member of the team. Rachel was skinny and thin and had lanugo hair on her arms and back. Her blood pressure was low (70/50), her pulse rate was slow (60 per minute) and her extremities were cold. She was reluctant to be weighed. Her weight in under-clothes was 38.5 kg (84 lbs) and her height was 154 cm (5' 2''). Information obtained from the GP a week later indicated that her blood tests including thyroid function tests were normal.

Case conceptualisation and formulation

Rachel showed all the typical features of anorexia nervosa – a relentless pursuit to lose weight by dieting and exercising, fear of fatness and distorted body image and amenorrhoea. It was difficult to determine the duration of the illness but it appeared that she had been losing weight over the previous year. She had severely cut down her food intake and been starving herself to attain her ideal weight of 65 lbs. She had a severely distorted image of her body and, more importantly, she was preoccupied with wanting to lose weight. She appeared to have lost a considerable amount of weight, especially during the last 3 months, resulting in physical symptoms like fainting and feeling cold. At this stage of assessment, it was not clear as to what factors contributed to the onset and maintenance of her anorexic behaviour. There did not appear to be overt family issues but a note was made to explore this later.

As a first step to assessment of anorexia nervosa, Rachel's weight and height were recorded on the weight-height-growth chart. Her percentage weight for height and age was calculated by looking at the tables (alternatively, this might be done using a slide ruler) and at a weight of 38.5 kg (84 lbs) she was found to be at 80% of average weight for her height and age.

Permission was requested for a school report. The school report, which arrived a week later, described Rachel as a conscientious and hardworking girl with lots of positive qualities, such as enthusiasm for schoolwork, interest in PE and good relationships with teachers.

Theoretical perspectives

Dieting is widespread in developed countries. Surveys of young people report that most of them have dieted at some time during their teenage years. For example, one Australian study of adolescents aged 12–17 years reported 38% of girls and 12% of boys as 'intermediate' to 'extreme' dieters. The prevalence of eating disorders is directly related to the rates of dieting behaviour (Hsu, 1996). Only a minority of adolescents who diet go on to develop an eating disorder.

Eating disorders are a phenomenon found in countries where food is abundant and the social pressures to be thin and attractive are immense. The combination of personal vulnerabilities and societal and cultural pressures are thought to lead to eating disorders. Individual risk factors for eating disorders include female sex, genetic vulnerability, perfectionist personality traits, low self-esteem and dys-functional family functioning. Precipitating factors may include comments by others about body size and shape or events leading to a fall in self-esteem ('narcissistic wound').

Anorexia nervosa should be distinguished from other causes of weight loss in children and adolescence. Common physical illnesses that lead to weight loss are diabetes, thyrotoxicosis and malabsorption syndromes such as coeliac disease. A particular condition that is sometimes confused with anorexia nervosa is selective eating. Some children and adolescents are extremely selective in what they eat. This often a lifelong habit and may cause poor weight gain and is often difficult to treat. In younger children feeding disorders are relatively common and need to be distinguished from eating disorders. Occasionally, anxiety and phobic disorders may interfere with food intake. Fear of sickness is a relatively common feature of anxiety in children and adolescents and may lead to significant restriction of food. It has to be noted that these conditions are not accompanied by the psychopathology specific to anorexia nervosa. The central feature that distinguishes eating disorders from other conditions involving abnormal eating and weight loss are the core anorexic cognitions that underlie the former (see later).

The prevalence of anorexia nervosa has been estimated to be around 0.7% in the 14–17 age group (Steinhausen *et al.*, 1997). It is about 8 times more common in girls than boys.

Anorexia nervosa is characterised by persistent efforts to achieve a low weight, often to the point of severe malnutrition, and is accompanied by specific psychopathology that includes a morbid fear of fatness and distorted body image. Unrelenting dieting usually leads to weight loss, which in turn leads to amenorrhoea. The diagnostic criteria for anorexia nervosa are given in Box 8.1. It is important to point out that clinically significant variants of anorexia nervosa are common. It is well recognised that around half of all subjects with eating disorders do not meet the full criteria for anorexia nervosa. In current classificatory systems these incomplete forms have been called 'atypical' anorexia (ICD-10) and Eating Disorder Not Otherwise Specified (EDNOS, DSM-IV).

Box 8.1 Key features of anorexia nervosa

- Refusal to maintain minimal body weight for age and height (i.e. weight loss or failure to make expected weight gain) leading to a body weight less than 85% than that expected.
- Self-induced restriction of food intake or other means of losing weight (such as self-induced vomiting, excessive exercising, use of laxatives or diuretics).
- Specific psychopathology including: extreme body image dissatisfaction, body image distortion, intense fear of fatness and denial of the seriousness of the current low body weight.
- Amenorrhoea (or delayed or arrested puberty in early-onset cases).

Although when presented with a young person with an eating disorder the diagnosis is rarely in doubt, it is important to be clear what constitutes an eating disorder and what does not. Not all cases of loss of weight are due to eating disorders. Some professionals dealing with children tend to subscribe to the belief that any unexplained weight loss in a young person is due to an eating disorder. This form of reasoning is open to two errors. First, it ignores the possibility that the loss of weight may be due to occult, yet undiagnosed physical disorders. Common medical causes of weight loss such as diabetes and throtoxicosis are easy to exclude, while rare causes of weight loss like coeliac disease may go undiagnosed for years. Second, to diagnose a psychological/psychiatric problem, absence of physical illness is not sufficient; there needs to be positive evidence of psychological/psychiatric dysfunction or disorder. Whereas weight loss and amenorrhoea may be due to a multitude of physical causes, the diagnosis of anorexia nervosa in the context of weight loss is made on the basis of presence of specific psychopathology. It is the presence of unambiguous abnormalities in thinking (anorexic cognitions) that distinguishes anorexia nervosa from other forms of weight loss.

The essential psychopathological features associated with anorexia nervosa are:

- Weight phobia: dread of fatness leading to drive for thinness; fixation on abnormally low 'ideal' body weight; any perceived increase in weight is received with panic and anxiety.
- Extreme body image dissatisfaction.
- Body image disturbance: overvalued ideas about body size and shape; feeling fat and ugly; overestimation of body size and shape of various parts of the body (abdomen, hips, thigh); denial of thinness.
- Preoccupations with weight and dieting: extreme interest in diets, food and cooking accompanied by reluctance or refusal to eat.

The central and specific cognition that is characteristic of anorexia nervosa (and bulimia nervosa) is the tendency of those with the illness to overevaluate themselves in terms of their weight and shape. All personal qualities and self-worth are judged entirely by their weight and the ability to restrict food consumption. Persons with anorexia nervosa are driven by their psychopathology to relentlessly persue measures to lose weight. The most common way is by restricting food intake. They may eat less during meals, take small portions, cheat at meal times, give up certain foods, measure what they drink and count the calories of what they eat. Inducing vomiting after meals and using laxatives are common. Many become adept at provoking vomiting and need less stimulation of the throat. Frequently, they overexercise to lose weight, a behaviour that is difficult to overcome. When their weight-reducing measures come to the attention of friends and family members, they may resort to extreme measures to deceive or cheat. For example, they wear loose clothes and many layers of clothing to cover their emaciated body, throw away or hide food or drink large quantities of water before being weighed. Often they deny the physical effects of starvation such as feeling faint, tired or cold.

Commonly patients with anorexia show perfectionist and obsessional traits, especially those involving food, diet and exercising. Ritualistic eating habits may be evident. Comorbid depression, obsessive compulsive disorder and self-injurious behaviour are frequently seen in subgroups of patients and present challenges for the management of such patients.

Although limiting food intake and using other weight-losing methods is the commonest presentation of patients with anorexia nervosa (called restrictive type), a subgroup of patients show marked bingeing and counteracting behaviours like purging or vomiting. The clinical profile of the bulimic-anorexic patients is somewhat different from the restricting anorexic patients. They tend to have been overweight before the onset of the illness, show more impulsive behaviours (such as deliberate self-harm) and have a worse prognosis than their restive anorexic counterparts.

Many of the behaviours shown by patients with anorexia nervosa may be indistinguishable from the effects of starvation seen in normal people. One of the most revealing studies into the effects of food restriction and weight loss, called the Minnesota Starvation Study, was carried out by Keys *et al.* (1950). Healthy individuals who were made to lose 25% of their weight were studied under laboratory conditions. They showed a number of unusual changes in their behaviour, cognitions and feelings. All subjects showed an extreme preoccupation with food and eating, and food became the main topic of their conversation. They smuggled food, became interested in cookery, menus and cookbooks. They spent most of their time planning how they would eat their allocated rations. Some hid their rations without eating. At the end of the experiment when they were refed and gained weight, most of the symptoms disappeared.

It is likely that, to a degree, some of the symptoms of anorexia may indeed be due to starvation. Self-starvation also leads to physical changes in the gut such as sluggish bowel movement and reduced motility of the stomach, both of which may make the subject feel full after small meals. This may set up a vicious cycle leading to food avoidance and weight loss.

Many psychological theories have been put forward to explain the onset of anorexic behaviour. None of these are specific to eating disorders and may as well be used as explanatory mechanisms for a number of adolescent mental health problems. There is certainly little empirical evidence to support most such theories. The common theories include the following:

- maturity fears, fear of growing up; wish to remain a child; regression
- sense of personal ineffectiveness and a wish to exercise control
- a wish to feel unique and different from peers; positive reinforcement through tasting success by losing weight
- escape from aversive and distressing life events often of an interpersonal nature
- psychosomatic families characterised by enmeshment, maternal overinvolvement and overprotection (Minuchin *et al.*, 1978).

Assessment of a young person with anorexia nervosa necessarily involves proper physical examination. Weighing the young person, preferably in underclothes, and charting the weight and height is essential. Height and weight should be plotted on standard growth charts for comparison to population norms. Body Mass Index (calculated by dividing weight in kilograms, by height in cms^2) has been found to be a useful index for assessment of weight deficits in adults. Usually a BMI below 17.5 is taken to indicate the anorexic range. BMI is not a linear constant in childhood and adolescents and may be unreliable, and calculation of weight to height is considered to be a better indicator. A Coles Growth Assessment Scale or slide ruler can be used to estimate the weight for height for the given age. A threshold of 85% of expected weight for height and age is used as the cut-off for diagnosing anorexia nervosa. Clinically the rate of weight loss may be more important than weight for height or BMI. Menstruation resumes at an average of 95% weight for height, but there is considerable variation around this.

The severity of anorexia nervosa is judged by the percentage weight for height and age, the rate of weight loss and the physical state. The physical complications include low blood pressure, slow pulse and peripheral oedema. Routine laboratory investigations should include serum electrolytes, blood count and renal function tests. Weights below 75% of average weight, physical complications and the presence of disabling psychiatric conditions are indications for inpatient treatment.

Outcomes for anorexia nervosa are not very optimistic. Only about half the adolescents with anorexia nervosa have good outcomes; 25% have intermediate outcomes and 25% continue to be seriously ill in terms of restoration of weight and social functioning; the mortality rate is about 5%. The common causes of death are starvation-related complications and suicide. Poor prognostic factors include greater weight loss, longer duration (more than six months), later age of onset, conflictual family relationships and comorbid psychiatric conditions.

Choice of treatment and management

The evidence base for the treatment of adolescent anorexia is limited. Although there are number of recommendations and guidelines, there a few randomised controlled trials. The NICE guidelines on treatment of anorexia nervosa (NICE, 2004) made on the basis of published evidence makes no Category A recommendations, i.e. those based on randomised controlled trials. NICE concluded that 'the research evidence base to guide decision making is very limited'. Consequently NICE makes only Category B recommendations (well conducted clinical studies but no randomised controlled trials) for treatment of anorexia nervosa.

There is now general consensus that family therapy is the most effective form of treatment for adolescents with anorexia nervosa. The long clinical tradition of family therapy interventions have been now been validated through a number of elegant clinical trials. The first efforts to include families in the treatment of anorexia nervosa began with the work of Salvador Minuchin in the 1970s. He and his team treated a series of 53 patients and provided data on their outcome and follow-up. Most patients were adolescents and treatment included inpatient care and some received individual therapy. However, the primary intervention was family therapy and they showed that 86% of patients had a successful outcome. Although the study was a case series and not a controlled trial, the remarkable success reported by Minuchin's team established family therapy as the backbone of treatment in adolescent anorexia nervosa.

The first controlled treatment study to build on Munichin's work was conducted by Russell and his colleagues (1987) at the Maudsley Hospital, London. This study compared family therapy with individual supportive therapy in a group of patients with eating disorders in whom the onset of the illness was before the age of 18. Eighty patients were first admitted to hospital for weight restoration and randomly allocated to the two treatment groups at discharge. Following one year of psychological treatment they were reassessed. The sub-group of adolescents treated with family therapy had a significantly better outcome than those who had individual therapy. A follow-up study five years later showed that 90% of those assigned to family therapy continued to do well on outcome measures while only 36% in the individual treatment group had a good outcome (Eisler et al., 1997).

In an outstanding second study of psychotherapy process research, the Maudsley group of workers (Eisler et al., 2000) carried out a randomised controlled trial in a group of 40 adolescents and their families using two forms of family interventions. One group was assigned to 'conjoint family therapy' (CFT) that involved the engagement of the whole family with the explicit aim of encouraging the parents to take control of re-feeding their daughter. The other treatment group received 'separated family therapy' (SFT) in which the parent and patient were seen separately to discuss strategies for achieving satisfactory eating, but without the opportunity for the therapist to intervene directly in the process of interactions between the parent and the child. One of the remarkable outcomes from the study was that only 10% of the subjects required admission and overall about 70% showed good or intermediate outcome (restoration of weight and return of menstruation) across both groups

However, when individual status measures were explored, there were further differences between the treatments. Symptomatic change was more marked in the SFT, whereas there was considerably more psychological change in the CFT group (Eisler et al., 2000). The counterintuitive finding that SFT, where there was an opportunity to work individually, did not produce better psychological functioning may be taken to mean that the family and patient benefited from discussing wider family issues around family beliefs and history and taboo subjects. On the other hand, in families with high levels of criticism towards the patient, the SFT may be a useful way of engaging families. When seen at the 5-year follow-up, irrespective of the type of family treatment, 75% of the patients were rated as having had a good outcome, 15% had intermediate outcome and 10% were seriously ill.

In the Maudsley approach, treatment of adolescent anorexia nervosa is carried out in three phases: an initial phase of re-feeding in which the parents are enabled to take control of the young person's eating, a subsequent phase of gradually handing over the control of eating to the adolescent and addressing important family issues and a third phase in which social and other disabilities resulting form the illness are addressed (Lock *et al.*, 2001). In the first phase the treatment is highly focused on behavioural change around eating and weight gain, rather than on the causes of the anorexia nervosa. The therapists emphasises the importance of changing eating patterns and increasing weight as the first step to recovery. He or she also strongly advises parents that their support and commitment are of critical importance and they can and must take up the task of re-feeding their child.

The second phase begins when the adolescent is approaching normal weight and eating behaviours have become normal. During this phase the parents slowly begin to turn over control of eating and related behaviours back to the teenager. The therapist helps parents identify when they feel ready and safe to begin this process. The aim of the third phase is to help the parents and patient make sure that any hurdles that may have developed as a result of anorexia nervosa are overcome. For example, due to the illness, an adolescent may have fallen behind in school, become socially isolated or grown more dependent on the parents. The therapist assists the family to identify and address these issues and then terminates treatment. An important development in the treatment of adolescent anorexia nervosa has been the manualisation of the Maudsley family-based treatment approach (Lock *et al.*, 2004). This has enabled the dissemination of the pioneering work of the Maudsley group and helped further research. Management of Rachel and her family was broadly based on this approach.

Another significant development in the treatment of anorexia nervosa is the randomised controlled study currently being undertaken in the North West of England called The TOuCAN trial. This study involves 215 subjects randomised to three treatment groups: treatment as usual by CAMHS, specialist outpatient and specialist inpatient treatments. The specialist outpatient treatment is an individual manualised programme using motivational interviewing and CBT approaches. The approach is unique in targeting the core belief system that underlies the disorder (Gowers and Smyth, 2004). The treatment subjects are currently being followed up at one and two years and the results are expected to be published in 2006.

Two other additions to the armoury of the clinician treating anorexia nervosa are motivational interviewing (MI) and multiple-family day treatment (MFDT). MI (Miller and Rollnick, 2002) is a unique interviewing technique based on the universal principle that change is normal. Essentially MI is a method of communicating with a person in a way that elicits the person's own reasons for, and advantages of, changing, rather than advising, prescribing or advocating change. It is particularly helpful with people who are reluctant to change or are ambivalent about changing. It has been shown to be effective in maintaining people in treatment for alcohol problems and addictions. Recently MI has found a place in motivating adolescents and families to adhere to treatment and overcome eating problems. It should be noted that MI is a technique for increasing compliance and not a treatment by itself.

MFDT is an intensive day programme for groups of families and adolescents in which families are encouraged to explore how the eating disorder and the interactional patterns of the family have become entangled (Scholz and Asen, 2001). Sharing of experiences among families and the intensity of the programme (meeting together for several consecutive days) makes it a unique experience for families. The proponents of the model claim that helping the families find their own solutions is the critical therapeutic factor in the model. Initial studies have reported high rates of success.

Management plan for Rachel

Explaining anorexia nervosa: At the end of the first assessment session, the parents and Rachel were told in no uncertain terms that she suffered from an illness called anorexia nervosa. The family had already come to the conclusion that Rachel had an eating disorder, having been told by the GP and talked to friends. They were told about the nature of anorexia nervosa, describing it as an illness rather than a defect or fault in Rachel or the family. The therapist took time to explain the nature of the illness and how it 'gets into' vulnerable young people and makes them do things that normal people do not do. The partially involuntary nature of Rachel's preoccupation with her body size and shape was described as demands placed on her by the illness. They were told that Rachel was grossly underweight. The weight chart was shown; it was explained to them that the average weight for height according to the charts should be 48 kg or 105.6 lbs. Currently Rachel was 80% of her weight, which was in the region of dangerously low. They were given a leaflet on eating disorders (Royal College of Psychiatrists, 2004) and were also asked to access internet sources.

The physical complications that arise from anorexia nervosa were described in some detail, including electrolyte imbalance and cardiac arrhythmias. The mortality rate associated with anorexia nervosa and the need for hospitalisation if it did not improve was impressed upon them. Holding up the weight charts, the therapist indicated that a fall to 75% of the body weight (36 kg or 79 lbs) would necessitate immediate admission to a regional unit. The main aim of this part of the discussion was to impress upon both Rachel and her parents the seriousness of the condition and to get the parents to take control of feeding Rachel. A target weight for her was set at 45.6 kg (103.5 lbs), which is 95% of her expected body weight. It was explained that this was well below her average or 100% weight (48.0 kg or 105.6 lbs). This was to reassure Rachel that she would not be allowed to become overweight. Moreover, research showed that most girls resumed menses at 95% of their average weight. The aim was to get her to put on at least half a pound (1 kg) a week. Her weight would be checked at every visit to the clinic.

Initially they were baffled by their daughter's unwillingness to eat and get well because it seemed 'so silly that a sensible girl like Rachel could not see that she was starving herself to death.' In the beginning of the family sessions, Rachel remained silent with downcast eyes and her sister was quiet and distant. Her mother did most of the talking, while her father appeared to be an authoritative figure.

Putting parents in charge: As parents they were charged with the task of getting her back to normality by getting her to eat. At the same time the therapist attempted to reduce any parental guilt by presenting the problem as something that had happened to their daughter rather than anything they may have done.

Equally, it was pointed out, it made no sense to blame Rachel for the illness; it would be like blaming the victim in the case of child abuse. The illness was the problem and not Rachel. Understandably her parents were frustrated at trying to get their daughter to eat and the therapist empathised with the dilemma that the parents were in. The therapist emphasised the need for getting Rachel to have 'normal meals'. This included three main meals and two snacks. Her parents were to supervise her during all meals and avoid arguing about food. The parents were to ensure Rachel stopped all physical exercises including jogging in her room. Until she gained sufficient weight she was to be kept at home.

Weekly family sessions were arranged and all the members were asked to take part. It was envisaged that the treatment would take at least 12 months, during which the initial sessions would be weekly. All sessions would last 50–60 minutes and the entire family was asked to attend. The first 15 minutes of the session would be spent individually with Rachel, during which time she would be weighed. She would have the opportunity to bring up any issues or concerns with the clinician before entering the family sessions.

In the second session Mrs Parkinson said that, after the previous session, her husband had become more authoritarian and shouted at Rachel at mealtimes. He had been getting angry with Rachel and asking her to 'pull up her socks' and be sensible. Her mother had found herself caught in the middle between her husband and Rachel. She had become the 'peacemaker', trying to reason with her husband and at the same time get Rachel to eat. Rachel's younger sister was protective of Rachel but was also easily annoyed by her and usually spent little time with her. All family members reported that they were disappointed with Rachel's lack of effort.

The therapist reiterated that it was the illness that was making Rachel resist their efforts to feed her rather than her wilfulness. It was the anorexia that was fighting back and not Rachel. The responsibility for getting Rachel to take an adequate amount of food was again placed on the parents. They were reminded of occasions when Rachel had been ill in the past and the parents had to feed her up during the recovery phase of the illness. It was up to them to make sure Rachel took an adequate diet. A large part of the early sessions were focused on attempts to decrease family criticisms of Rachel by helping them to understand how little control Rachel actually had of her eating behaviour. Family strengths of caring, commitment and support for Rachel at times of illness were emphasised. In the first few sessions the family struggled to understand the illness as something separate from Rachel and it was pointed out they were fighting Rachel, rather than fighting the illness. Rachel was able to articulate her concerns at this stage, saying that her parents' criticism and blame made things worse for her and caused her to resist her food intake. It was emphasised that the parents had to learn to control their emotions, especially at mealtimes, and take a calm, but firm, attitude to encouraging Rachel to eat.

During the family sessions they were asked to resist all temptations to make critical comments about Rachel and try to adapt non-critical ways of intervening with Rachel to increase her food intake. They agreed amongst themselves to reduce their criticisms to reasonable levels. Rachel's sister, Tanya, proved to be an asset during family sessions. She had caused several arguments with her sister in the past but during the sessions she started defending Rachel and supported her sister by pointing out that some of their parents' criticisms were unfounded and unfair. For example, Tanya told the therapist that she knew how hard it was for Rachel to eat but her parents were 'constantly at her', talking about food all the time. She suggested that the parents stop talking about food outside mealtimes and take a more detached attitude. Tanya agreed to monitor the 'emotional temperature' at home and bring it to everyone's attention if it was too high. Looking at her father she jokingly said, 'I am the temperature monitor.'

In later sessions Rachel was able to tell the family and the therapist that her greatest fear was that she would become fat and obese. This was one of her core beliefs that dominated every other aspect of functioning. The family tried to reassure her that

1 she was not fat by any standards
2 she could weigh herself regularly to ensure that she did not 'overshoot the mark' and
3 her mother could keep a close watch on her weight.

The therapist observed that at the moment it was not helpful to challenge Rachel's belief, for no amount of reasoning could make her change it. She had to come to the conclusion herself. It was more productive to concentrate their efforts on getting her to eat a reasonable diet. They were reminded that talking about things did not always produce the desired effect; action was more important. At this point Tanya interjected and said, 'An ounce of action is worth more than a pound of talk.' The therapist agreed with her and quoted an African saying, 'Talking about pumpkins does not make them grow!'

A good part of some of the sessions was spent discussing how members of the family communicated their desires, wishes and preferences. For example, how did they show love in the family? What methods did they use to elicit caring responses? What was the role of food in the family, who prepared meals and who was most upset if meals were not ready? Rachel pointed out that in the past going to bed without eating had been a particularly powerful way of showing her anger at her mother. Her parents were surprised by this. Discussions around the part food played in the family brought up a number of issues. Mr Parkinson had always insisted on having 'proper meals' at the table. For him it was how he was brought up and it represented a united family. The children had different views. They wanted to have 'TV dinners' as most of their friends did. Mrs Parkinson agreed with the children and felt that her husband was too inflexible in his ways and while she was reconciled to them, the children were not. It was pointed out that for the first time she was not playing the role of the peacemaker. This part of the session was animated and generated a lot of ideas.

During the first few months of treatment, Rachel was stopped from attending school and the parents took turns in taking time off work to stay with Rachel and to make sure that they could monitor her food intake. Gradually over a period of time Rachel began accepting her parents' efforts to monitor her food intake. All exercising was stopped for the time being. In one of the sessions Rachel observed that it was not helpful for her parents to be watching her during mealtimes. She complained that she felt that they were 'putting her under a microscope'. She also protested that after she finished eating her mother would ask her to have an extra portion of one or other food item. The mention of 'a little more' irritated Rachel and added to her sense of powerlessness. Instead, she wanted her mother to prepare her plate just like everyone else's and trust her to finish eating it. The parents agreed to this. During this phase of treatment, there was a discussion about Rachel's feeling that her independence was severely curtailed by the family. She said that her parents, especially her mother, chose all her clothes and dictated what she should and should not do at home.

Family interventions: This led to a discussion about autonomy versus dependence in adolescence. Both Rachel and Tanya were asked to give a list of things which they were dependent on their parents for and a list of things that they did not want to be dependent on their parents for. The parents were made to comment on the list presented by each of their children. The aim of the discussion was to promote age-appropriate autonomy for the children, particularly for Rachel, who appeared to feel the lack of autonomy acutely. The parents agreed that it was easy for them to overstep the mark and try to control most aspects of Rachel's life. The therapist encouraged them to talk about how each of them would indicate to the other their displeasure at feeling dominated by the other. Her parents jokingly admitted that there were times they too felt that their adolescent daughters were trying to run their lives. At this point, treatment was focused on negotiation of new patterns of relationships within the family whilst accepting that the re-feeding process must go on.

During the next few weeks Rachel was gaining weight at the rate of about one pound a week. Her eating disorder symptoms remained and she agreed that it was a struggle for her to eat but was now reconciled to having three regular meals a day. She found the two snacks difficult to accept but was doing enough to keep gaining weight. Her overall mood was much better and she was enjoying life more. She was much less irritable and visibly happier than at the start of the treatment. She reported that her energy levels were better and physically she felt fitter. She said that at the beginning of treatment she kept thinking about food 90% of the day and three months later it had been reduced to 40% of her day. She was not exercising. At this time she started going back to school and had enjoyed reconnecting with her friends. She was also going out with friends but she was agreeable to coming back home for the meals. She had been allowed to serve her own meal if she wished to but her parents made sure that she took a normal serving and was not excluding particular items of food. With each small success, Rachel was given more responsibility over serving and eating her own food, including cooking it. But it was made sure that her eating was supervised by her parents, albeit in a non-intrusive way.

As Rachel gained weight, other issues in the family came to the fore. Rachel felt her father was overbearing and dominated the household. For example, he liked the temperature in the house to be on the cool side. This meant that the rest of the family felt so cold that they had to wear jumpers whenever he was at home. Her sister agreed with Rachel and launched into an attack on her father. Mrs Parkinson had to come his defence. The therapist pointed out that she was falling into the role of the 'peacekeeper' and wondered how she felt about the issue. She agreed that the house was cold for all of them but it was his house and he was entitled to enjoy the house after a hard day's work. A major part of some sessions was spent discussing gender roles and the power structure within the family and boundaries between parents and children. Many structural therapy techniques described by Salvador Minuchin *et al.* (1978) were employed to enable them to understand each person's designated role within the family and explore what they wanted to see changed. Mr Parkinson was initially reluctant to be drawn into discussion about family issues. He viewed therapy as treatment for Rachel and when the focus shifted to the family, he was distinctly uncomfortable about discussing family issues. He missed attending one appointment and appeared rather sceptical about therapy. The therapist reiterated that the objective of the second part of the therapy was to address family issues so that Rachel could be helped to make a quick and lasting recovery.

As Rachel became more in control of re-feeding herself the parents started complaining of her general behaviour and 'attitude'. The family had noted that Rachel had been becoming more assertive and, in fact, a little aggressive and demanding in her dealings with the family. She was tending to come home late, claiming that her peers were spending their time away from home and also wanted to bring her friends home. The parents complained that when her friends visited her, the house was 'overrun' by them because Rachel allowed them to do what they wanted in the house, especially if her parents were not there. The therapist observed that it was not unusual for young people recovering from eating disorders to become 'too independent' and test the limits of their freedom. Her mother was reminded about her own adolescence when she did similar things just to assert her autonomy and independence. The therapist observed that these issues were the 'normal adolescent' problems that most parents and young people face. Eventually the two sides negotiated a way forward.

In some of the later sessions issues of school and career were discussed. Rachel had performed well in her examinations, having made up for the schooling lost during the illness. Rachel had decided to change direction and become a psychologist! This came as a great relief to the therapist because formerly she had wanted to be a gymnast which meant she would have to pay more attention to her weight and food intake.

Progress and outcome

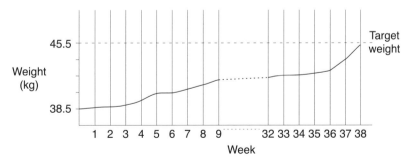

Figure 8.2 Rachel's weight chart.

After a faulty start Rachel gained around a pound of weight a week. She had completely stopped exercising. Her anorexic thinking, however, continued, though it did not dominate her life. Her weight gradually improved over a 12-month period (*see* Figure 8.2) and at the time of discharge her weight was 47.7 kg (105 lbs) and her height was 156 cm (5′ 2½″), placing her at 96% of her average height for weight, height and age (correcting for her age and height; she was one year older and her height had increased by half an inch). She had resumed menstruation. There were no particular areas of conflict in the family and her parents became supportive once they had come to understand the nature of the illness. Her level of body dissatisfaction, although better, was not completely abolished, but her pattern of eating had been restored to normal, even though she was careful about what she ate. At the time of discharge she was not excluding any particular items of food; in fact she was enjoying eating ice cream and cake, having developed a sweet tooth. She was more relaxed about her eating and the therapist was gladdened to hear that she had started eating chocolates and 'junk food' (a sure sign of recovery)! Although she did go swimming, it didn't seem to be excessive and was quite within the normal range. In the case of Rachel most of the prognostic factors were favourable apart from the duration of illness. There were no co-morbid psychiatric conditions like depression, she did not have binge eating nor did she induce vomiting.

Comments

Admittedly, for anorexia nervosa, Rachel's case was an easy one. After a shaky start the family mustered all their resources to help Rachel overcome her difficulties with eating. The disease model was acceptable to the family and there was little denial, a feature seen with some 'difficult' families. Rachel too proved to be psychological-minded and used the initial quarter of the sessions well. The family was initially under a lot of stress, mainly as a result of the diagnosis and the difficulties in getting Rachel to eat, but proved to be surprisingly flexible and was prepared to be reflective as to how they functioned as a family.

The treatment of Rachel broadly followed the Maudsley model. Although the introduction of the treatment manual had been a welcome development, implementing methods found in manualised treatments present their own difficulties. According to the manual the family meal is an important aspect of treatment. The therapist was not comfortable with this aspect of treatment and preferred to use verbal reports of mealtime behaviour.

Ideally the family should have been seen in a family therapy clinic. Unfortunately, at the time Rachel was seen, the CAMHS team did not have a family therapist or family therapy service. An alternative would have been for two therapists to see the family. But the service was depleted of staff and it was left to the clinician with responsibility for the case to do the best he could in the circumstances – probably not an unfamiliar situation in many CAMHS. The service, however, did have an auditable protocol and procedure to ensure safe good clinical practice.

Given the potential for physical complications, most eating disorder cases need to be treated as a matter of urgency. Clinicians who deal with such cases need to be skilled in the management of families and adolescents and know when to ask for help from inpatient services. There are difficulties in accessing inpatient beds for patients with anorexia nervosa. Given the shortage of inpatient psychiatric beds in regional Tier IV services, clinicians working in the community often seek admission to private units. This puts extra strain on families and young people, not to mention the costs to the NHS. Not many specialised inpatient services are available for this group of patients either. There is an ongoing debate as to whether Tier IV services should have separate specialised beds for eating disorders, but financial considerations have dominated the issue and are unlikely to be resolved in the near future.

Box 8.2 Research on adolescent anorexia nervosa shows that . . .

- Adolescent anorexia nervosa is a serious illness with a prevalence estimated at 0.1% in 11–15-year-old girls and 1% in 16–18-year-old girls; partial syndromes are twice as common.
- Family interventions are the methods of choice; they produce improvement in about 75% of cases.
- The main principle underlying family treatment is to encourage parents to take charge of the young person's eating.
- In families with high levels of criticism of the young person, separate sessions with parents and the adolescent (separate family treatment) have been show to be more effective.
- Those with severe weight loss (<75% of expected weight), physical complications and co-morbid severe depression need inpatient treatment.
- Approximately half the adolescents with anorexia nervosa have good outcomes; 25% have intermediate outcomes and 25% continue to be seriously ill.

References

Eisler I, Dare C, Hodges M *et al*. Family therapy for anorexia nervosa: the results of a controlled comparison of two family interventions. *Journal of Child Psychology and Psychiatry*. 2000; **41**: 727–36.

Eisler I, Dare C, M Russell *et al*. Family and individual therapy in anorexia nervosa: A 5 year follow-up. *Archives of General Psychiatry*. 1997; **54**: 1025–30.

Gowers SG, Smyth B. The impact of motivational assessment interview on initial response to treatment in adolescent anorexia nervosa. *European Eating Disorders Review*. 2004; **12**: 87–93.

Hsu LKG. Epidemiology of eating disorders. *Psychiatric Clinics of North America*. 1996; **19**: 681–700.

Lock J, Le Grange D. *Help Your Teenager Beat an Eating Disorder*. New York: Guildford Press; 2004.

*Lock J, Le Grange D, Stewart AW *et al*. *Treatment of Anorexia Nervosa: a family based approach*. New York: Guildford Press; 2001.

Keys A, Brozek J, Henschel A *et al*. *The Biology of Human Starvation* (2 vols). Minneapolis, MN: University of Minnesota Press; 1950.

Miller WR, Rollnick S. *Motivational Interviewing: preparing people for change*. 2nd edn. New York: Guilford Press; 2002.

Minuchin S, Rosman BL, Barker L. *Psychosomatic Families: Anorexia nervosa in context*. Cambridge: Harvard University Press; 1978.

Polivy J, Herman CP. Diagnosis and treatment of normal eating. *Journal of Consulting Clinical Psychology*. 1987; **55**: 635–44.

Royal College of Psychiatrists. *Eating Disorders in Young People. Mental health and growing up*, Fact sheet 24, for parents and teachers. London: Royal College of Psychiatrists; 2004.

Russell GFM, Szmukler GI, Dare C *et al.* An evaluation of family therapy in anorexia nervosa and bulimia nervosa. *Archives of General Psychiatry.* 1987; **44**: 1047–56.

Scholz M, Asen KE. Multiple family therapy with eating disordered adolescents. *European Eating Disorders Review.* 2001; **8**: 4–18.

Steinhausen HC, Winkler C, Meier C. Eating disorders in adolescents: a Swiss epidemiological study. *International Journal of Eating Disorders.* 1997; **22**: 147–51.

Chapter 9

Hyperkinetic Disorder

Strangely, the referral came from the service manager of the CAMHS team. A formal complaint had been made to the Chief Executive by a parent. Her son Ben, aged 10, had been referred by his GP and his name had been placed on the CAMHS waiting list, which stood at 9 months. He had been seen in the service two years ago. His behaviour was considered to be difficult both at school and home and was getting worse. The parents had been seen a number of times for 'parent counselling'. They had attended a few appointments and, later, dropped out. However, the problems had not got any better and in fact he was close to exclusion from school. Parents had approached the GP and asked Ben to be referred again to the service. On this occasion he had been seen by a consultant psychiatrist but was not followed up because the psychiatrist had left the service. On enquiring they had been told that Ben had been placed on the waiting list. His mother had complained that the delay was unreasonable and wanted to know why he had been kept waiting. He was getting into trouble at school and his behaviour at home was equally difficult. They needed help now.

The service manager had investigated the matter and found that the complaint was indeed valid. Following the departure of the consultant, it had taken considerable time for a new consultant to be appointed. In the meantime, the team was under considerable pressure. Consequently, a long waiting list had built up. The service manager felt that Ben should be seen as soon as possible.

Clinical presentation and background

Ben and his family were offered an appointment. Ben, his brother and parents attended. There was an atmosphere of unease in the meeting. It was felt that it was important to clarify what the family expected from the meeting. Were they hoping to pursue the complaint and want answers to questions like why the case had been put on the waiting list and so on or did they want the session to focus on clinical issues? Both parents were clear about what they wanted: they wanted Ben assessed because he was close to exclusion at school and his behaviour at home was just as difficult. They had had an uphill struggle with the local education authority in getting him help with his difficulties in reading and writing. After a great deal of struggle over a period of four years, he had been assessed by the education psychologist. It had been agreed that he had severe specific reading difficulties (dyslexia) and was receiving some help at school.

The main problem now was his behaviour at school and at home. He would not sit still or play on his own. He got bored easily with anything he did such as watching TV or playing computer games. Whatever activity they got him engaged in did not last for more than 5–10 minutes and he would be on to another task. The parents found it difficult to find enough things for him to do. He needed constant adult attention. He was 'all over the place' and he would climb the stairs and hang out of the rails. He got overexcited when family friends came home and would run around, creep under chairs and, eventually, start physically pulling either of his parents asking them to do things he wanted. He had pushed his mother's hand while she was holding coffee, spilling it over her hand.

According to the mother, when taken out, 'He never walks, he always runs'. The parents had to hold him by the hand whenever they took him out. He ran away at the slightest chance and parents had to go looking for him. Sometimes he ran off and hid himself and on a few occasions he had got lost. He was not aware of danger and would run across the road without looking. On the way to school he looked for empty cans to kick around and, for him, it was a game to run around kicking them. When taken to the supermarket he ran around and tried to play hide and seek. He would hide himself in the clothes rack and upset things on the shelves. On several occasions he had had temper tantrums in the shops where he had thrown himself on the floor kicking and screaming. His parents had stopped taking him out to shops anymore. His behaviour at school was said to be very disruptive and the mother had been called to school several times a week. He had been hiding under chairs, getting under the teacher's table and been boisterous and unruly. At the after-school club he had climbed over the fence trying to escape. The parents brought a brief written report from school. It read as follows:

> As you are aware Ben was transferred from Stage 1 to Stage 4 when it was confirmed that he was dyslexic. Following this the school worked on an individual education plan (IEP) with Ben and has received help and advice from the pupil support service. However, despite the effort and work put in by the staff he has not shown noticeable progress. He is disruptive in class and tries to avoid class work. He experiences frustration regularly during written activities and becomes stubborn and anxious. On Monday Ben physically attacked another child with a pair of scissors. He marked the child just above the eye. He had to be 'safely' restrained by the class teacher and another adult. The children in his class witnessed the incident and a great many were frightened. At the after-school club my staff reported that Ben tipped a cup of squash over another child's head. When staff tried to discuss the incident with Ben, he totally disregarded them, ran outside and without the use of physical restraint it was impossible to stop him. He is a likeable and friendly boy who has marked difficulties in literacy skills. There are continuing difficulties in concentrating and applying himself to tasks. His general behaviour in class could frequently be very disruptive. The behaviours of concern occurring on a daily basis typically include: shouting out, making inappropriate contributions to class discussion (seeking attention from peers), interfering with other children (e.g. poking, kicking), fiddling inappropriately with instruments (e.g. overhead projector) and repeated tapping.

Developmental history

Ben's mother had made notes about his development and the difficulties they encountered (presumably she was used to being asked questions about Ben by various professionals). Excerpts of it are given here:

'Ben was born four weeks early and had to be readmitted to hospital as he had neonatal jaundice and was treated with ultraviolet light. He was a very active baby during the day, but slept quite well at the night. He was somewhat late in learning to speak and it was considered that this was because his brother who was 3 years older than him spoke for him. His difficulties began as soon as he was able to walk. As a toddler he seemed quite reckless and he did not sleep very much during the day. He was very lively and was into things around him, exploring, meddling and touching; he started climbing at every opportunity. He had to be carefully watched all the time because he would try to put his fingers into electric sockets, the gas fire and any cracks in the wall. We had to take extra precautions to make the house safe because we had had no such problems with his older brother. He would get up the stairs at every opportunity and we had to make sure that the stair gate was locked. I struggled to put Ben into his pushchair and put on the straps – he would get out at every opportunity. Thinking back, we felt it was the first noticeable problem, but at that time we thought of him as a curious child.

When he was around 2 years, on one occasion Ben was found on the flat roof of the house throwing bricks. Ben would run across the road without looking, if there was something interesting on the other side of the road. He always wanted to walk, and if we put the straps on him he would dangle off them. When Ben was a toddler most hairdressers refused to cut his hair because of his unruly behaviour. He would have to be held, as he kicked and screamed all the time he was in the chair. He was fine immediately before and after the haircut. This went on for a number of years. We had lost him on shopping trips, he would wander off when our backs were turned. When he was taken to the shops he would push things off shelves, run around the shop and become hyperexcited. He was a nightmare when standing at the checkout. He could not simply wait for our turn. He would meddle with things on the shelf, ask for sweets near the checkout (supermarkets have the policy of keeping sweets and chocolates at the checkout to tempt us to buy them) and start interfering with other people's items.

Ben got bored with his toys quickly and needed to be constantly entertained, or he would get into mischief. He would watch his favourite television programmes as long as they were not too long, but when others, especially his brother, had their programmes on Ben would initially become fidgety and restless; thereafter he would start standing between his brother and the television and start acting the clown. Obviously this led to arguments and fights between the two of them. Usually one of us would take him away from the scene. We thought it was sibling rivalry and attention-seeking behaviour. Things got more difficult when he started school. He was boisterous and upset some of the other children. In the reception class I began to be called into school to discuss Ben's behaviour. The calls from school were so frequent that it became very embarrassing for me to be called in constantly in front of all the other parents.

Ben did not make much progress when he started to read and write and his behaviour got worse. He mixed up the b's and d's, p's and q's and wrote his name as a mirror image. I asked his teacher in the reception class if Ben could have dyslexia but she reassured me that it was not unusual for children of his age to make such writing errors. The teacher was more concerned with his behaviour. When he started in year one at school, he had a different teacher who was newly qualified. She suspected that something was wrong but did not know what and wanted the SENCO to be involved. She spent some time with Ben and his teacher but attributed all his difficulties to his behaviour. He was placed on Stage 1 in the special needs register.

Meanwhile Ben was becoming rejected by his peers. Invitations to children's parties and birthdays began to dry up and slowly Ben was becoming socially isolated. We realised that we would have to do something ourselves. When he was in Year 2 his new teacher told me that Ben had got very upset when he could not do a piece of written work and sat there crying in class. By now it was clear to us that he was finding writing difficult. A friend advised us to get him tested for dyslexia privately. I got a report from an independent source that confirmed my suspicion that Ben indeed had dyslexia.

The Year 2 teacher was very good with Ben and knew that he had the capability of doing well in the SATs. She sat next to him when he did the SATs to keep him on task and he did very well in the test. We felt that the teachers who looked beyond Ben's behaviour managed to get the best out of him. With the report from the dyslexia institute we managed to get Ben moved from Stage 1 of the special needs register to stage 3. When he started in the junior school he continued to struggle with reading and writing and I insisted that he be moved to Stage 4 and be statemented. We took up the matter with the LEA. The teachers, although supportive, did not think I would succeed. After six months of struggle he was statemented and received 3 hours of extra help during school hours.

Ben was good at making friends but most of them kept off Ben because of his behaviour. In spite of all the difficulties he caused, we would describe him as an affectionate child. He was not aggressive and held no grudge. We feel that he was not deliberately defiant rather that he needed excitement all the time and the breaching of rules in the classroom or at home was not malicious but the result of unthinking actions. He is by nature an active boy; he has always been active from the time he woke up to the time he went to bed. Ben ran around a lot and enjoyed climbing. We felt that he simply had more stamina than other children. He tried to get interested in football but was not very successful. He liked to draw pictures, but they were usually rushed and looked untidy. He had been rather clumsy and was prone to falls. He was late in learning to ride a bike.'

Family history: The family consisted of his parents who had been married for 14 years, Ben, who was 10, and his brother, who was 12-plus. His brother had Crohn's disease, a chronic bowel disease, which made him tired and feel depressed at times. Ben and he did not get on very well. Apart from the problems with the two boys there did not appear to be other family stresses. There was no history of autism, learning disability or other psychiatric disorder in the family. Ben's father was a self-employed electrician and did not feel that he could turn down work. Consequently he worked long hours. His wife was rather resentful that during his spare time he ran a scout troop. This left the mother to deal with the children, the problems at school and run a home. There was little support from the extended family.

Examination: During the family interview, Ben was quiet for the first few minutes and answered questions willingly and appropriately. He drew a picture of the Simpson family. But he soon became curious about the things in room and got off the chair and started wandering around, touching and meddling with things on the table. He would comply with his mother's requests for a while and sit down to play with the toys in the room but soon got off the chair and started exploring. After a while he started crawling under the table. At this point he had to be removed from the room by his father. The rest of the history was obtained from the mother and another appointment was made for Ben to be seen on his own. The parents were given the Conners' Parent Rating Scale and asked to complete it before they attended the next session. With parent's permission, the class teacher was asked for a report and also requested to complete the Conners' Teacher Rating Scale.

When seen on his own Ben was well spoken and appeared to be quite aware of his difficulties in reading and writing. He said that the kids in his class were mean to him and called him names. He did not care about them or what they said. He was not interested in being popular. He would rather get back at them. He agreed that he got involved in skirmishes with them. But often they got back together and were friends again. He said he was good at art and PE. When asked to write down something about himself and his three 'magic wishes', he wrote the following:

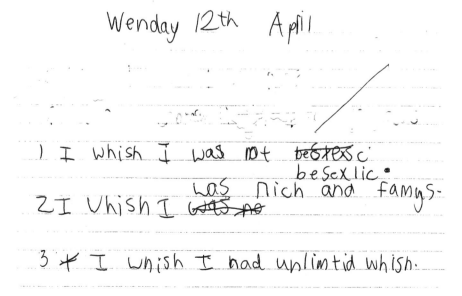

Figure 9.1

Ben held an uninterrupted conversation for a little more than ten minutes. Thereafter he wanted to explore the items on the table. On being asked to return to the chair he came back, did some more drawing and talking but soon went on to explore the bookshelf and started fiddling with the books. Then he discovered a soft toy in the corner of the room and went under the table to look for more toys. He was seen playing with the toy while under the table. The cycle of talking, drawing, exploration and unfocused activities continued for some time. During the period of examination he was distracted several times by noises outside and went over to the window to see what was going on. On two occasions he got up from the seat and began to walk around the room as if looking for other things to do. When asked to join in doing a jigsaw puzzle, he was initially interested and started on it with enthusiasm, but within three minutes and as the task became harder he became visibly bored and soon gave up claiming that he was not very good at 'silly games'. The clinician attempted to get him to tell a story using dolls or drawings. After a good start, he lost the plot and got distracted. And when asked to do some more drawing (an activity he liked) he became disinterested and wanted to know whether he could leave.

During the fifteen minutes he was in the room on his own, he was co-operative, polite and well mannered. He asked a lot of questions about the clinic and the objects in the room. He did not show much fidgetiness but was keen to do things rather than talk about things. He said he did not like his brother because he called him names. Although he did believe that his brother had Crohn's disease, he felt his brother was making a big fuss about it.

School report: With permission from the parents the clinician spoke to his class teacher by telephone. Her description of Ben was of a boy of average or above average intelligence who was in many ways likeable. But his behaviour was unpredictable and his response to other kids was, at times, erratic. For example, he had kicked a girl for reasons that the teacher could not understand. During class time he was frequently out of his seat and found every excuse to leave his seat. However, on a one-to-one basis he was amiable, co-operative and did more work than in a group. The teacher agreed to send a more detailed report and fill the Conners' Teacher Rating Scale. The school report read as follows:

> Attendance: Autumn term 100%; Spring term 99.25%.
>
> Behaviour – Structured time (e.g. class): Ben constantly fidgets during instructions to lessons and has difficulty listening to teacher instructions. He finds it difficult to remain on task unless he is working on his laptop computer. He is frequently out of the seat and rarely sits still. He will taunt other children and interrupt them whilst they are speaking during whole class or group discussions. On a one-to-one he is receptive and well behaved and responds well to adults. He fails to complete assignments frequently.
>
> Behaviour – Unstructured time (e.g. break times): break times are causing problems. Many of Ben's original friends are now unwilling to play with him for a variety of reasons. For example, Ben may kick other children. Other children find his behaviour in the playground unacceptable and this frequently leads to skirmishes, resulting in Ben being sent back into school to sit outside the headmaster's office until he calms down.

Attainment: His difficulties in reading and writing had been recognised for some time. He was reviewed by the education psychologist. The following is an extract from his report: 'On a standardised test of word recognition skill (WORD: Basic Reading) at chronological age 10 years 4 months, Ben's performance placed him in the lowest 4% of his age-population with an approximate age equivalent score of 7 years 3 months. On a standardised test of prose (Neal Analysis of Reading Ability) Ben's performance for *accuracy of reading* placed him in the lowest 4% of his age-population, with an approximate age equivalent of 6 years 11 months.'

Relationships – Adults: this is variable. On a 'good day' Ben responds extremely well to adults and is eager to please; his manners are good and he is keen to talk to his class teacher. On a 'bad day' he is very unresponsive, will not follow instructions and is rude to staff in front of other people.

Relationships – Peers: this is variable too. Other children are becoming less tolerant of his 'erratic' behaviour and Ben is aware of this. He has punched/kicked other pupils although afterwards he is apologetic. He is close to a couple of female pupils in his class but these are often the children he frequently falls out with.

It is generally agreed that he needs more one-to-one support to reach his full potential and we would welcome your support in getting the help he requires.

Conners' Rating Scales

The parents and teachers had completed the Conners' Rating Scales – Revised (S). These are scales containing 27 and 28 items respectively. Each behaviour is rated on a 0 (not true at all) to 3 (very much true) scale. The total scores for the four domains (oppositional, cognitive/inattention, hyperactivity and Conners' ADHD index) are plotted on a graph enabling them to be compared with norms adjusted for age and sex. In Ben's case the scores were more than two standard deviations in all four domains in teacher ratings. The teacher ratings were also much higher than those of the parents. While teachers rated inattention highest, parents scored highest on hyperactivity (*see* Figure 9.2).

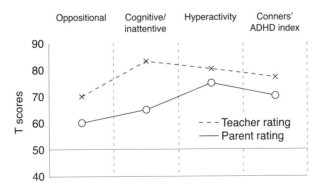

Figure 9.2 Profile of ratings on Conners' scale.

Case conceptualisation and formulation

Ben exhibited most of the typical features of Hyperkinetic Disorder (HKD). The descriptions of his behaviour obtained from several sources indicate that he showed the three cardinal features of HKD: impulsivity, hyperactivity and inattention. These features were seen in more than one situation – school, home, clinic and after-school club. The onset of the difficulties had been around the age of two years. Thus the clinical features fulfil the criteria for a diagnosis of Hyperkinetic Disorder. Yet it is important to exclude other possible reasons for such behaviour. A similar clinical picture may occur in a number of conditions or situations:

1 **Normal variation:** The features that constitute hyperactivity are traits that are seen in the normal child population and show variation from low levels of activity to extreme overactivity. Children with difficult temperaments are usually restless, intense, distractible and moody, overactive and have problems adjusting to changes. Longitudinal research has shown that without intervention a difficult temperament can be a precursor to later behaviour difficulties (*see* Chapter 1). Such children who are overexcitable, exuberant and over-enthusiastic may be mistakenly diagnosed as showing features of HKD, especially if parental control is poor.

2 **Poor parental control:** Parents are the main agents in teaching appropriate behavioural regulation, self-control and discipline to children. Research has repeatedly demonstrated that parenting practices make a considerable contribution to early difficulties in behaviour in children. Inconsistent parental discipline, harsh punishments and poor supervision play a significant role in the development and maintenance of child behaviour problems including overactive behaviour. When this also includes little positive parental warmth and little involvement with the child and poor monitoring of the child within and outside the family, the outcome is likely to be problematic for the child. Adequate parental control of children is likely to be compromised under conditions of poor parental commitment to parenting and psychiatric disorders in parents, especially depression and severe marital problems.

3 **Oppositional defiant disorder and conduct disorder:** Distinguishing Hyperkinetic Disorder from ODD (*see* Chapter 1) and conduct disorder (CD) requires careful examination of the behaviours of the child and parents and calls for clinical expertise. The uncontrolled behaviour of the child with HKD is qualitatively different from the wilful and sometimes malicious behaviour of children with CD. Observation of the child in various settings, information from several sources and the absence of significant parenting problems are crucial in making the distinction between the two conditions.

4 **Attachment disorder:** A risk factor for development of poor behaviour control in children is the quality of parent/child attachment. Attachment refers to the quality of child/parent relationship and has to do with how available and sensitive and responsive the parent is to meet the child's emotional needs. Attachment difficulties in infancy predict behaviour difficulties in middle childhood. For example, mothers who are unresponsive to their infants have been found to have children with more significant levels of disruptive behaviour during their middle school years relative to mothers who are

initially responsive to their infants (Wakschlag and Hans, 1999). These interactions become habitual over time. Many children who have experienced disruption in parenting early in their lives (e.g. looked after children) show hyperactive and inattentive behaviour and it is unclear how these behaviours are related to insecure attachment.

5 **Learning (intellectual) disability and autism spectrum disorders:** Many children with developmental problems exhibit hyperactive and other behaviours that mimic the features of HKD. Caution needs to be exercised when making a diagnosis of HKD in such children. This is not to say that the categories HKD and of LD or ASD are mutually exclusive. Indeed, research shows that children with developmental disabilities are more likely to have HKD. Research has consistently shown that children with HKD are more likely to show neurodevelopmental delays of various domains, including speech and language and fine motor co-ordination or dyspraxia. The issue of comorbidity is discussed later.

6 **Child abuse and neglect:** Physical abuse or extreme forms of coercive parent/ child interactions have been linked to childhood behaviour problems, including hyperactive and inattentive behaviour, in both cross-sectional and longitudinal research. Many neglected children show features indistinguishable from those of HKD.

It is important in every case of suspected HKD that the clinician systematically analyses the findings from the history, examination and information from school and other sources to exclude the above conditions before making a judgement about whether or not the child could be diagnosed as showing HKD. Such a decision is made more difficult by the fact that, as a rule, in child mental health risk factors tend to co-occur. A child with a difficult temperament or learning disability may have parents who themselves have personal and social difficulties and the presenting features may suggest the picture of HKD. More importantly, comorbidity, i.e. the concurrent occurrence of two or more disorders in the child, is relatively common. It is as likely that children with HKD have conduct disorder, autism or attachment problems as they have asthma or diabetes.

In the case of Ben, although the parents and teachers found him difficult to manage and probably contributed in some measure to the continuation of the problem, there did not appear to be other parental or environmental factors that contributed significantly to the clinical picture. Everyone agreed that he was of average intelligence. Undoubtedly the specific reading retardation (dyslexia) was a significant factor in causing difficulties at school. In general, parental management of Ben was thought to be reasonably good. Observations in the clinic and the history as well as reports by the teachers confirmed this. However, there appeared to be a number of family factors that may have contributed to or maintained his difficult behaviour. The two boys were intensely competitive, the level of the father's involvement in the family, especially in disciplining Ben, was marginal, and the mother was left to struggle with all the problems the children presented. His brother's bowel problems needed medical attention and no doubt made Ben feel less special. There were also indications of much oppositional and defiant behaviour both at home and school. In spite of these family issues, it was insufficient to explain the entirety of the clinical presentation. Hence it was decided that the primary diagnosis was HKD. It was acknowledged that there was a certain amount of learned oppositional and defiant behaviour. The following formulation was made.

From the information that was available from the history, examination and the school report, it was reasonable to conclude that Ben showed features of Hyperkinetic Disorder. The description of his behaviour at home (excessive running, climbing, restlessness and meddling with everyday objects) was a manifestation of his overactivity, while his difficulties in concentration and task completion together with distractability (e.g. getting lost) is best seen as inattentive behaviour. Impulsivity was evident in his unthinking (not being able to wait his turn, and reckless (e.g. running across the road)) behaviour. It was clear that he showed the features of Hyperkinetic Disorder. The triad of features that constitute Hyperkinetic Disorder – overactivity, inattention and impulsivity – are given in Box 9.1. Ben appeared to have developed these features from the age of two or so. The triad of difficulties had been evident in different situations (home, classroom, playground, after-school club and shops), i.e. it had been pervasive across situations. Moreover, the family was under extreme stress, his school was finding it difficult to manage him and he was close to exclusion from school. He also had dyslexia which added to his problems at school. There was no evidence of autistic features or other developmental disorders. Ben was considered to be of average intelligence. He had had mild motor clumsiness (dyspraxia) which had got better over the years. Based on the above information the severity of HKD and related features were rated on a scale of 0 to 10 as follows: Hyperactivity (8) Inattention/Distractibility (7) Impulsivity (8) Aggression (3) and Oppositionality (5).

Box 9.1 Key features of Hyperkinetic Disorder (HKD)

The symptoms have to be persistent and be consistent with the developmental level of the child as well as cause impairment in family, individual or academic functioning.

- Inattention:
  - difficulty in sustaining attention in tasks or play activities
  - not listening when spoken to directly
  - avoiding, disliking or being reluctant to engage in tasks that require sustained attention such as schoolwork or homework
  - failure to pay close attention to details or making careless mistakes in school and other work
  - failure to follow through instructions or finish schoolwork and other activities
  - getting distracted easily
  - difficulties in organising tasks and activities, e.g. getting ready to go to school
  - losing things necessary for tasks, e.g. pencils, books, homework book
  - forgetting daily activities.
- Hyperactivity:
  - fidgeting or squirming in seat
  - leaving the seat in the classroom when expected to be seated

---

- – running around or climbing excessively and inappropriately
- – unduly noisy or difficulties in engaging in leisure activities quietly
- – 'on the go' most of the time 'as if driven by a motor'
- – talking excessively.
- Impulsivity:
  - – difficulty awaiting one's turn
  - – blurting out answers even before questions have been completed
  - – interrupting or intruding on others often (e.g. butting into conversations or games).
- Symptoms present in two or more settings (e.g. school, home, clinic).
- Onset of symptoms before the age of 7 years.
- Presence of significant social or educational impairment.

Theoretical perspectives

Most young children are, by nature, active, energetic, impulsive and flit from one activity to another. This is especially so in preschool children and, with age, these traits and behaviours show marked decline. Abnormally high levels of over-activity, impulsivity and inattention lead to difficulties in behaviour control at home and school. In the primary school child this is most evident in structured situations and on tasks that require effort and concentration. Hyperkinetic disorder indicates persistent developmentally inappropriate levels of inattention, hyperactivity and impulsivity, which cause functional impairment in the child. The constellation of traits included in the description of HKD is present in the child population as a continuum of severity.

The dimensional view of HKD holds that the traits of hyperactivity, impulsivity and inattention are normally distributed in the child population and very high levels of these characteristics may lead to functional impairment. Thus, according to the spectrum concept of HKD, the difference is quantitative rather than qualitative and HKD represents the pathological extreme. Different classificatory systems use different cut-offs, which often leads to confusion, especially when interpreting research findings. The US concept of Attention Deficit Hyperactivity Disorder (ADHD, DSM-IV) is a broader concept than the European concept of Hyperkinetic Disorder (HKD, ICD-10) and includes a large proportion of children who would be considered disordered by European psychiatrists. HKD is a narrower category describing a subgroup of ADHD. European literature on the subject makes this distinction explicit in their publications. For example, the NICE (2000) guidelines on the use of medication in ADHD acknowledges this difference when it states, 'Methylphenidate is recommended for use . . . for children with *severe* ADHD' (implying HKD; emphasis added). Figure 9.3 illustrates dimensional and categorical concepts of hyperactivity-impulsivity-inattention.

Diagnostic criteria for the two groups differ in that:

1 the diagnosis of HKD requires evidence of inattention while it is not a necessary condition of the diagnosis of ADHD
2 ICD-10 insists on pervasiveness of all three groups of symptoms across

(a) Categorical approach to classification.

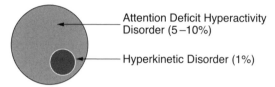

(b) The dimensional concept of normality, ADHD and HKD.

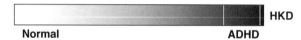

(c) Distribution of hyperactivity-inattention-impulsivity traits in child population showing the proportion of children who may be diagnosed with ADHD and HKD (not to proportion).

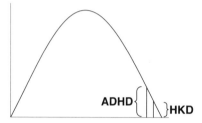

Figure 9.3 The European concept of hyperkinetic disorder and the North American concept of ADHD. Hyperkinetic disorder is a narrower concept than ADHD and has more stringent criteria.

situations (home, school and other situations) whereas DSM-IV states that the criteria be met in 'at least one situation' and

3 presence of comorbidity such as anxiety, depression or other psychiatric disorders (except conduct disorder) is an exclusion criterion in ICD-10 when making a diagnosis of HKD; this is not the case when using DSM-IV criteria.

It is all too common for clinicians, reviewers and researchers in the UK not to specify whether they are dealing with HKD or ADHD. Given the widely different research bases and correlates it is important to be clear as to the subject that one is discussing. The following account and the rest of the chapter refer to HKD rather than to ADHD unless indicated.

The point prevalence for HKD is about 1.5% in primary school age population (Swanson *et al.*, 1993). Estimates of prevalence of ADHD, as would be expected, are higher and vary from 4 to 20%, but the generally accepted figure is around 5%. The US Center for Disease Control and Prevention (CDC) estimated that 7% of children aged 6–11 had ADHD. A survey at the Mayo clinic in 2002 revealed that 7.5% of school age children showed ADHD. Both ADHD and HKD are more common in boys than girls (M:F ratio 3:1).

The precise causes of HKD are unknown. Both heredity and environment contribute to the aetiology of HKD. The occurrence of HKD in relatives of probands is higher than in the general population. Based on twin studies the trait of hyperactivity-impulsivity has been show to be highly heritable (about 80%). Twin studies also show that the contribution of shared environment contributes little to the traits (as little as 5%). Approximately 15 to 20% of the variance in hyperactivity-impulsivity-inattention traits has been attributed to nonshared (nongenetic) factors. HKD is more common in the low socioeconomic group. The mechanisms responsible for the causation of HKD are unclear. Symptoms of HKD are seen in many developmental disorders including generalised learning disability and autism spectrum disorder.

The nature of the principal psychological abnormalities or deficits that are associated with HKD (and ADHD) have been extensively studied over the last half century or more. But, to date, there is little agreement among researchers as to how the psychological mechanisms that are central to HKD are best understood. First, in spite of its name, there is little objective evidence of a deficit in attention in children with ADHD (and HKD). Second, the psychological construct of attention is not a unitary concept. It comprises at least three elements: selective attention, sustained attention and attentional shift. There is little consistent evidence of impairment in any of these components of attention in ADHD. Third, it is unclear what particular psychological functions are measured by conventional tests of attention such as continuous performance tests.

A number of other psychological mechanisms have been studied and much theorising has occurred around impairments in executive functions, especially behavioural inhibition. Executive functions refer to higher brain functions that involve planning, initiating and monitoring mental activities. Behavioural inhibition is the ability to inhibit prepotent responses, stop ongoing responses and delay execution of behaviours and is considered to be part of executive functions. Proponents of these theories hypothesise that specific deficits in these mechanisms are responsible for the triad of impairments seen in children with ADHD, but hard evidence is sadly lacking.

The same is true of neurological theories of its causation. Although advocates of biological theories refer to HKD and ADHD as neurodevelopmental disorders, there is little evidence to support the neural aspect of the disorder. Studies of cerebral brain flow, evoked response measures, and brain imaging have produced few replicable findings. Functional neuroimaging studies do not agree on which structures are involved in detail. Underfunctioning of the cortico-frontal cortex and the basal ganglia demonstrated in some studies may add support to theories that suggest deficits in executive functions.

The diagnosis of HKD in made entirely on clinical grounds. Clinical assessment has to take into account information obtained from:

1 history from the parents
2 direct observation of the child during the family interview and individual session; getting the child to do standard exercises such as writing, drawing and playing which make demands on his capacity for sustained attention
3 teacher reports and observations (some clinicians undertake observation of the child at school) and
4 scores and profiles obtained on a standard rating scale such as the Conners' Rating Scale.

Integration of information obtained from these sources is essential both for diagnosing and estimating the severity of the symptoms. The various steps in the clinical assessment of HKD are summarised in Box 9.2.

Box 9.2 Clinical assessment of HKD

1 Careful history from parents; amongst others focusing on HKD symptoms.
2 Direct observation of child in during family interviews and individual sessions; observation of child doing observer directed tasks such as writing, drawing (freehand drawing, drawing to tell a story), play (free play and on tasks demanding a high degree of attention, e.g. jigsaw).
3 Teacher reports (written), telephone discussion or face to face meetings.
4 Direct observation at school, if necessary.
5 Results of Conners' (or other) Parent and Teacher Rating scales and their interpretation.

Integration of information obtained from the above to enable one to answer the following questions:

1 Are the features a manifestation of something else (differential diagnosis)?
2 How severe is the HKD in the domains of hyperactivity, inattention and impulsivity? Rate oppositionality, aggression and learning disability, if significant.
3 Is there any significant comorbidity (ODD, CD, etc.)?

A number of rating scales are available for assessing the severity of HKD and ADHD. Of these the best known and most commonly used one is the Conners' Rating Scales Revised. It is important for clinicians using such rating scales to be able to administer, score, and interpret the results properly and accurately as well as appreciate their limitations. The procedures for using the scales are available in the technical manual that accompanies the rating scales. The scales are relatively easy to use and, unlike other psychometric measurements, do not need special training. It is one of the commonest scales used in CAMHS and is therefore described in some detail here.

Conners' Rating Scales (CRS-R; Conners, 2001): These consist of three types of scales: the parent, teacher and a self-rated scale for adolescents. There are many versions of CRS. The short versions of the instrument are more commonly used because of ease of use. The parent short form consists of 27 items and the teacher's short form of 28 items and take about 10–15 minutes to administer.. The CRS-R is a suitable instrument for reporting on youths aged 3–17. Normative data for the revised version comes from a large community-based sample of parents, teachers, children and adolescents conducted in several sites in the United States and Canada on more than 8000 children. Responses are given on a 4 point scale from Not at all true (Never, Seldom), Just a little true (Occasionally), Pretty much true (Often, Quite a bit) and Very much true (Very often, Very frequently). The scales are useful in screening, monitoring treatment, in research and as an aid in direct clinical/diagnostic work.

The four sub-scales in the parent short form are:

1 oppositional (6 items)
2 cognitive problems/inattention (6 items)

3 hyperactivity (8 items) and
4 ADHD index (12 items).

Raw scores are of limited value on their own. Transferred on to the profile form, the raw scores are converted to T-Scores. The profile form gives the T-Score for different age groups and male and female sexes separately. T-Scores enable one to put the CRS-R raw scores into context of the general population.

T-Scores are the standard scores that are calculated from raw scores such that each scale will have the same mean 50 and standard deviation of 10. T-Scores allow each obtained score to be compared to the same reference value. Raw scores are converted to T-Scores by plotting them on the appropriate CRS-R profile form. T-Scores maybe interpreted as follows:

- >70 (>2 standard deviations): Markedly increased indicating significant problem
- 66–70: Moderately increased; may indicate significant problems
- <60: Not significant.

Proper interpretation of the CRS-R results is important. After completion of the form the following steps should usually be followed:

1 Assess the validity of CRS-R results. Before proceeding to the interpretive stage it is important to consider whether the input from the raters, i.e. parents or/ and teachers, are valid. Many parents and teachers may produce misleading responses to items for a number of reasons; how well they know the child and how well they have understood the questions are important. All self-rated measures are open to a number of biases, including the following:
  a Random responding: This can occur when the rater is poorly motivated or has not understood the items properly. Contradictory patterns of answers are consequently produced.
  b Response bias: Parents who want the child to have a diagnosis of ADHD may intentionally bias their responses and present an overly pathological picture by marking 'in the extreme'.
  c Inconsistent responses: At times responses contradict each other and this may reduce the validity of the scores.
2 Examine the profile overall in terms of sub-scale scores. Scores that are elevated above 60 or 65 are thought to indicate problematic functioning. Examination of the four sub-scales in the short form may indicate the various areas of functioning that are problematic. Elevation in one scale but not in others should make one question the diagnosis of ADHD. By definition for ADHD to be present, elevation in the following sub-scales needs to be seen; hyperactivity, cognitive problems/inattention and hyperactivity index. Conners considers the ADHD index to be the best indicator of whether a child is likely to have an attentional problem. But he is also careful to emphasise that high scores on the ADHD index identifies children 'at risk' from a diagnosis of ADHD. Further discussion of the scales and their scoring and interpretation are given in the manual (Conners, 2001).
3 Integrate findings from parental accounts of behaviour, clinical examination, school reports, and the results of Conners' teacher and parent rating scales.

It should be emphasised that these and other scales are used to *rate* the severity of symptoms and are not intended to be used to *diagnose* the disorder. HKD is primarily a clinical diagnosis although scores from the rating scale may be used to confirm the clinical impression. Over-reliance on rating scales to make diagnoses is a common error, especially among those new to the field.

Comorbidity: Like in most child mental health problems comorbidity is common in HKD. Studies show that the most common co-occurring problem is oppositional defiant/conduct disorder. In such instances the treatment of HKD needs to be supplemented by robust measures to address conduct issues. Other common developmental disorders that may accompany HKD are autism spectrum disorders, specific and general learning disabilities, speech and language disorders and dyspraxia (motor clumsiness). Contributions by each of these disorders to the presenting problems often vary in degree. When other developmental disorders significantly contribute to the presenting problem, the condition has been termed Complex Developmental Disorder.

Choice of treatment and management

In common with most mental health problems in children, the treatment of HKD requires multimodal management. Medication as well as psychological interventions with the family and school is necessary to produce optimal outcome for the children (Taylor *et al.*, 2004).

Medication: There is now incontrovertible evidence that in children with HKD central nervous system stimulant medications produce marked improvement in their symptoms and in educational and social functioning. In their review of 'what works for whom' Fonagy and colleagues state that, 'the beneficial effects of stimulants for the primary symptoms of inattention, hyperactivity and impulsivity have been confirmed by more than 100 trials of medication' (Fonagy *et al.*, 2002). The National Institute of Clinical Excellence (NICE, 2000) guidelines unequivocally state that methylphenidate (trade names: Ritalin, Equisam) be used as the first line of intervention in severe ADHD (severe ADHS is equivalent to HKD). A review of several studies by Swanson *et al.* (1993) found that 70% of children with HKD responded to medication with stimulants and that the effect size was in the order of 0.8.

The MTA study (The MTA Cooperative Group, 1999), is the most ambitious and detailed study of effects of medication and psychosocial interventions undertaken so far on children with ADHD. (Note that study used the wider US definition of ADHD.) It was a 5-year study of multimodal treatment of a large population of children (N = 539) with ADHD set up by the National Institute of Mental Health in the US. Treatment was randomly allocated to four groups of children:

1 a carefully constructed medication regime
2 intensive behavioural management with parents, child and school
3 a combination of medication and behavioural interventions and
4 standard care provided by community teams.

It should be pointed out the psychosocial interventions were intense and consisted of 27 sessions. The main finding was that combined medication and psychosocial interventions were *not* superior to medication alone, a finding that has disappointed many and caused some controversy. Medication alone was more powerful and effective than intensive behaviour therapy. However, they found that the dose of medication in the combined intervention group was lower than that in the medication alone group. The superiority of medication to behavioural interventions is even more striking when the results were reanalysed using criteria for children with HKD.

NICE guidance (2000) on the use of methylphenidate state that 'Methylphenidate is recommended for use as part of a comprehensive treatment programme for children with a diagnosis of severe Attention deficit/Hyperactivity disorder (ADHD). 'Severe ADHD' is broadly similar to a diagnosis of Hyperkinetic Disorder (HKD)'.

Methylphenidate is a central nervous system stimulant. Paradoxically it has a 'calming' effect on many children who have HKD, reducing impulsive behaviour and the tendency to 'act out', and helps them concentrate on schoolwork and other tasks. The means by which methylphenidate helps people with ADHD are not well understood. Internationally, methylphenidate is a Schedule II drug under the Convention on Psychotropic Substances. Surprisingly methylphenidate produces few serious side effects. The common side effects are sleep disturbance and temporary dimunition in appetite.

Psychosocial interventions: In spite of the above findings many consider parent training based on behavioural principles to be an important and useful part of management. A number of studies have drawn attention to the usefulness of parent training for this group of children but the psycho-educational element and the understanding of the behaviour from a different perspective may be the crucial factors in bringing about change in parents. There are many models and approaches to parent training (*see* Chapter 1). European clinical guidelines (Taylor *et al.*, 2004) suggest that the following components of parent training programmes are more suitable for families with HKD children:

- address specific behaviour problems on behavioural principles (antecedents, behaviour and consequence)
- enhance positive interaction between parents and child through dedicated play time and providing positive consequences for good behaviour
- use token systems to improve specific behaviours
- use effective negative consequences to reduce frequent problem behaviours and time out for serious rule violations.

School and classroom interventions: Behavioural interventions based broadly on the behavioural principles mentioned above have been employed in school settings to manage the specific behaviours this group of children exhibit. Such programmes improve academic performance, behaviour and peer interactions.

Diet: There is little scientific evidence to incriminate particular foods or additives in the causation or aggravation of hyperactive/impulsive behaviour.

Management plan for Ben

A management plan guided by the earlier formulation of Ben's difficulties and grounded in the evidence base outlined above was devised. It consisted of the following:

1 prescription of stimulant medication
2 parent education and behavioural interventions for specific behaviours and other family issues.
3 liaison with school with the explicit purpose of
  – discussing HKD in general, and its impact on Ben's behaviour
  – supporting the school to get extra help to manage Ben's behaviour
  – emphasising the need to address the reading and writing difficulties (dyslexia) in their own right to help Ben's academic achievement.

Medication: Ben was started on methylphenidate (Ritalin) at a dose of 5 mg in the morning and 5 mg at noon. The possible side effects of the medication as well as the expected and desired effects of it were discussed. The parents were reassured that the medication was not addictive; if necessary it could be withdrawn quickly and would not produce withdrawal effects. They were given literature on HKD and methylphenidate (Royal College of Psychiatrists, 2004a, 2004b). After a week the dose was increased to 10 mg in the morning and 10 mg at noon. Within a few weeks parents reported a dramatic improvement in Ben's levels of concentration and attention. The teachers had seen a similar change. He was completing tasks and was able to focus on the task at hand for longer periods. He was easier to manage at home. He could be taken out to the supermarket and, in fact, went on a camping trip with his father a month later. His parents were amazed at the degree of improvement and felt a great sense of relief. They were able to spend time together as a family without having to separate Ben from the rest as they had done earlier.

   The dose of Ritalin was monitored closely. Eventually a maintenance dose of 20 mg in the morning, 20 mg at noon and 10 mg at 4.00 pm was agreed upon. It was made clear that although medication would help in reducing the symptoms it was not a cure. Hence it was important for them to learn new methods of managing him and make allowances for his difficulties. There was some improvement in his behaviour but he was still snappy and prone to unpredictable behaviour, especially if he was provoked. There were occasional incidents at school when the parents were sent letters.

   Intervention with parents: The main aims of the parent sessions were to

1 help them understand the nature and the problems associated with HKD and adapt their behaviour to suit Ben's difficulties
2 get better at managing Ben's oppositional behaviour and
3 address other family issues.

The parents were told about the sort of difficulties that children with HKD have. Because of their limited attention span children with HKD needed short spells of activities rather than long drawn-out ones. For example, if they took Ben out shopping, they had to make sure that it was completed within a reasonable time period. Moreover, he had to be kept engaged in the activity by giving him a task to do. The tendency for children with HKD to seek excitement was explained to them, stressing the importance of helping him to learn to calm down, especially before bedtime. These children crave excitement and if none is available they tend to create it by interfering, talking back or provoking others. This had to be understood as a specific difficulty the children have rather than wilful bad behaviour. The parents were encouraged to read on the subject and given literature on managing children with HKD. Basic parent management skills (described in Chapter 1) were discussed, including attending to good behaviour and ignoring bad behaviour. They were also advised to give the credit to Ben for any improvement they observed rather than ascribing it to the medication.

Attempts were made to get Ben's father to take more part in managing the children. In parents-only sessions the difficulties in managing children with HKD were explained. Ben's mother expressed her frustration in dealing with it all on her own. She said that she found it very draining to keep Ben under watch all the time, go to school every time there was a problem and manage the day-to-day activities. She wanted her husband to share some of her burdens. The impact of his brother's Crohn's disease on the family was also brought up for discussion. It was clear that the family was under considerable stress and Ben's father agreed to play his part in supporting his wife.

Liaison with school: An informal meeting was held with Ben's class teacher and the SENCO to explain HKD and its implication for teachers. They were pleased that Ben was receiving help from CAMHS. They said that they had all along known that Ben's problems amounted to much more than his specific learning difficulties but did not know what it had been. They described Ben's behaviour as unthinking rather than deliberately defiant. Strategies for managing children with HKD were discussed. The SENCO had had experience in dealing with children with HKD in her previous school and had lots of ideas about how there should be a whole school approach to managing children with such problems. They also felt that Ben needed more help with his reading and writing. The clinician agreed to write to the LEA supporting their request for increasing the number of hours of extra help Ben received. The teachers were particularly anxious about his transfer to secondary school when he turned 11. It was agreed to keep each other informed of Ben's progress.

Progress and outcome

Ben's symptoms showed remarkable improvement after starting on medication. His behaviour improved a great deal both at home and school. The parents felt that he was a different boy. They also felt that they understood him better. There were occasional 'incidents' at school when Ben would lash out at one of his friends but there were no major setbacks. He could be taken out to the shops and even had invitations for birthday parties. He joined scouts and went out with his father camping.

When the Conners' rating scales were repeated three months later after the dosage of medication had been stabilised the scores showed a reduction to near normal levels (T-scores < 55). But on the impulsivity domain the reduction was less marked (T-score 60). According to his parents, hyperactivity had been reduced by almost 90%, impulsivity by 60% and inattention by 80%. But he continued to be somewhat unpredictable when he was provoked by fellow pupils. He was more compliant than before and his teachers were pleased with his behaviour.

Predictably, the improvement in reading and writing was less pronounced. The very fact that he had been diagnosed with HKD made the LEA take more notice of his difficulties and the number of hours of individual help at school was increased to 12 hours a week. A strong case was made for him to be transferred to a secondary school within the LEA which had a special dyslexia unit. There was a lot of competition for admission to the school because the number of places was limited. His parents worked hard and he was ultimately successful in securing a place there when he was 11 years. The SENCO at the new school was told about the past problems. Ben turned out to be one of her favourite pupils and he benefited a great deal from the special input from the dyslexia unit. Schooling was not without its problems. Every now and then he got into trouble for minor transgressions and got punished. His parents felt that having a diagnosis made him more vulnerable to blame; whenever things went wrong he was more likely to be punished than the other children.

Medication was continued for 30 months and a joint decision was made to withdraw it. It was withdrawn gradually over a period of 4 weeks. Over the next few months his behaviour was closely monitored at home and school. At the time of discharge Ben was 14 years. He had decided to become a graphic designer because of his interest in art and computers.

The parents were happy with his progress. At the time of discharge they could not help but wonder how things could have been different had a diagnosis been made sooner, perhaps when he was eight or earlier. His mother said, 'I had suspected that he had dyslexia when he was in reception class and it took four years before it was officially recognised and he got help for it. When he was in Year 2 (7 years) I knew that he had a problem although I did not know what it was. By the time he received a diagnosis of HKD and treatment for it he was past his 10th birthday. It was already too late. All this time we were made to feel that we were bad parents. By this time a lot of damage had occurred and the situation was ever deteriorating. It would have been easier to pull back earlier before Ben had developed set patterns of behaviour. It takes moments to ruin a child's reputation and many months/years to retrieve it – if at all.' Ben's mother has become an active member of the CAMHS user group and acts as an advocate for children with HKD and other mental health problems.

Comments

This chapter has adhered to the European concept of HKD rather than the US concept of ADHD. But some of the medication trials referred to are from children diagnosed with ADHD. The general consensus is that these findings have more applicability to HKD where the symptoms are more severe.

The diagnosis and treatment of HKD evokes much emotion especially among non-medical members of the multidisciplinary teams. Taken as a syndrome that responds significantly to medication, it is a useful concept. There is no doubt that stimulant medication improves the core symptoms of HKD; their effect on aggression and non-compliance are marginal. They also positively influence peer–child and parent–child interactions as well as academic productivity performance/functioning. The dramatic turnaround after commencing on stimulant medication in the behaviour of children with HKD has to be seen to be believed. Anyone doubting this has only to see first hand a child who is properly assessed and treated with stimulant medication to accept that HKD is a useful working diagnosis. The contentious issue is not the effectiveness of medication, but *on whom* to use medication. Since the diagnosis of HKD is a clinical one based on extant literature and personal experience, the threshold for making the diagnosis varies from clinician to clinician and there is the danger of overdiagnosing or underdiagnosing the condition.

Difficulties arises when the picture is not so clear-cut as in the case of Ben or is compounded by comorbidity especially with oppositional and conduct problems or where the response to stimulants is partial. In such instances the outcome may not be clinically significant and many clinicians tend to 'get stuck' with cases that show little improvement, yet the parents do want the children to be on medication. In such instances greater attention needs to be paid to psychosocial interventions, particularly parent training programmes. Often this is more easily said than done because a small subgroup of parents see medication as the entire answer to the problem and absolve themselves of any responsibilities for the management of the children. Also a small proportion of children with HKD do not respond or respond poorly to stimulant medication.

A growing small minority of parents insist that a diagnosis of HKD be made on their child, having convinced themselves that the behaviour problems are the result of HKD and see medication as *the* solution to all the problems including parenting problems. Although clinicians may be clear that medications are not to be used as a 'quick fix' or to satisfy a stressed parent or teacher, in clinical practice they often come under heavy pressure to prescribe, and even face complaints from dissatisfied parents.

For the unwary clinician, the more common error is *not* to consider other possible reasons for the impulsive and hyperactive behaviour of children. A good example of environmental conditions that produce hyperactive and inattentive behaviour is severe child neglect. There is now sufficient evidence that neglect and poor attachment produce clinical pictures very similar to those of ADHD. This has been convincingly demonstrated in a naturalistic study by Rutter and others. The English and Romanian Adoptees (ERA) study is a seminal piece of research in developmental psychopathology and, amongst others, has important implications for our understanding of inattentive/hyperactive behaviour. This is an ongoing study that involves a group of 165 children who had experienced extreme privation and were adopted from Romania before the age of 42 months. They were compared with normal controls at 4 years and 6 years on a number of social and personal domains of functioning and psychopathology. Although there was no single pattern or syndrome that characterised these children, three overlapping groups could be delineated (Rutter *et al.*, 2001): attachment problems (21%), inattention/overactivity (25%) and quasi-autistic features (12%)

The authors point out that nearly half of the inattentive/overactive group also showed attachment problems. These findings, together with other research that shows inattention/overactivity is common in children reared in residential homes and those looked after, strongly suggests that the care-giving environment is an important factor that contributes to inattentive/hyperactive behaviour in children. As Rutter points out in this study, 'it remains to be seen whether the clinical picture of inattention/hyperactivity in these children is the same as in more "ordinary" varieties of attention-deficit or Hyperkinetic Disorders' (Rutter *et al.*, 2001).

Box 9.3 Research on Hyperkinetic Disorder shows that . . .

- About 1% of children of school age show features of Hyperkinetic Disorder (HKD), and boys are three times more likely than girls to show these characteristics.
- The hallmarks of HKD are hyperactivity, impulsiveness, and inattentiveness that are pervasive and occur across two or more situations (e.g. home, school and other situations) and have been present from before the age of seven years or earlier.
- There are no reliable laboratory, radiological or psychological tests that clearly identify HKD. Hence the diagnosis is made on clinical grounds.
- The US concept of Attention Deficit Hyperactivity Disorder (DSM-IV) is a broader concept and refers to a wider group; more than 5% of children exhibit features of ADHD.
- Central nervous system stimulants such as methylphenidate have been shown to be highly effective treatment for the symptoms of HKD.
- In the MTA study on ADHD, treatment with medication alone was shown to be superior to intensive psychosocial interventions.

References

Conners CK. *Conners' Rating Scales – Revised, Technical Manual*. New York: Multi-Health Systems; 2001.

* MTA Cooperative Group. Fourteen month randomized clinical trial of treatment strategies for attention deficit hyperactivity disorder. *Archives of General Psychiatry*. 1999; **56**, 1073–86.

National Institute for Clinical Excellence (NICE). *Guidance on the Use of Methylphenidate (Ritalin, Equasym) for Attention Deficit/Hyperactivity Disorder (ADHD) in Childhood*. Technology Appraisal Guidance – No.13. London: NICE; 2000. Available at: www.nice.org.uk/page.aspx?o=11562.

Royal College of Psychiatrists. *Mental Health and Growing Up*. 3rd edn. Stimulant medication for hyperkinetic disorder and attention deficit hyperkinetic disorder. Fact sheet 5, for parents and teachers. London: RCOG; 2004a.

Royal College of Psychiatrists. *Mental Health and Growing Up*. 3rd edn. Stimulant medication for hyperkinetic disorder and attention deficit hyperkinetic disorder. Fact sheet 6, for parents and teachers. London: RCOG; 2004b.

Rutter M, Kreppner JM, O'Conner TG. Specificity and heterogeneity in children's responses to profound institutional privation. *British Journal of Psychiatry*. 2001; **179**: 97–103.

Swanson JM, McBurnett, Wigal T *et al*. Effect of stimulant medication on children with Attention Deficit Disorder: A 'review of reviews'. *Exceptional Children*. 1993; **60**: 154–62

* Taylor E, Dopfner M, Sergeant J *et al*. European clinical guidelines for hyperkinetic disorder – first update. *European Journal of Child and Adolescent Psychiatry*. 2004; **13**(Suppl): 1/17–1/30.

Wakschlag LS, Hans SL. Relation of maternal responsiveness during infancy to the development of behaviour problems in high risk youth. *Developmental Psychology*. 1999; **35**: 569–79.

Chapter 10

Obsessive compulsive disorder

Dear Team

I would be most grateful if you could see this 16-year-old boy with worsening behaviour problems for the past 18 months. His problems centre on his room at home and relate to his reactions when people enter his room. For example, when his sister enters his room he gets irritable and angry and has outbursts. This also extends to him sitting in the car. He prefers to keep a distance from other people and insists on sitting away from the others. His grandfather was admitted to hospital under a Section of the Mental Health Act with problems of self-neglect and paranoia. He died six months ago. He does not describe himself as being very close or spending a lot of time with his grandfather.

Speaking with Matthew alone, he is concerned about his behaviour and the stress he is putting on his mother. The impression I get from him is that he would like to stop behaving the way he does. There has been no family trauma or major illness, other than problems with his grandfather. There do not appear to be any particular family issues that are relevant. He attends regularly for football training. There are no signs of thought disorder, delusions or hallucinations.

I am not sure whether this is obsessive compulsive disorder or some other form of behavioural problem. Both Matthew and his mother are happy to have something done about it. I would value your opinion and advice.

Many thanks for your help.

Yours sincerely

Dr Smith

Even before the referral could be discussed at the team intake meeting, a second letter arrived the same week.

Dear Team

May I request you to expedite the appointment for this 16-year-old boy who has been having behaviour problems for the past 18 months.

He is particular about his cleanliness and does not allow anyone to even visit his room. He will not allow his sister to touch him. He is also not willing to travel in a car with his sisters. I am told that his paternal grandfather had similar problems. His mother feels that the problem is getting worse day by day and he often gets upset and angry. In view of his worsening symptoms I would be grateful if you could see him as early as possible. Some of the behaviours certainly seem certainly odd. For instance, he will not get into his parents' car but he will get into a work van or taxi. I wonder whether these behaviours are indications of a psychotic illness.

Yours sincerely

Dr Smith

Clinical history and background

Matthew and his family were offered an appointment the next week. The family consisted of Mr and Mrs Jones, and Matthew (16 years) and Kimberley (13 years). Early in the first interview it became clear that the main problem was Matthew's excessive washing, which took quite a lot of time and caused great inconvenience to the family. For example, before he went to the toilet he would vacuum the carpet all the way from his room to the toilet. He would do this several times before he entered the bathroom. Following this he would clean the bathroom floor, sink, bath and commode and use large quantities of antiseptics to do so. Thereafter, he would shower himself and this would take up to an hour. He would not use a towel to dry himself but would rather stand in the toilet until he was dry. Before coming back to the room he would wear particular clothes and vacuum his way back into his room. These rituals happened every day and it took more than two to three hours in the morning to complete. The family was baffled by Matthew's behaviour at home because he could use the toilets at school and public places without much difficulty although he did not particularly like them.

Matthew's problems were causing problems in the family. Other members of the family had to wait outside the bathroom until Matthew finished cleaning the bathroom and washing himself. He vacuumed the carpet in his room three times a day and took more than 10 minutes to complete each session. This had led to arguments in the family because Mrs Jones could not use the vacuum cleaner when she wanted. Recently she had bought a second vacuum cleaner so that she did not have to argue with Matthew. His sister, Kimberley, was particularly angry as she felt that Matthew was being selfish and did not care for other people's convenience and comfort. Two days before the assessment session, Matthew had a massive argument with his sister for having spilt talcum powder on the bathroom floor. He had shouted at her, saying that she was making him do more work and he was getting exhausted doing the cleaning in the bathroom. Kimberley had retorted by saying that all his cleaning was unnecessary and, in any case, he must be 'mad' to be doing cleaning all the time. She had been in tears, gone to her parents complaining that something needed to be done about Matthew because he was getting 'loony'. Following this incident they had rung up the GP to get him to expedite the appointment.

Of late Matthew had started to sit away from others and got angry if any member of the family touched him, even if it was by accident. For example, on the way to school he would sit in the corner of the car seat and if Kimberley touched him by accident he would get irritated and angry and shout at her. At home he would sit further away from the rest of the family so that there was no chance of them touching him. This happened mainly with family members and when outside the house he was not particular about being touched by others, so much so that most of his friends did not know about his 'habits'.

Mrs Jones felt that while cleaning, Matthew was very anxious and uptight. He did it repeatedly and seemed never satisfied with the outcome. He felt exhausted at the end of the cleaning sessions. He had broken down several times, saying that it was getting to him. The parents had spoken to him about the futility of repeated cleaning and washing and pointed out how time-consuming it was. But Matthew had been unable to stop his 'habits' of washing and cleaning.

Matthew felt the excessive cleaning and washing had started about two years ago. Initially it involved showering himself for long periods of time, and over the months he had felt that the bathroom needed cleaning. He was not satisfied with cleaning it once and was always unsure at the end of each cleaning session whether he had left any dirt behind. He, therefore, kept cleaning it numerous times until he was certain that he had removed all dirt. The family recollected that Matthew had always vacuumed the carpet in his room from the time he was given a separate room. Initially, they were pleased about how clean he kept it and how well arranged and ordered the things in his room were. Over the past 18 months, however, he had spent long periods of time cleaning his room and rearranging things in there. They were surprised that his 'habits' had not affected his friendships or schoolwork.

Developmental history: Matthew was a planned pregnancy and there had been no complications during pregnancy and childbirth. Mrs Jones described Matthew as a delightful baby. He was early in talking, walking and toilet training. As a toddler he was curious and more advanced than those of his age in his nursery. They had always been proud of Matthew. He had no separation problems when he started nursery and, later, school. He had been early to read and write. The teachers loved him because he was bright and always full of ideas. He had always had good school reports. He was good in PE and sports, especially football. He had a good group of friends with whom he went out and socialised. They had no complaints about his behaviour. They described him as a responsible young man who was loving and close to the family. In fact, they could not find any reason why he should have been seen in the CAMHS.

Matthew had been somewhat a perfectionist from a young age. He always completed his schoolwork on time and was always punctual. He wanted the family to be punctual as well, so much so that they remembered that as a five-year-old he would nag his parents if they did not keep to time. Kimberley said that he would be very upset if for any reason they were late in going to school. Often he tried to organise Kimberley and get her to do things in time. He was careful with money and as early as seven years he saved his birthday money and accumulated it in a saving account! His schoolbooks were always tidy and neat. He had neat and good handwriting. His homework was well laid out and presented, with lots of underlying and side lining. They described him as an all rounder who was good in all subjects at school, as well as in sports. He had never shown any behaviour problems and, in fact, he was quite compliant. This was all the more reason that they were puzzled by the difficulties that Matthew showed. They felt that Matthew tried his best to resist showering and washing but he could not help himself. Apart from an operation to correct undescended testicles, Matthew had been a healthy boy and there was no significant medical history.

Family history: Mr and Mrs Jones had been married for the last 18 years. They were proud of their two children, both of whom they described as loving and caring. Both were good in their studies. Mr Jones had been employed as a manager in a local firm but had been made redundant five years previously. He had been depressed on a number of occasions and following the redundancy had a prolonged episode of depression, which required inpatient treatment. He had been on antidepressant medication for a long time but had been weaned off it over the last year. Mrs Jones felt that he had not completely recovered from his depression and, consequently, she had taken over the responsibility of running the home and the family finances. She worked as an administrative secretary in the local council. Matthew's paternal grandfather had been known to engage in excessive cleaning, washing and was particular about who he let into the house. He died six months ago and, as far as they knew, had not received any treatment for his difficulties. Mr Jones too was a person who could not tolerate disorder and untidiness and everyone in the family said that he had always insisted on cleanliness.

Mental state examination: When seen on his own, Matthew was outspoken about his difficulties. He was a tall boy, with an athletic body build. He had just started shaving. His hair was short and he was neatly dressed. He was somewhat anxious at the beginning of the interview but a few minutes into it he seemed to relax and talk about his difficulties without much hesitation. Matthew said that he was quite aware that his washing and cleaning 'habits' were excessive and caused a lot of inconvenience for the family. He said, 'Not that I enjoy doing them; in fact, I hate cleaning'. But he could not prevent himself from cleaning the toilet and showering himself several times a day. When the time came for him to go to the toilet, he could feel that he was getting more and more tense and had a sense of mounting anxiety build up in him. Cleaning the carpet and the toilet made him feel better but after doing it once, he felt that it was not properly done and, therefore, he kept repeating the action over and over again. The same applied to showering himself. After the shower he felt that he was not clean enough. He would apply soap to himself several times and wash the soap away and yet felt unclean. Therefore, he would shower himself repeatedly; sometimes after coming out of the shower he would go back again to make sure that he had cleaned every part of his body. He did not want to dry himself with a towel because the towel appeared dirty to him.

What would happen if he did not get rid of the dirt? He was not sure, but he could not relax until he felt he had got rid of all the dirt. He was also concerned about 'catching dirt' from others, especially his family members. When asked about what specifically bothered him about the 'dirt', he was unsure. He had no concerns about germs or catching specific diseases, rather it was the general notion of dirt that made him vacuum the carpet, clean the toilet and shower himself repeatedly. He said that the cleaning and showering were getting worse and he was becoming more and more intolerant of the people at home. He tried his best to keep as far away from them as possible. For example, if any member of the family touched him, he felt that there was dirt in their fingers. He did not allow other people to come into his room for the same reason. He knew that he would start vacuum cleaning the carpets in his room if anybody entered. More recently he had started shampooing the carpet in his room but he thought his mother had not yet come to know about this.

When asked about any other unusual 'habits' he may have, he said he wanted things arranged in a particular order, especially furniture, books and CDs in his room, and he found it difficult to tolerate disorder. He said the curtains in his room had to be drawn in a particular way and the pillows arranged in a specific manner. He also had magic numbers, such as 666, which he considered to be unlucky. He would, therefore, not read page number 666 in a book or if he came across the figure 666 he would try and change it to 667 or some other number. Matthew denied having unwanted repeated thought apart from vague thoughts of dirt and being dirtied by others. He was quite sure that he did not have any particular obsessional thoughts prior to the cleaning or washing behaviours apart from the fear of dirt. He said these happened as if they were automatic. Resisting them made him very upset and jumpy. In short, the washing and cleaning compulsions were not preceded by obsessional thoughts. More specifically, he had no intrusive thoughts about harm to self or to others.

The rest of the mental statement examination was unremarkable except for his mood which appeared somewhat low, especially when talking about his problems. However, there was some variability in his mood, for when he talked about neutral subjects such as PE and football he brightened up and was very hopeful that he could make a future in sports. Matthew's sleep and appetite were good. He has not lost any weight recently, although he felt exhausted and depressed after performing the cleaning rituals. When he went out with his friends he forgot his problems and could enjoy their company and the activities.

He was good at schoolwork but wanted to be a football player. He had a good group of friends, which included both girls and boys. They visited each other, went to music concerts and the cinema. He described himself as an outgoing person. But he kept his 'habits' to himself and was glad that they had not affected his friendships. In fact, he had kept it a secret from everyone outside the family. Although he had been quite depressed, he felt that the depression was related to the difficulties he had.

Formulation and case conceptualisation

Matthew presented with compulsions that were severe and distressing. Matthew was particularly distressed by his need to clean his room and carry out the washing rituals which disrupted family life and occupied a major part of the time that he spent at home, especially in the mornings. The obsessive compulsive behaviour had started around the age of 12 and there did not seem to be any particular precipitants to the problem. His compulsions were situation-specific and were confined to the home; he functioned reasonably well outside home and his schoolwork and peer relationships were not affected by the obsessions and the compulsions. There was no evidence of other mental health problems commonly associated with obsessive compulsive disorder (OCD) such as Tourette's syndrome. His compulsions involved other family members causing them great inconvenience as they tried to accommodate his 'habits'. It was obvious his mother was colluding with him for 'the sake of peace'.

The differential diagnosis in Matthew's case included the following:

1 **Major depressive disorder:** As mentioned above, Matthew's depression appeared to be a reaction to his obsessive symptoms rather than the cause of it. His appetite and sleep were good.

2 **Autistic spectrum disorders:** Many children and young people with autistic spectrum disorder show preoccupations and stereotyped behaviours. Though most textbooks refer to such behaviours as obsessions these are qualitatively different from obsessions but may be confused with OCD. There were no developmental delays or features of autism in Matthew's case.

On the basis of the information that was available it appears reasonable to conclude that Matthew's problems were best characterised as OCD. More specifically, the contents of his obsessions and compulsions included the following:

1 **Cleaning and washing compulsions:** The normal routine of showering and washing in the mornings appeared to trigger in Matthew high anxiety and thoughts related to dirt. This lead to excessive cleaning and showering, until he was sure that he had got rid of all dirt. The resulting reduction in anxiety appeared to be perpetuating the compulsions.
2 **Ordering compulsions:** Matthew wanted things in his room arranged in a particular way and spent a lot of time arranging and rearranging items.
3 **Obsessional thoughts:** These thoughts were about fear of dirt that accompanied the above compulsions. But Matthew was not sure of whether these thoughts were responsible for the above compulsions.

As a part of the assessment, in a subsequent session the Children's Yale-Brown Obsessive Compulsive Scale (CY-BOCS; Goodman *et al.*, 1986) was used to rate his symptoms. The CY-BOCS is a clinician-rated instrument that assesses obsessions and compulsions. It has two sections, a screening part that covers the common obsessions and compulsions and an assessment section that is used to rate obsessions and compulsions separately in terms of time consumed, distress, interference, degree of resistance and control (the scale may be found in March and Mulle, 1988). While filling CY-BOCS, it was noted that he also had hoarding compulsions that he had not mentioned before. He pulled out from his pockets various articles: buttons, pieces of paper, pebbles, a bullet, safety pins, numerous bottle tops and other items that he 'collected'. His parents were not aware of his hoarding habits. In Matthew's case the composite score for obsessive compulsive symptoms was 27 (a score of 24–31 is considered to reflect severe symptomatology and 32–40 extreme OCD).

As for the aetiology, in the case of Matthew there was high genetic loading for OCD. His grandfather appeared to have had OCD and there was evidence of some obsessional traits in his father. Matthew's OCD had a profound effect on the family and disrupted family life and the family appeared to be unwittingly helping to maintain the washing rituals by accommodating themselves to his difficulties (e.g. getting up early in the morning to use the toilet) and at times by colluding with him (e.g. buying large quantities of disinfectants).

Theoretical perspectives

Most, if not all, children exhibit age-dependent rituals and habitual behaviours. For example, young children like things done in a particular way or insist on elaborate bedtime rituals or have stereotyped play (e.g. lining up cars). These disappear by middle childhood and are replaced by collecting things, hobbies and focused interests. The main function of developmentally appropriate 'obsessions' seem to be about mastery and control as well as feeling a sense of security. In contrast to developmentally appropriate obsessive behaviours, OCD occurs somewhat later and appears 'bizarre' to adults and other children.

Obsessions and compulsions: Obsessions are persistent and recurrent intrusions into the consciousness of unwanted thoughts, impulses or images, despite the individual's recognition of their senseless nature and resistance to them. Obsessional thoughts are generally accompanied by emotional distress, high anxiety and disgust. Obsessions have the following characteristics:

- They are accompanied by a subjective sense of compulsion and a degree of lack of control.
- They are recognised as unwanted, absurd, senseless or silly, i.e. the person has insight into it.
- The subject recognises that the obsessions are the product of his own mind and not imposed from without (this distinguishes them from psychotic phenomena).
- The person attempts to resist, ignore or suppress the thoughts.

Contemporary definitions of obsessional phenomena emphasise five core features: intrusive quality and the unintentional nature; unacceptability and the associated negative affect; subjective resistance and the urge to be rid of them; uncontrollability and the difficulties in suppressing them; and ego-dystonicity (inconsistency with one's basic values or being uncharacteristic of the individual) (Clark, 2004). In children the degree of resistance and ego-dystonicity are said to be poor because of their immature cognitive development.

Usually the word obsession is reserved for thoughts and compulsions for the acts.

Compulsions are repetitive, purposeful, and intentional behaviours that are performed in a stereotyped way or in accordance with certain rules. The behaviour is designed to neutralise or prevent discomfort or some dreaded event happening; the person recognises that his or her behaviour is excessive and unrealistic. For example, persons who have fears of contamination may repeatedly wash their hands. In many cases they take on a ritualistic form such as doing things in a particular order or repeating an action for a fixed number of times. It is generally agreed that in children the degree of resistance and the level of insight may be low, or even absent.

The form of these mental phenomena (i.e. obsessions and compulsions) should be distinguished from their content. The contents of the obsessional thoughts, impulses and images are usually repugnant or of a bizarre nature and typically involve themes of

1   harm befalling close members of the family
2   aggression toward others
4   sexual thoughts and blasphemous or sacrilegious thoughts.

The usual contents of compulsive behaviours include cleaning, checking, arranging, putting things 'just right' and counting. The common obsessions and compulsions are listed in Table 10.1.

Table 10.1 Common obsessions and compulsions

Obsessions	Compulsions
Contamination	Washing
Harm to others	Checking
Aggressive themes	Touching
Sexual ideas/urges	Counting
Scrupulosity/religiosity	Ordering/arranging
Need to tell, ask, confess	Hoarding

One of the few studies to examine the phenomenology of OCD in children was done by Swedo *et al.* (1998). They analysed the obsessions and compulsions of 70 children and adolescents prospectively. There was a striking similarity between the clinical presentation of OCD in children and in adult patients. The common obsessions were concern with dirt or germs (40%), something terrible happening (fire, death/illness in loved one; 25%), symmetry, order and exactness (17%), scrupulosity (religious obsessions; 13%) and forbidden, aggressive or perverse sexual thoughts, images or impulses (4%). The common compulsions were excessive washing, bathing or grooming (85%) repeating rituals (e.g. going in/out door, up or down; 38%), checking (doors, locks, route; 48%) and ordering or arranging (17%).

Teachers and peers are usually unaware of the problem because the patients often have partial control of the symptoms. Parents find it difficult to understand the child because the child is able to suppress the rituals at school or with friends but 'has' to do them at home. Most children and young people with OCD initially conceal their obsessions and rituals and are notorious for being secretive about the contents and severity of their obsessions for fear of being labelled mentally ill. During the interview it is common for them to refer to obsessions as 'silly thoughts' without disclosing what the silly thoughts are about. Often they under-report the obsessions and compulsions they experience through embarrassment or fear of ridicule. In such situations it is useful to provide them with a list of common obsessions and compulsions and ask them to indicate the ones they have. The first part of CY-BOCS provides a list of common obsessions and compulsions that can be read out to the young person, making it easy for him or her to indicate their presence.

In some subjects certain stimuli trigger the obsessional thoughts or rituals. One 16-year-old boy reported aggressive and sexual thoughts whenever he saw images of children on the television. Another 15-year-old boy had intrusive thoughts of stabbing his mother whenever he saw knives or scissors. Most take great precaution to avoid stimuli that provoke obsessions and compulsions. For example, the 15-year-old boy mentioned above wanted his parents to check his school bag several times in the morning to make sure he was not carrying any sharp objects to school for fear using them against his PE teacher.

The word 'obsession' tends to be used loosely by many and should be distinguished from other related phenomena such as preoccupations, ruminations and overvalued ideas. The term 'preoccupation' is used to describe engrossment, absorption and excessive attention to particular thoughts or activities. The term 'rumination' refers to thoughts that reoccur usually about past events. In contrast to obsessional thoughts, the contents of ruminations are actual or imagined events and are commonly more controllable. In depression for example, ruminations are common. Overvalued ideas refer to strongly held *beliefs* about self or the external world that are invested with enormous personal significance. Distorted body image in a person with anorexia nervosa (*see* Chapter 8) and the strong belief which a person with body dysmorphic disorder (see later) holds, that her nose is too ugly, are examples of overvalued ideas. Though such individuals strongly protest to the accuracy of their beliefs, they usually entertain the possibility of error, albeit as a distant possibility. Unfortunately many tend to refer to these mental phenomena as obsessions.

Occasionally OCD symptoms may mimic psychotic symptoms. Some children and young people find it difficult to describe the obsessional thoughts and may refer to them as voices; often obsessional images are described as 'seeing things'. The following case illustrates the difficulties encountered in distinguishing OCD from a psychotic disorder:

Brendon, a 15-year-old boy was referred by the GP on account of his odd and bizarre behaviour. He had been accusing his mother of trying to poison him. He insisted on reading the labels of every item of food he ate and wanted to know their expiry dates. At night he would wake her up to ask if the food that she had given him had been poisoned. He also spoke of voices in his head that told him to do things. In a number of instances he had been verbally aggressive towards his mother, so much so that she was frightened of him and often gave into his demands. When seen by the GP he was agitated and said that voices in his head told him to attack his mother. The GP wondered whether Brendon experienced hallucinations and delusions. On taking a detailed history it became clear that Brendon had recurrent unwanted thoughts. Although he called these voices, he agreed that these were in his head and were indeed his own thoughts. The thoughts involved harming his mother, or some harm befalling her (such as accidents). Additionally, he had a fear of contamination, especially a fear of spoilt food. Therefore he checked the food he ate and wanted reassurances from his mother that the food was safe to eat. He was diagnosed as having OCD but was found to be unsuitable for CBT. His obsessions and compulsions improved a great deal after three months of treatment with SSRI medication.

Obsessive compulsive disorder (OCD): Obsessions are a feature of many psychiatric disorders including depression and schizophrenia. But the most common clinical condition associated with obsessions and compulsions is OCD. OCD is an anxiety disorder that involves recurrent, distressing, unwanted thoughts (obsessions) and repetitive, ritualistic behaviours (compulsions) that interfere with ordinary activities and day-to-day life. OCD can be severely handicapping; the symptoms can spread to interfere with the person's social and personal functioning and involve the entire family. The syndrome of OCD is much more common in children and adolescents than once believed. Studies have shown that the overall prevalence of OCD in children and adolescents is around 1% (Flament *et al.*, 1988). Nearly 80% of adult OCD cases have their onset before the age of 18. The mean age of onset of childhood OCD is 10 years (Swedo *et al.*, 1989). Childhood OCD is more common in males than females. In boys OCD tends to be prepubertal in onset, whereas girls are more likely to develop it during adolescence.

The familial nature of adult OCD has been demonstrated in a number of studies. About 10% of adults with OCD have a first degree relative with the OCD. Early onset OCD, i.e. OCD that starts before the age of 16, has a stronger genetic aetiology. Studies show that about a quarter of young people with OCD have a close relative with similar problems. Comorbidity is common and the commonest disorder associated with OCD is tic disorder, including chronic motor tics, and Tourette's syndrome. Depression is common in OCD and may be either a reaction to the distressing experiences of the illness or may coexist with it. It is worth remembering that obsessive ruminations and frank mood-congruent obsessive thoughts are common in clinical depression. OCD is often comorbid with other anxiety disorders.

The cognitive behavioural conceptualisation of obsessions hold that it is not the intrusive thoughts *per se* that cause distress and neutralising actions, rather their interpretation (metacognitive appraisal) that make the obsessive thoughts so powerful and problematic. Several dimensions of incorrect interpretations of obsessional thoughts have been described:

- the assumption that anxiety produced by the thoughts is unmanageable
- overestimation of importance of the obsessional thoughts
- exaggeration of sense of responsibility for various events
- overestimation of seriousness of the consequences if neutralising actions are not carried out
- the need to achieve perfection
- thought action fusion.

Thought action fusion refers to the perception that thought is equivalent to action, i.e. the belief that thinking something is the same as doing it. For example, the obsessional thought 'I will stab my mother' is considered to be equivalent to actually hurting or killing the mother. In short, the person with such intrusive thoughts holds himself equally responsible for thinking as for acting.

Contemporary cognitive appraisal theories of OCD propose the chain of events leading to obsessions and compulsions as follows: triggering external stimuli → unwanted mental intrusions → faulty appraisal → mounting anxiety → neutralisation responses/compulsion → anxiety reduction and perceived loss of control → unwanted mental intrusions and so on.

A number of studies carried out in normal populations have shown that irrational and unwanted thoughts are common in normal people. While a 'normal' individual is able to dismiss such thoughts, the persons with OCD find it difficult to distance themselves from them; instead they dwell on them and come to imbue them with personal significance (e.g. 'I must be an evil person to think of harming my mother').

Recent brain imaging studies in children and adults with OCD have demonstrated an increase in the size of basal ganglia structures, and regional cerebral blood flow studies have shown an increase in metabolic activity in the basal ganglia and prefrontal cortex. Following treatment with medication or CBT the basal ganglia have been shown to return to normal size and metabolic activity return to normal levels in those patients who have been responsive (Rosenberg and Hanna, 2000). These and the findings from genetic studies support the current view that OCD is a neuropsychiatric disorder.

PANDAS: Recently a subgroup of paediatric OCD called PANDAS (paediatric autoimmune neuropsychiatric disorders associated with streptococcal infection) has been described. The onset of PANDAS follows infection with group A beta haemolytic streptococci and has a dramatic onset with obsessions and compulsions that meet the criteria for the diagnosis of OCD. The onset is during the prepubertal period and follows an episodic clinical course in response to infection with the offending streptococci (Swedo *et al.*, 1998). PANDAS has been the subject of intense study, especially in the US, and has led to much speculation about the neurological substrate in the aetiology of OCD.

Body dysmorphic disorder (BDD): This is a mental disorder which involves disturbed body image. The central feature of BDD is that people who are afflicted with it are excessively dissatisfied with their body because of a perceived physical defect. An example would be a adolescent girl who is extremely worried that her nose is too big, although other people don't notice anything unusual about it.

BDD is thought to be similar to but not the same as OCD. BDD and similar conditions have sometimes been described as OCD 'spectrum' disorders. In BDD the psychopathology is one of intense preoccupation with one or more body parts, rather than it being an obsession or compulsion, and is best characterised as overvalued ideas. Curiously, the treatment for the condition includes CBT and SSRI drugs, although the response is less than that for OCD. The following case illustrates this.

Emma was a 14-year-old girl referred to CAMHS for 'not communicating, not attending school and losing her temper with her mother'. Emma had not been attending school for more than a year, reportedly because of a long history of bullying. Later she disclosed that her major concern was her appearance, specifically her nose, skin and hair. Her main preoccupation was with her nose. She was convinced that it was too long and big and ugly. The 'disgust' she felt about her nose had led her to avoid all social interaction. Her GP had referred her to a plastic surgeon for possible surgery. Her preoccupation with her skin led to her using a host of camouflage to cover her face and use a vast amount of make-up to get it to look right. This usually took several hours. She refused to go out if her hair was not perfect. She rarely went out on her own and on one occasion when she had been out with her mother she had seen a reflection of herself in a shop window which made her so anxious that she had insisted on going back home. She was not keen on CBT and was treated with SSRI medication. There was an overall improvement over a period of a year and her preoccupation with her nose became less and she was able to go out more. The turning point came when, with the help of a youth worker, she attended an interview for a beautician course in college, and was selected. She has since been attending college and, although very self-conscious, is no longer preoccupied with the way she looks. Medication was withdrawn after 14 months.

Treatment choice and management

OCD is a heterogeneous disorder and young people with OCD vary in the nature and severity of OCD symptoms. There is now considerable evidence for the efficacy of two types of treatment for the core symptoms of OCD in children and adolescents: CBT and medication. The research base for drug treatment is more extensive than that for psychological therapies. These may be used alone or in combination depending on the case.

Cognitive behaviour therapy for OCD: It is generally accepted that the first-line treatment of OCD in young people should be CBT, given that it is as effective as medication and has far lower relapse rates. March (1995) reviewed 32 studies of varying designs that used CBT in OCD and concluded that although empirical evidence for the efficacy of CBT was rather weak, available evidence suggested that CBT was the treatment of choice in children and adolescents with OCD. CBT for OCD encompasses two treatment strategies:

1   exposure with response prevention (ERP) and
2   cognitive therapy (CT).

ERP is based on the finding that anxiety usually abates after sufficient duration of contact with a feared stimulus. Thus subjects with fear of contamination must remain in contact with objects considered to be dirty or 'germy' until their anxiety is extinguished, a process called habituation (*see* Figure 10.1). The main principles of ERP are:

1   Construction of a stimulus hierarchy and careful planning of the exposure exercises, breaking them down into small, manageable steps.
2   Identifying fearful predictions and preparing a 'tool kit' to be used to cope with fearful thoughts; doing exposure without credible strategies would scare the client away.
3   Getting clients to stay on task until anxiety abates and habituation occurs; this may take up to half an hour or more.
4   Repeating each exposure; doing it once is not sufficient.
5   Carrying out the exposure tasks as frequently as possible (homework tasks); 'practice makes perfect'.
6   Dealing with each step in the hierarchy in a planned, progressive fashion.

CT usually takes the form of changing faulty beliefs such as overestimation of danger if the rituals are not carried out, exaggerated sense of responsibility and inflated importance of obsessional thoughts. Experts believe that ERP is the optimal therapy for OCD, while CT may provide additional benefits by directly targeting dysfunctional beliefs and improving compliance. With CBT about 60% of young people with OCD could be expected to make symptomatic and longer lasting improvement.

Medication for OCD: There is extensive empirical literature that demonstrates that potent Selective Serotonin Reuptake Inhibitors (SSRIs) are an effective treatment for adults with OCD. Large systematic trials with SSRIs in adults with OCD have reported impressive results. Typically, the subject shows improvement over a period of 6–10 weeks and may continue to improve over the first 3 months of drug treatment. A number of SSRIs have been shown to be effective and safe in children and young people. The only drug licensed in the UK for OCD in children and adolescents is sertraline.

The paediatric OCD treatment study (POTS, 2004) carried out by March *et al.* is considered to be the definitive study in this group. POTS was a multicentre randomised controlled trial involving 97 children between the ages of 7 and 17 with OCD. The study was designed to compare the effect of CBT alone, sertraline alone, combined treatment (with CBT and sertraline) and placebo. Outcomes were measured for symptom severity (on CY-BOCS) and remission rates. The main findings were as follows. On symptom improvement, combined treatment was found to be better than CBT or sertraline alone, and CBT and sertraline when used alone did not differ statistically from one another. Remission rates were: combined treatment 53.6%, CBT alone 39.4%, sertraline alone 21.4% and placebo 3.6%. The POTS stands out from other trials in that it was investigator-initiated (rather than by the pharmacological industry) and the patients involved in the trial were typical of those seen in clinics (there were no exclusions). The basic message from the study is that paediatric OCD responds best to a combination of CBT and medication; sertraline alone is less effective than CBT alone, i.e. while medication is effective, it is not as effective as CBT-containing treatments; and it is no longer acceptable to just rely on medication as monotherapy.

It is now generally accepted that the first-line treatment of OCD in young people should be CBT. Reflecting the above findings, NICE guidelines state that: 'for a young person (aged 12–18 years) with OCD and severe functional impairment if there has not been an adequate response to CBT . . . the addition of an SSRI to ongoing psychological treatment should be offered' (NICE, 2005).

Management plan for Matthew

The CBT for Matthew's OCD was designed to target his two main symptoms:

1 vacuuming his room and
2 avoidance of touching.

For Matthew, the sequence of events appeared to be that when he was in his room (the stimulus), thoughts of dirt were triggered which were overestimated and exaggerated. This led to mounting anxiety and distress. Matthew attempted to reduce the distress by vacuuming the room (neutralising behaviour) repeatedly to reduce his anxiety levels. The obsession also led to avoidance behaviours such as preventing others entering his room or avoiding being touched by others. This was explained to the family and Matthew using Figure 10.1.

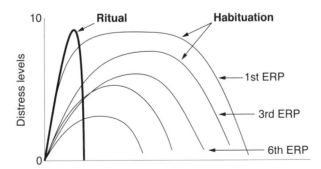

Figure 10.1 The principle behind ERP. Rituals reduce anxiety dramatically and hence reinforce and maintain compulsive behaviours (thick line). Exposure to the anxiety provoking stimulus produces reduction in anxiety if maintained long enough leading to habituation.

It was decided to use CBT initially as the main form of treatment for Matthew. The aim of treatment was to help Matthew overcome his fear of dirt and reduce the ritualistic vacuuming. The ordering and checking compulsions were to be addressed in the later part of the course of treatment. The hoarding behaviour was not considered a major problem and was not addressed directly. The treatment was carried out according to the following steps. Although described under different headings for the sake of clarity, some sessions included more than one of the steps.

Family sessions: The purpose of the family sessions was to

1 explain the nature of OCD
2 reduce family involvement in his compulsive behaviour and
3 enlist the parents' help in the ERP sessions.

Obsessional thoughts were normalised and compared with other perfectionist traits that everyone had. OCD was explained to them as a temporary 'wiring problem' in the brain due to a chemical imbalance in the circuit. Matthew was said to be getting 'false danger signals' from the brain very much like a smoke alarm that goes off for no valid reason. The impact of the problem was mapped and the chronic nature of OCD was emphasised. It was pointed out that OCD cannot be cured but it could be controlled if Matthew and the family were motivated and put in some hard work to overcome it. The vicious cycle of anxiety, compulsion/avoidance was explained. More specifically, the parents were asked not to take part in the rituals or be a party to them. His mother was to gradually stop buying detergents and antiseptics for him.

Next the principles of treatment outlined above were explained to them, emphasising the need to carry out homework exercises regularly. The football metaphor was used to illustrate this: if you want to be good at something you need to practise it often as possible. It was agreed that the initial exposure exercises would be chosen collaboratively.

The principle of ERP was compared to the way the body gets habituated when one takes a swim in cold water.

Two strategies were used to motivate Matthew to take an active part in the treatment process. The first was to map the impact of OCD on his day-to-day life. The therapist asked him to relate how the OCD had dominated his life so far. Matthew was helped to make a list of various impairments and difficulties that resulted from OCD. He was then asked to visualise how his life would be if he woke up the next day and found that his OCD had gone. The second was to 'externalise' OCD as something that was outside him that invaded him when he was vulnerable. OCD made him do things he did not want and over the years he had got used to giving into it and it had now come to dominate his life. The question was how could he re-establish control over it. Next the CY-BOCS ratings were discussed and the target obsessions and compulsions were identified. Matthew and his family were given information on OCD.

Cognitive training: Matthew said he found it difficult to identify the thoughts that occurred before the cleaning compulsions and he felt that his compulsive behaviours were automatic. The need to pause and think about the period preceding the compulsions was discussed. He was asked to make a note of any thoughts, beliefs or ideas that came into his mind before he started the cleaning. In the following session Matthew declared that he was unable to pinpoint any thoughts that led to the cleaning apart from feeling dirty or not clean enough. Although this contradicted the clinician's cognitive hypothesis, Matthew's account of his experiences had to be taken seriously. After all, he was the best witness of his experiences and not the therapist. Consequently, the therapist decided to rely less on the cognitive approach and put greater emphasis on the behavioural or ERP aspect of treatment.

It was important for Matthew to learn some trick to keep OCD from over-powering him. He was asked for a nickname for OCD and to give form to it by drawing it. He drew an ugly blob and called it 'ABCD'. Whenever he was tempted to carry out a compulsion he was to use self-talk and tell himself, 'It is ABCD; it's trying to trick me'. He was to keep watch for the thought traps that ABCD set up and be aware of ABCD's way of making him exaggerate the threat when his anxiety mounted. He learnt to relax and do deep breathing exercises to keep 'ABCD' away from his system and to fight anxiety.

Exposure with response prevention (ERP): The principles underlying expo-sure with response prevention were discussed and written down in detail. A hierarchy of exposure tasks to overcome cleaning rituals were worked out. Matthew was to start with reducing the amount of time he spent doing each of those activities in a stepwise fashion, until he was able to do them once a week. Matthew chose the target behaviours and indicated the anxiety levels for each. The first target behaviour (Target A) was vacuuming the carpet and the second one was practising touching family members (Target B). It was agreed with Matthew that this was to be done in 6 steps and take three days for each step. A stimulus hierarchy was drawn up collaboratively, indicating the level of distress for each step (*see* Table 10.2). The main aim was to shorten the ritual and later reduce the number of times it was carried out. He was to use the techniques he had been taught to keep ABCD thoughts out of his system. In order to help facilitate the exposure exercises he was to use the cognitive 'tricks'. The exposure exercises were discussed with the family. The parents were to encourage him with exercises. Matthew was given a diary to record his performance and his level of anxiety ratings (on a 0–10 scale) each time the task was performed. He was also reminded about the need to keep himself detached and not believe what ABCD told him to do.

Table 10.2 Hierarchy of exposure with response prevention for Matthew

Step	ERP task for repeated vacuuming of room	Anxiety levels (0–10)
Step 6	Reduce to once a day (5 minutes)	9
Step 5	Reduce to twice a day (5 minutes)	8
Step 4	No repeats; time spent 5 minutes	5
Step 3	Reduce time spent to 10 minutes	5
Step 2	Halve the number of times	4
Step 1	Delay by 10 minutes	2
Start	Vacuuming in opposite direction	2

An initial 'practise' exposure exercise was carried out in the clinic with the assistance of the therapist. Although Matthew's cleaning rituals were worst when he was at home, he did admit to discomfort and anxiety when using toilets outside the home. He was made to go to the toilet in the clinic, use it and then wash his face. Matthew estimated that his anxiety levels would get as high as 8 and that he was likely to wash his hands and face numerous times and take up to

10 minutes to complete the whole exercise. The trial exposure exercise was designed to reduce the time he spent cleaning himself. He was forbidden to wash the toilet and was given 3 minutes to complete the exercise. Matthew was surprised that he had come out of the toilet before 3 minutes and had not washed his hands as many times as he had expected. He said his anxiety levels had risen to 6, but had soon come down. He was asked to repeat the exercise some time later. But on this occasion he was to spend even less time. Matthew was able to carry out this task successfully. He said he spent the time looking at his face in the mirror, doing his hair and flushing the toilet. The anxiety levels had been high (6) at the beginning and had come down steeply to 2.

Matthew claimed that the exercise was an easy one because his difficulties were mostly when he was at home. Nevertheless, the clinician-assisted trial was used as an illustration of an ERP exercise. The next step was for him to carry out the ERP exercises according to the hierarchy, beginning with the one at the bottom of the ladder, i.e. vacuuming in the opposite direction.

When reviewed the next week it was clear that he was trying hard but finding it difficult to progress along the steps in the treatment programme, on Target A (vacuuming). The hierarchy was revised breaking down the steps into smaller, more manageable ones and by giving him more time to master each step. Further discussion took place about not allowing the OCD thoughts to overpower him and for Matthew to make repeated positive self statements. He did better on Target B (touching) and was able to sit, touch and ultimately hug his mother and father. A new target behaviour was agreed upon. Target C consisted of contrived exposure to touching 'dirty' items and a stimulus hierarchy was drawn up. Over the next three weeks and with great effort, Matthew was able to keep to the new Target A behaviours but found that as the tasks got more demanding he was getting tired out, anxious and exhausted. He said he was getting more depressed and felt that he could not go out with his friends because the tasks had sapped him of all energy.

After six weekly sessions, Matthew's progress in therapy was discussed with Matthew and his family. There was a clear decrease in the symptoms, as evident from the level of anxiety that Matthew experienced in doing the exposure tasks. He was spending 5 minutes daily on vacuuming his room and was carrying the washing to the washing machine (Target C). But Matthew's progression along the hierarchy of tasks had slowed down. He was unable to move to the next step in the hierarchy. He was quite dispirited by the failure to make any further progress. The more important ritual of cleaning and showering could not be addressed. When it came to emptying the dustbin he said he went into a 'melt down'.

Medication: At this stage medication was considered in order to help with the progression in the tasks. Following a detailed discussion with himself and his parents, it was decided to use an SSRI drug to help Matthew with the tasks. The role of medication, they were told, was to assist the ERP exercises rather than to replace them. They were told that the drug took some time to bring about its effect; one would expect improvement to begin in about two to four weeks time. Matthew was prescribed sertraline, starting with 50 mg daily and increasing to 100 mg in a week and, if there were no significant side effects, to increase it further to 150 mg daily.

In the meantime, Matthew was seen weekly and new targets were agreed upon. Three weeks after commencement of medication Matthew reported appreciable improvement in his level of anxiety when he engaged in exposure tasks and felt confident enough to move to the next step in the hierarchy. He also said that his concerns about orderliness and symmetry had got less and there was a distinct overall improvement in his symptoms. A new stimulus hierarchy was constructed to address the washing and cleaning behaviour. Drawing from the experience of the vacuuming task, on the cleaning and washing behaviours the therapist was cautious and helped Matthew break down the task into smaller, less ambitious steps. Although this prolonged the course of treatment, the strategy proved to be successful. His parents agreed that there had been an overall improvement.

Progress and outcome

Eventually Matthew completed all the ERP tasks. Six months after commencing ERP Matthew was almost completely free of washing, cleaning and ordering compulsions. The CY-BOCS score at this time was 10, i.e. in the mild range of severity. His relationship with his sister had improved a great deal. Although he insisted on having his privacy he was not averse to her occasionally entering his room. He was able to tolerate disorder and untidiness. He was spending up to 20 minutes in the bathroom in the mornings. The family was surprised at the dramatic turnaround in Matthew and gave him all credit for the efforts he had made to get the programme to work.

Medication was continued after the CBT programme ended. Altogether Matthew was on medication for 10 months. Given the marked improvement in symptoms it was felt that medication could be withdrawn at the end of six months or so. But around this time he was sitting for GCSE examinations and a decision was made to continue the medication until the stress of the examinations was over. Medication was withdrawn gradually and he was closely monitored for recurrence of symptoms. This was an anxious time for Matthew (and the therapist). In previous sessions the possibility of occasional setbacks had been discussed. This was reinforced during booster sessions. Methods of coping with recurrence of symptoms were discussed. In the event, during withdrawal of medication no relapse occurred. Medication was reduced further over the next six weeks and stopped altogether with no adverse outcome. At the six months follow-up there was no evidence of the original OCD symptoms. Matthew and the therapist kept in contact with each other through Xmas cards. Five years on, the improvement has been maintained and he has remained symptom-free. He has taken to professional football and his name has been in the sports column of the local papers.

Comments

What worked in Matthew's case, CBT, medication or combination of the two? Undoubtedly the CBT programme did not produce the sufficient improvement expected. This may have been due to a number of reasons. First, the way the therapy was conceptualised and executed could be criticised on a number of counts. In the hands of a clinician better trained and experienced in CBT the results might have been better. The first stimulus hierarchy was certainly over-ambitious and unrealistic. Second, the program was probably not modified sufficiently when improvement stalled. Third, therapy relied almost exclusively on ERP and the cognitive therapy element in the programme was limited. Alternatively, it could be argued that the severity of the OCD symptoms warranted combined treatment from the onset.

Use of medication in conditions like OCD is not controversial. In children there is a tendency to avoid medication wherever possible, even though the safety and efficacy of many drugs including SSRIs are in no doubt. In situations where CBT is not possible due to lack of motivation or other factors, medication may be the only option. In others, where CBT produces partial improvement, the addition of an SSRI may make a substantial difference. Medication can also provide a window of opportunity for beginning psychotherapeutic work in some instances. Sometimes starting on medication may have the opposite effect: the patient and the family (and the therapist) may rely entirely on medication and become passive partners in the treatment process.

A frequently encountered problem in the treatment of OCD is non-compliance. Clinicians working with this group are familiar with clients in whom therapy never takes off because of lack of co-operation. All too frequently homework assignments are not completed, diaries are not kept and patients fail to attend CBT sessions. Motivating patients to carry out the exposure exercises is a crucial aspect of treatment and may need more consideration than some therapists give to the issue. Clinicians are used to working from their 'secure bases' in clinics and therapy rooms. Action-oriented methods including group activities and home visits to promote exposure exercises need to be explored. Recent research shows that very intensive (daily) group-based CBT programmes are more effective than routine interventions.

Box 10.1 Research on OCD in children and adolescents shows that . . .

- OCD is common in children and adolescents, with prevalence estimates of around 1%.
- The mean age of onset is around 10 years; boys outnumber girls.
- There is little difference between paediatric and adult OCD in terms of symptoms, course and treatment.
- Two types of treatment have been shown to be effective: CBT focused on OCD symptoms and SSRI medication.
- The mainstay of CBT is exposure with response prevention (ERP); cognitive techniques facilitate ERP exercises. The effects of CBT are longer lasting than those of medication.
- Medication using SSRIs has been shown to be effective, safe and useful. Combined treatment with CBT and SSRIs produce better results.

References

* Clark DA. *Cognitive Behavioral Therapy for OCD*. New York: Guilford Press; 2004.

Flament M, Whitaker A, Rapoport J *et al*. Obsessive compulsive disorder in adolescence: an epidemiological study. *Journal of the American Academy of Child and Adolescent Psychiatry*. 1988; **27**: 764–71.

Goodman WK, Price LH, Ramussen SA *et al. Children's Yale-Brown Obsessive Compulsive Scale (CY-BOCS)*. New Haven: Yale University Press; 1986.

March JS. Cognitive-behavioral psychotherapy for children and adolescents with OCD: A review and recommendations for treatment. *Journal of the American Academy of Child and Adolescent Psychiatry*. 1995; **34**: 7–18.

* March JS, Mulle K. *OCD in Children and Adolescents: a cognitive-behavioural treatment manual*. New York: Guilford Press; 1988.

NICE. *Obsessive-compulsive Disorder: core interventions in the treatment of obsessive-compulsive disorder and body dysmorphic disorder. Clinical Guidelines 31*. London: NICE; 2005. Available at www.nice.org.uk/CG031.

* Pediatric OCD Treatment Study (POTS). Cognitive-behavior therapy, sertraline, and their combination for children and adolescents with obsessive-compulsive disorder. *Journal of the American Medical Association*. 2004; **204**: 1969–76.

Rosenberg DR, Hanna GL. Genetic and imaging strategies in obsessive compulsive disorder: potential implications for treatment development. *Biological Psychiatry*. 2000; **48**: 1210–22.

Swedo SE, Leonard HL, Garvey M *et al*. Pediatric autoimmune neuropsychiatric disorders associated with Streptococcal infections: the first 50 cases. *Journal of American Psychiatry*. 1998; **155**: 264–71.

Swedo SE, Rappoport JL, Leonard H *et al*. Obsessive compulsive disorder in children and adolescents: clinical phenomenology of 70 consecutive cases. *Archives of General Psychiatry*. 1989; **45**(4): 335–41.

Chapter 11

Somatisation

The paediatrician looking after Charlotte had been concerned for some time about her repeated admissions to the paediatric ward. On this occasion she had been admitted to the paediatric ward for difficulties in walking and weakness of legs. The current admission was precipitated by a fall that Charlotte had sustained while at home. Charlotte and her mother insisted on admission to the paediatric ward because Charlotte's weakness of the legs had been getting worse. Charlotte was well known to the ward staff, this being her sixth admission. At the time of admission she was in a wheelchair and quickly settled into the ward, making friends with other patients and becoming somewhat overfamiliar with the nursing staff. She had to be taken to the toilet in her wheelchair but otherwise appeared well. The nursing staff were struck by her lack of concern for her physical symptoms and apparent cheerfulness in the ward. The paediatrician had investigated her thoroughly. A number of X-rays, myelograms and MRI scans had been done. There had been no demonstrable abnormalities.

On examination there was no wasting of muscles in the lower limbs. There was some weakness of the legs but the findings had been inconsistent. On some occasions power in her legs had been reasonably good and at other times quite poor. The most striking feature was her difficulties in walking. Charlotte swayed from side to side and needed support if she was made to walk. Her gait was wide-based and unsteady. She could not stand for more than a couple of minutes. She had been referred to the regional paediatric neurological unit by the paediatrician in the past. She was admitted to the unit for more than 12 weeks and had a course of physiotherapy and rehabilitation. Although there had been slight improvement, Charlotte continued to have weakness of her legs and was wheelchair-bound. She was being followed up at the regional centre on a regular basis. The paediatrician was convinced that organic causes had been ruled out but was at a loss as how to manage her further. The ward staff had made discreet enquiries about any stresses that Charlotte may be experiencing but there appeared to be none. Both Charlotte and her mother were convinced that she suffered from a physical illness that had not yet been diagnosed. They wanted further investigation to 'get to the bottom of it'.

Clinical presentation and background

At this juncture the paediatrician wanted to discuss the case with a CAMHS worker. A meeting was held in the ward in which the paediatrician and the nursing staff outlined their concerns. From their perspective, physical causes for Charlotte's symptoms had been excluded. They felt the sooner she could get off the wheelchair and go back to school, the better it would be for Charlotte. The paediatrician had discussed with them the referral to CAMHS. Following the discussion she and her mother were seen briefly on the ward to get an under-standing of their perception of Charlotte's problems. Charlotte's mother was somewhat confused as to why they were being seen in a psychiatric clinic and was not sure how a 'psychologist or psychiatrist' could help Charlotte. It was put to them that the paediatricians would continue to see Charlotte and, in the mean-time, the CAMHS clinician would work with them to find out how he could help Charlotte. They were offered an appointment in the outpatient's clinic.

When seen in the clinic as an outpatient Charlotte was on crutches. She and her mother were seen together for the first assessment session. She entered the room with crutches, holding on to her mother. Although the clinician had read Charlotte's medical notes including the correspondences from the paediatric neurologist and made a summary of them, the first session was spent on getting a detailed history of her illness.

History: Charlotte had been quite well until two years ago, when she had an attack of flu. The illness lasted for about one week, with fever, cough and muscle pains. She was treated by her GP and although her fever subsided, Charlotte found that she was weak and dizzy when she tried to get out of bed. Over the next two weeks the dizziness got worse whenever she tried to get up from bed or when she turned her head. She saw her GP again and was told that she may have vertigo following the infection and was treated with some tablets. Charlotte felt somewhat better and went back to school a week later. By now she had been away from school for four weeks and on the first day of return to school some of her peers had asked her why she had been away from school and made remarks like, 'You have been skiving from school, haven't you?' There had also been some teasing, and towards the end of the day, Charlotte had been feeling dizzy, weak in her legs and had collapsed. She was taken to the sick room and was seen by the school nurse. School telephoned her mother and asked her to take Charlotte home. The next day Charlotte spent most of her time in bed and felt dizzy and light headed every time she tried to get up from bed. This went on for three days and she was seen by the GP at home and referred to the ENT department. The GP had wondered whether Charlotte had a form of vertigo that caused her dizziness and unsteadiness.

It took two weeks for her to be seen by an ENT surgeon. During this period Charlotte had improved to an extent and was able to walk around the house but continued to have spells of dizziness. The ENT surgeon examined her and did some tests and after a period of investigation, which lasted for about four weeks, he could not find anything abnormal in Charlotte's ears that could account for her dizziness. Over the next two weeks Charlotte's dizziness improved but she found it difficult to balance herself on her feet. She was swaying from side to side when she tried to go to the toilet and had to hold on to her mother. At this time she had a first admission to the paediatric ward. Her mother was getting worried about the weakness of the legs and her inability to walk without support. At this time Charlotte could walk with the help of her mother and while in the ward she needed the support of her mother or a nurse to go to the toilet. She was investigated for possible neurological illnesses; a number of blood tests and X-rays were done. These investigations proved normal. More investigations were ordered and Charlotte was discharged home. At home she continued to be nursed by her mother. She spent most of her time in her bed but needed help when she wanted to go to the toilet. The family had installed a TV in her room and Charlotte spent the next few months mostly in her room watching TV and being visited by relatives. She was taken for further investigations at the local hospital. The tests were extensive and included more blood tests, X-rays, CT scans and, later, MRI scans. There was no abnormality detected in any of the tests.

She was then referred to the regional specialist paediatric neurological unit. She was seen there by a paediatric neurologist and was admitted to hospital and further tests were carried out. A course of rehabilitation was arranged while in hospital and Charlotte had physiotherapy with a group of young people similar to her. Most of the other patients in the ward and those in the physiotherapy group had damaged their spinal cord, either through accident or tumours or other illnesses. Charlotte was one of the most physically able young people in the group. Although she benefited a great deal from the rehabilitation programme she continued to be unsteady on her feet and had to use crutches to support herself. Following 10 weeks of rehabilitation and inpatient treatment, she was discharged. At the time of discharge the family's understanding of the illness was that Charlotte suffered from idiopathic paraplegia. Physiotherapy was arranged at the local hospital but by this time Charlotte had got disillusioned with programme of rehabilitation and physiotherapy and preferred to do the exercises that she had learned at hospital herself. She diligently carried out the exercises every day at home.

By now 18 months had passed since her first admission to the paediatric ward. Charlotte had not attended school for more than a year. Home tuition was arranged and she had two hours three times a week and school sent her work regularly. Charlotte was keen on completing her work and, surprisingly, kept up with her schoolwork. Her family had been advised to join the Paraplegia Association. Charlotte and her mother attended their meetings. She was the only young person in the group, as most of the patients were much older and had suffered from accidents, back operations and more serious illnesses. Although Charlotte's mother found it very helpful in understanding difficulties of people with paraplegia, Charlotte found the meetings depressing because she had little in common with the others in the group.

At this point they requested a wheelchair and Charlotte started using it to go out with her mother. Although she did not have dizziness this time, Charlotte could not walk. At home she used crutches to get to the toilet or asked her mother to help her. Her mother had been a care assistant in an old people's home and was, therefore, used to caring for disabled people. She was glad that she could help Charlotte at home but found it difficult to balance her work commitments and looking after Charlotte. Therefore she gave up her job and became a full-time carer for Charlotte. The family was receiving Disability and Carer's Allowance.

Developmental history: Charlotte was born at full term and the delivery was normal. She was an easy, if placid, infant. He mother had suffered from postnatal depression, but had not realised it at that time. She was not sure how long the depression lasted and quipped 'It has never left me'. Charlotte's developmental milestones were normal but she was prone to chest infections. 'With her I spent most of the time in the GP surgery', she said. Asked to elaborate on it, she said that the only person who listened to her at that time was her GP and she used to visit her frequently because of Charlotte's chest infections.

Family history: The family consisted of Mrs Banks and her three children Tanya (21), Tony (19) and Charlotte (16). Mr Banks had been an 'alcoholic' and

Mrs Banks had left him some time ago. Tanya had moved out of the house recently. A number of family members had suffered from various physical illnesses (see later).

Examination of Charlotte: When Charlotte was seen on her own during the next session, she was still using crutches and had difficulties sitting in the chair and getting out of it. When asked about her difficulties in walking and balancing herself, she said that her legs felt heavy and wobbly. She could not bear weight on them. However, she had no numbness or loss of sensation in her legs. Getting in and out of bed, using the toilet and washing herself were the biggest problems and she needed her mother's help. Because of her difficulties in using the stairs she had her bed in the living room. She spent most of the time watching television, reading and doing her schoolwork.

Charlotte was a tall girl with short hair. She was co-operative and keen to talk of her illness. She said she had got used to the disability and had found ways of coexisting with it. She had a keen interest in history and found the Discovery channel on television interesting and educational. Asked about what she missed most, Charlotte said she missed her sister and friends. She would like to go out with friends. Now she depended on her mother to take her out. She was using the wheelchair when they went out. She was sad that her friends had not visited her and stopped telephoning. She was not optimistic about improvement in her condition. She felt that the doctors did not understand what was wrong with her. 'Nobody knows what it is', she said. She did not admit to feeling depressed. Her appetite and sleep were good.

School Report: Permission was obtained to ask for a school report. Excerpts from the report from her class teacher said: 'Charlotte is a bright and hard working pupil. We are all saddened to hear of her illness. Despite of her problems she manages to complete her assignments and her homework. She had been a model pupil and a valuable member of the class. She has a good group of friends. She is polite and respectful. Academically she has been outstanding and she is undoubtedly 'university material'. She is an all rounder and is good in most subjects, especially maths. However, she does not seem to think much of herself and lacks self-confidence. She is a relatively quiet pupil in class. She had been subjected to some bullying in the past, but this has been sorted and Charlotte has been asked to bring any such problems to our attention. As far as we are aware there has been no bulling this year. Her mother has kept us informed of her medical problems and we would do everything possible to help her when she returns to school'.

Case conceptualisation and formulation

Charlotte presented with dizziness, weakness of legs and unsteadiness of gait over a period of about eighteen months. Exhaustive medical investigations had been carried out and had proved to be negative. A period of inpatient stay in a tertiary unit had confirmed the absence of physical illnesses but had produced little improvement in her symptoms. In mental health literature unexplained medical symptoms have been referred to loosely as 'psychosomatic illnesses'. The implication here is that psychological factors rather than a physical condition are responsible for the presenting symptoms. It is now generally accepted that all physical conditions have psychological dimensions and all psychological disorders have physical dimensions. Hence the word psychosomatic has fallen out of favour. A more common term used to describe the phenomenon of somatic presentations of psychological difficulties is somatisation (see later).

In ICD-10 the partial or total paralysis of limbs for which no medical cause exists is called conversion disorder. In conversion disorders the presence of one or more symptoms or deficits affecting voluntary motor or sensory functions suggests a medical condition but there is no evidence for physical causation. With Charlotte this was clearly the case. Exhaustive investigations had been carried out and all the tests had been negative. Two paediatricians including a paediatric neurologist were of the opinion that there was no evidence of a physical illness that accounted for her symptoms.

Diagnostic guidelines for conversion disorder stipulate that there should not only be no evidence of a physical disorder, but also the presence of a convincing psychological reason for the onset and maintenance of the symptoms. The appearance of symptoms in Charlotte did not coincide with any specific major trauma, life event or overt stressor. However, the onset of the difficulties appeared to have followed a minor illness in Charlotte. Dizziness and weakness are common in any fever or viral infection. These symptoms appear to have been given an undue degree of importance by Charlotte and her mother. The family had a history of numerous physical illnesses and it was likely that physical symptoms evoked a lot of anxiety in the family and elicited excessive caregiving from the mother. It is noteworthy that Tanya, her older sister, had left home immediately before Charlotte developed the symptoms which may have made her mother focus on Charlotte to a greater extent than previously. Secondary gain arising from parental attention and school non-attendance may have contributed to the maintenance of the sick role and reinforced symptomatic behaviour.

A number of case studies on children with somatisation reveal that such children are high achievers. They tend to set themselves high standards and strive to please adults such as teachers and parents. It was hypothesised that Charlotte had a need to continue the sick role in order to obtain relief from pressures to succeed and anxieties about facing minor lapses in performance at school. At the time of assessment it was not clear whether this was the case. A mental note was made to explore this in individual sessions with Charlotte. Some of the factors that contributed to Charlotte's difficulties are shown in Figure 11.1.

Theoretical perspectives

Medically unexplained somatic symptoms are common in children and adolescents. These usually consist of minor aches and pains (e.g. headache, abdominal pain or feeling sick) which are perceived by parents to be related to worries about friendships, school or family issues. Commonly parents respond to such complaints by comforting, ignoring or reassuring the child and normally children learn to cope with stressful situations without having to resort to complaining about physical symptoms.

Occasionally, the somatic symptoms may persist and become bothersome and disabling. Somatisation is the tendency to experience, conceptualise and communicate mental states and distress as physical symptoms or altered bodily function. Somatisation is best regarded as a process rather than a syndrome or

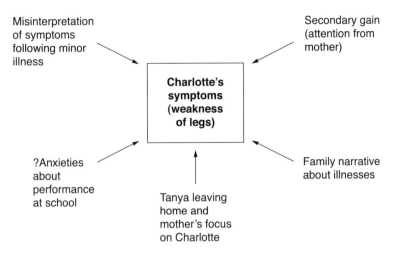

Figure 11.1 Factors contributing to somatisation in Charlotte.

diagnosis. Research shows that disorders involving somatisation are common and often cause severe distress and handicapping, and are costly, both for the Health and Social Services, and the patient. The symptoms commonly result in gain, either though relief and avoidance of underlying conflict and anxiety (primary gain, negative reinforcement), or by eliciting caring responses from others (secondary gain, positive reinforcement), or both. Repeated medical consultations and hospitalisations as well as 'doctor shopping' are common as are extensive medical investigations. The symptoms (or elaboration of symptoms of pre-existing disease) may serve several conscious and unconscious purposes:

- Perpetuating the gains of the sick role (see later)
- Avoiding conflict engendering situations
- Evading the challenge of developmental tasks
- Eliciting caregiving behaviour.

Among children and adolescents non-organic somatic symptoms are common, but diagnosable conditions are rare. One study reported that 11% of girls and 4% of boys in a community sample aged 12–16 reported distressing somatic symptoms. However, only about 1% meet the full criteria for somatisation disorder. In psychiatric classificatory systems unexplained somatic symptoms are included under the umbrella term Somatoform Disorders. The main features of this group of disorders are repeated presentation of physical symptoms in spite of repeated negative findings and reassurances by doctors that the symptoms have no physical basis. In contrast to factitious disorders and malingering, the physical symptoms are not intentional. The various disorders included under the broad category of Somatoform Disorders differ in the two classificatory systems, DSM-IV and ICD-10, and has lead to much confusion. The more clinically relevant conditions are as follows:

- (Psychogenic) pain disorder: persistent, severe and distressing pain that cannot be explained fully by a physiological process or physical disorder (e.g. headache, recurrent abdominal pain).
- Conversion disorder: motor or sensory symptoms suggesting a neurological or

medical condition that cannot be explained on the basis of an underlying physical condition.

* Somatisation disorder: chronic multiple physical symptoms with no physical basis.

In children showing somatisation most research has been carried out in three clinical groups:

1 **Recurrent abdominal pain (RAP):** Recurrent abdominal pain is one of the commonest 'functional' disorders seen in primary care and paediatric clinics. About 10% of children of school age have been shown to have RAP. The commonest presentation is in middle childhood and most cases resolve with symptomatic treatment and reassurance. Follow-up studies into adulthood show that abdominal pain persists into adulthood in about a third of the cases and that many cases predict adult emotional disorders. Adult studies show that visceral hypersensitivity may contribute to the abdominal pain.
2 **Psychogenic headache:** Non-organic headaches are common in prepubertal children and are usually managed at a primary care level.
3 **Conversion disorder**: Formerly called 'hysteria', this refers to symptoms involving the motor or sensory systems that suggest a neurological condition for which psychogenic factors are thought to be responsible for the origin or maintenance of the symptoms. The symptoms are not fully explained by a medical condition and investigations are negative. The term conversion originates from the Freudian theory that unpleasant and intolerable psychological affects resulting from conflicts can be transformed into certain physical symptoms. Typically the presenting symptoms in children are paralysis, paresis (weakness), gait disturbance or non-epileptic seizures. Usually the symptoms correspond to the patient's notion about the illness. It is this inconsistency between the presentation and known symptoms of the illness that provides the clue to the diagnosis. It used to be said that patients with conversion symptoms showed less than the amount of expected distress (*le belle indifférence*) but this has been shown to be true only in a minority of children.

For the paediatrician the diagnosis of conversion disorder is by a process of exclusion. Elimination of physical causes is never an easy task because rare conditions may manifest as bizarre symptoms and common diseases may present with atypical features. Moreover, children with psychological problems can develop physical illnesses. The nightmare scenario for the paediatrician is to label a condition 'functional' when, in fact, there is an underlying organic condition. Anxiety about the possibility of organic causes is often responsible for the medical over-investigation that some children with conversion disorders are subjected to.

Pseudo (non-epileptic) seizures: Children and adolescents with medically unexplained fits are sometimes referred to CAMHS. Distinguishing pseudo-seizures from epileptic seizures is fraught with difficulties, because intense emotional states can precipitate true fits. Moreover, both types of seizures may occur in the same child. In non-epileptic seizures the pattern of movements does not show a regular and stereotyped form of seizure; there is no incontinence or injury; and the tongue is not bitten. However, the typical epileptic fit may not be seen in some forms of true seizures such as frontal or temporal lobe epilepsy. The following clinical features of non-epileptic attacks are thought to be especially helpful: poorly co-ordinated thrashing, back arching, eyes held shut, head rolling and pelvic thrusting. Combined EEG and video monitoring has been found to be useful in most instances. Stores (1985) has written a useful account of clinical and EEG evaluation of epileptic and non-epileptic seizures.

Illness exaggeration: Not uncommonly patients exhibit disability and functional deficit out of proportion to the effects of the illness. Although in many cases amplification of symptoms may be conscious and wilful, in others it is unconscious. As mentioned above, it is not uncommon for some children with diagnosed epilepsy to exhibit pseudoseizures as well. In short, conversion symptoms may co-occur with organic symptoms. Another common scenario is when the disability resulting from the disease is far in excess of that which can be accounted by the illness alone.

The feature common to all the above conditions is somatisation, i.e. the presence of physical symptoms that suggest a medical condition, but the medical condition either is not found or does not fully account for the level of functional impairment. There is also commonly an overlap between documented physical illness and somatisation where the existing illness or injury can serve as a trigger or nidus for a somatic elaboration. Somatisation is best understood as the expression of psychological distress through somatic symptoms or, as Brian Lask (1989) has called it, 'the child talking with his body'.

Many sociologists have made a valuable contribution to our understanding in making a distinction between several types of health-related behaviours:

Health behaviour: This refers to a behaviour aimed at preventing disease (e.g. eating a healthy diet)

Illness behaviour: This refers to the way an individual in the 'sick role' perceives, evaluates and acts upon symptoms. There is considerable variation in this behaviour. One person may be stoical, another dramatic; one may communicate distress verbally, another physically.

The sick role: Once a person decides that he or she is ill, the person must decide how he or she is going to act. The sociologist Talcott Parsons introduced the concept of the sick role in 1951. He suggested that, when suffering from an illness, an individual behaves in order to facilitate recovery by, for example, being absent from work, avoiding normal social contacts and responsibilities and seeking medial help. This social state is known as the sick role and is a temporary role into which all people, regardless of their status or position, may be admitted from time to time. When people accept the sick role they are granted two privileges: (1) A sick person is exempt from social responsibilities. For example the sick person will be excused from performing normal social duties such as attending school or work. (2) A sick person cannot be expected to take care of himself or herself. He or she is in a condition in which he or she has to be 'taken care of'. The person is therefore exempt from responsibility for his or her own state. At the same time they are expected to accede to certain obligations: (1) A sick person is obliged to get well as soon as possible ('I must get back to work/school') and (2) a sick person should seek medical advice and co-operate with medical experts whenever the severity of their condition warrants it. Being a patient also involves accepting one's dependency on others and receiving instructions and health related advice (loss of autonomy).

Abnormal illness behaviour: This refers to the perception of illness when there is no obvious organic cause (Pilowsky, 1997). This maladaptive mode of perceiving, evaluating, and acting in relation to one's own state of health manifests as disease conviction, denial of personal or family problems and an unwillingness to attribute the cause of the disorder to psychological factors. It involves inappropriate and maladaptive attempts to be granted the benefits of the sick role without meeting the necessary obligations.

Aetiology: Usually a number of aetiological factors contribute to the onset and maintenance of somatisation features.

Child factors: The typical profile of children with somatisation disorders is that of a high achiever who is introverted and conscientious. A significant proportion of the symptomatic children are described as 'golden children', i.e. high achieving, compliant and perfectionist. Conversion symptoms often follow minor illnesses and these children appear to have a need to continue the sick role in order to obtain relief from pressures to succeed and anxiety about facing failure. Their families have high expectations of them which are internalised by the children. This creates a form of chronic stress and fear of failure.

Family factors: In the literature on conversion disorders in children and adolescents two distinct family patterns have been described. First, there is a pattern of 'chaotic social circumstances' in which multiple family members are symptomatic and suffer from psychopathology and obvious social stresses. The second group of families are characterised by high expectations of achievement, high levels of anxiety about illness and a tendency to dismiss significant life events from the past. It is not uncommon to find an aggregation of a variety of chronic physical illness in a number of members in the family unit and the wider family who act as models for the child's symptoms.

Many family factors can encourage or support somatising behaviour. Some families allow only a language about physical experience; children receive attention for physical pain but not attention for emotional pain. This approach conditions children to experience any need or problem as physical and physical symptoms become their language for a range of experiences and the currency for family communication. Moreover, such families share a pattern of interaction that seeks to avoid emotional pain. Minuchin *et al.* (1975) characterised the 'psychosomatic family' as one where there is (1) enmeshment, (2) overprotection, (3) parental disharmony, (4) rigidity and (5) a pattern of dysfunctional communication, lack of conflict resolution and use of the sick child in conflict avoidance.

Environmental factors: One way in which children who find themselves in a predicament from which escape is not possible manifest their helplessness through somatisation. Adverse experiences and life events are more common in somatising families and range from bullying to sexual abuse.

Treatment choice and management

Approach: The management of chronic somatisation calls for special skills and strategies, which are required whenever these patients are seen, both in primary care and in specialised medical settings. Chronic somatisers tend to resist appropriate treatment because they regard themselves as physically, and not mentally, ill. Good management facilitates the acceptance of treatment, including psychiatric referral when necessary. The approach has to be flexible, depending on the patient's response, but the principles of good management are the same, whatever the setting, and the skills involved can be clearly identified. Bass and Benjamin (1993) list a number of skills that are necessary for good management of chronic somatisers:

- Identifying psychosocial cues
- Setting limits for investigations
- Providing unambiguous information about findings
- Avoiding spurious diagnosis
- Being honest with the patient.
- Providing patient and family with a credible alternative explanation for the process by which physical symptoms arise in relation to anxiety.

Successful engagement and treatment with CAMHS professionals depend on planned and well thought out referral strategies. Before commencing psychological treatments, it is important that a number of issues be addressed:

1　All investigations should have been completed; the patient and the family should be told that treatment is conditional on no further investigations being carried out. This usually takes a period of negotiation with the patient and the family.
2　That the referring clinician emphasises the need to address symptoms rather than the cause of it ('care rather than cure'). The model of rehabilitation is eminently suitable for this group of patients. A stress vulnerability model is useful as well but most families and patients deny any stress in their life. It is important to make sure that the patients do not feel blamed for their condition.
3　It is important to provide the patient with face saving strategies and 'escape with honour'. Patients with chronic somatisation problems suffer as much as those with organic problems. Any credible explanation that helps the child and the parents to consider alternative explanations or provides a framework for understanding the problem is a helpful way of working with this group of clients.
4　Preparing the family and the child for psychological treatment may need time and usually involves a gentle process of engagement and rapport building. During this period the clinician may have to attend to external issues such as education, peer contacts and recreational activities for the patient.
5　Carefully planned handover of patient by the paediatrician to the therapist is of utmost importance because families with a somatising child strongly feel that they do not have a psychosocial problem. Such families are frequently resistant to seeking psychological help. The referrals, therefore, require patience, careful planning and much thought on the part of the referring paediatrician.

Because somatising patients initially do not accept the emotional component of their problem, collaboration by the therapist with the physician plays a crucial role in the treatment of somatising families. Somatisation is a problem that mandates the application of the bio-psychosocial, family systems approach. Unfortunately many physicians have been taught and socialised to be somatically fixated in their approach to medicine – that is to focus exclusively and inappropriately on somatic aspects of a complex problem. This mirrors the attitude of the somatising patient who experience most of their problems as physical. Patients often believe that the doctors do not understand them, cannot find out what is wrong, and seem not to want to care for them. The unhelpful cycle of events that led to Charlotte's referral to CAMHS is illustrated in Figure 11.2 and is an example of poor, but common, practice. Ideally the referral needs to be made early in the course of the cycle.

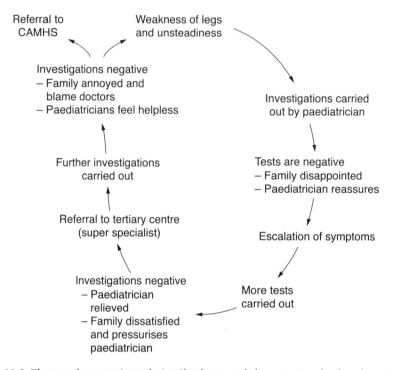

Figure 11.2 The psychosomatic cycle in Charlotte and the process of referral to CAMHS.

In general, there is a paucity of research on somatisation disorders in children and adolescents. There are few randomised controlled trials using psychotherapy for treatment of psychosomatic illnesses available in the literature. A rehabilitation approach is likely to be effective in working with such patients and families because it addresses many of the issues that lead to treatment resistance. It stresses return to usual activities as quickly as possible together with strategies to help the adolescent relinquish the symptoms through physical methods such as physiotherapy and other face-saving means, and has been found to be useful (Lask and Fosson, 1989). However, by far the most important therapeutic factor is engaging the family and the child in the treatment process.

Management plan for Charlotte

Liaison with the paediatricians: At the time of referral the medical care of Charlotte was being shared by the paediatric neurologist at the tertiary centre and the paediatrician at the local hospital. Before taking the referral the case was discussed with the paediatric neurologist and the paediatrician. The neurologist appeared quite frustrated that Charlotte and her family were not accepting of the findings of the investigations and continued to insist doing more and more tests. He was quite sure that all obvious physical causes had been excluded. Charlotte had had graded physiotherapy but the improvement was minimal. When she had been discharged from the regional centre she was still using crutches.

It was felt that it was important for the paediatric neurologist to be involved in her care while she was being seen in CAMHS. The objective of the exercise was to reassure the family that contact with medical services was not contingent on development of new symptoms. When this was explained within the framework of a continuing care model rather than a 'cure' model, the paediatrician was more accepting of this method of working. It was agreed that no more tests and investigations would be carried out but Charlotte would attend the neurology clinic for regular review.

A similar discussion took place with the paediatrician who referred Charlotte. He had taken a peripheral role in her management and was content to leave it to the paediatric neurologist to manage her in the future. However, the CAMHS clinician emphasised the need for a common approach to the management of Charlotte. This included not admitting her to the ward and not ordering anymore investigations. It was agreed to keep him and the neurologist informed about her progress in therapy. Over the following months Charlotte and her mother were seen in CAMHS together and each of them were also seen individually. Two workers from CAMHS were involved, one exclusively for individual work with Charlotte and the other for family and parent work. Initially the sessions were scheduled at weekly intervals and later fortnightly sessions were held.

Family sessions: For the first three sessions the family were seen by both clinicians. The main aims of the first few family sessions were to engage the family in treatment and focus on functional improvement. It was anticipated that it would take some time before the family could join in treatment. Extra care was taken to avoid getting into discussions about the cause of the problem. It was evident in the first session that both Charlotte and her mother were rather sceptical about the role of the CAMH clinicians although they were polite and compliant. The clinicians outlined the purpose of the meeting as helping Charlotte to cope with her difficulties.

It was considered important to convey that the therapists took the family's illness story and their experiences of medical involvements seriously. To this end, in the very first session a detailed history of the onset and course of Charlotte's difficulties was obtained making sure to ask each of them of their perceptions and experiences of the problem. They were allowed to tell their story as each of them experienced each step in the course of the disorder leading to admissions to the ward and the various investigations carried out. During these conversations the clinicians deliberately used medical language.

Next the impact of the problem on Charlotte's schooling, peer and family relationships were explored in considerable detail. At the time of the first assessment session Charlotte had not been to school for over a year. She had been very upset and offended that her friends had not kept in touch with her. At the beginning of her illness they had been supportive and visited her in hospital and at home. But over the months they had gradually lost interest in Charlotte and drifted away from her. She considered the 'betrayal' by her friends as more hurtful than her difficulty in walking.

At the conclusion of the first family session the therapist observed that Charlotte's problems had brought out the best in the family and generally made the family come closer together. Obviously, everyone was making sacrifices – mum had sacrificed her job and time and become almost a full-time carer and Charlotte had had to sacrifice her schooling and friends. The fact that no serious condition had shown up in investigations was characterised by the clinician as 'good news' providing hope for the future.

A major part of a subsequent family session was spent on eliciting the family's illness history. From the history obtained at the initial assessment it was evident that a number of family members had had various physical ailments. This was explored further through engaging the family in drawing a genogram.

The family consisted of Mrs Banks and her three children, Tanya (21), Tony (19) and Charlotte (16). A number of family members had or continued to suffer with various physical illnesses. Tony had suffered with epilepsy from childhood and was currently on medication. Yet he continued to have occasional fits. He was at college doing a part-time course. Before Charlotte was born her mother had had a miscarriage. Charlotte was described as a healthy and vibrant baby with no particular illnesses during her childhood. Mrs Banks suffered with severe migraine attacks and was on medication. One of her brothers had mild cerebral palsy and epilepsy but was coping well. Her father had suffered with a number of physical problems from early adulthood and taken early retirement because of ill health. She described him as a 'compulsive hypochondriac'.

Mrs Banks separated from her husband four years ago. He had had an alcohol problem for some time and previous to the separation he had started drinking heavily and become violent towards his wife. Mrs Banks also had a 21-year-old daughter, Tanya, from a previous relationship. Tanya had mild cerebral palsy with some weakness in her left leg and left arm. She also had tremor of the left hand which she found embarrassing. She had moved out of the house to live with her partner two years ago. Charlotte was said to be very close to her and continued to visit her frequently in spite of Charlotte's difficulties in walking.

The therapist remarked that given the number of physical problems in the family, each member was coping with their difficulties remarkably well and wondered aloud 'What would it take for Charlotte to cope with her problems as Tanya and Tony did?' This led to a discussion about how Tanya and Tony managed their problems. Each of them had gone through a phase of investigation, hospitalisation and invalidity but over the years they had been able to overcome their disabilities and forge ahead. The session ended with a discussion about the 'fighting spirit' in the family members. All the children, Tanya, Tony and Charlotte, were described as 'copers' who, in spite of their problems, were psychologically strong enough to make the best out of life.

An event that occurred around the time of the onset of Charlotte's illness was Tanya's move from home to independent living with her boyfriend. Although the family described this as a positive transition, there was no doubt that Charlotte perceived it as a loss because of her close relationship with Tanya. Interestingly, neither Tanya nor her mother described the separation and divorce from Mr Banks as a significant life event.

A clear picture was emerging by the end of the family interviews. The family was riddled with a number of family illnesses, most of them chronic. The experience of the family with the medical care system had been far from satisfactory. The maternal grandfather, considered the patriarch of the family (in spite of his 'compulsive hypochondrias'), had not received sufficient care and attention from the medical establishment during the terminal phase of his illness. His death and Tanya's departure from home appeared to have created a void for Charlotte and her mother. The onset of Charlotte's problems seem to have then taken their minds off the traumatic events in the family and 'kept them busy' focusing on Charlotte's symptomatic behaviour, which in many ways mirrored the experience of her grandfather at the hands of the medical professionals.

Individual sessions with Mrs Banks: Charlotte's mother was seen individually in a number of sessions. The aim of the sessions was described as 'to understand ways of helping Charlotte to cope with her difficulties'. From the very beginning it was conveyed to Mrs Banks that it would be more fruitful to think about ways of helping Charlotte to cope with the symptoms rather than trying to find out a cause for the problem. After discussing her concerns for Charlotte over a number of sessions, the therapist concentrated on finding out how Mrs Banks's role had changed since Charlotte's difficulties began.

Initially, Mrs Banks was guarded in what she said and gave defensive answers. Mrs Banks agreed that although she had given up her job and virtually become a full-time carer (receiving Carer's Allowance from the Benefit's Agency), she was increasingly finding it difficult to look after Charlotte. She said that it was physically and emotionally draining for her to be with Charlotte 24 hours a day and look after her every need. She admitted in a half hearted way that Charlotte was coming to depend on her too much and was getting to expect her to do things that Charlotte could reasonably manage well on her own.

To open up the subject of burden of care, the therapist commented about some of the other families he had seen where, although the parents were caring and loving, a point came when they became resentful of the demands placed on them. It was pointed out that the other side of dependency was hostility. But how could one be angry with a child who is supposed to be ill or disabled? The therapist wondered whether Mrs Banks had had a similar experience. The purpose of the discussion was to give permission to Mrs Banks to talk about the emotional difficulties that she encountered as a person in caring for Charlotte. Mrs Banks reluctantly agreed that it was both physically and emotionally draining for her to be looking after Charlotte. She got quite irritated by Charlotte's behaviour at times but had to suppress her anger because it would be 'cruel' to be hostile towards a disabled child. When asked how she coped with such frustrations and anger, Mrs Banks said that she hardly had a life for herself.

She described her ex-husband as a very dependent man. He got her to take over the management of family finances and running of the house. Apart from his work he took little part in taking responsibility for the family. Attending to the children's medical problems, school-related matters and other social matters were left to her. He requested frequent nurturing from her because of recurrent backache. Initially she enjoyed the responsibility and the trust he had placed in her but soon found that it had become an exhausting task. She came to resent her role as a caregiver and this led to frequent arguments between the two. She said that during this period she felt trapped and helpless. She got very depressed and was treated with antidepressants prescribed by her GP. It took a lot of courage to put an end to the relationship and make the separation final. After the final separation from her husband she felt quite relieved and in charge of her life and was enjoying the independence. Then Charlotte started falling ill. Now that Charlotte was dependent on her, she felt that life for her had come a full circle and that she had fallen back into the role of full-time carer.

The therapist discussed the need for her to look after herself after being overwhelmed by the demands that were being made on her by Charlotte and the rest of the family. Referring to her description of not having a life for herself it was pointed out to her that it was important that she developed something outside the family obligations to 'recharge her batteries'. Mrs Banks said that she felt guilty whenever she tried to spend some time on her own activities or be out of the house. She mentioned that she had recently developed a relationship with a man but did not want Charlotte to know about it because she was unsure as to how Charlotte would react. He had been quite sympathetic towards Mrs Banks and the difficulties she faced with looking after Charlotte, but Mrs Banks was unsure about Charlotte's reaction to it and, therefore, had not made any commitments to him.

Mrs Banks had many strengths. She was good at managing the family, financial affairs and all the medical appointments of all the children. The therapist described her as 'a super mum'. She had sacrificed her life and currently had put herself at Charlotte's disposal. Whilst this may be a good short-term strategy, in the long run it was exhausting and Mrs Banks was paying a heavy price. The question was to find out ways and means of doing things that made her feel fulfilled but this would invariably involve doing less for Charlotte. It was important that she did not feel guilty when she did things in pursuit of her own self-interest. Although she seemed to be somewhat uneasy and uncomfortable about the idea, she agreed to think about it.

Over the next few sessions Mrs Banks reported that she had decided to 'take time off from Charlotte' on some evenings and spend the time with her friends, including her man friend. She was surprised that when she had explained it to Charlotte, she was quite understanding of it and had made no particular objections to it. To make it easy for Charlotte, she had taken Charlotte to her sister's when she went out. But her hope was that Charlotte would spend her time at home whilst she went out.

Mrs Banks struggled with the idea of 'something being wrong with Charlotte' and kept bringing up the subject repeatedly in her individual sessions with the therapist. It was, therefore, felt important to redefine the 'illness' in terms that permitted recovery and healthy functioning. The therapists introduced the concept of 'threshold' to Mrs Banks (and Charlotte) and explained that in order for a sensation such as pain to be felt, it had to reach a certain level or threshold before the brain could perceive it. The threshold for each sensation varied from person to person. An example of a pain reaction to an injection was cited. Each person would react to the same injection with different degrees of pain. In the case of Charlotte, the messages from and to her leg muscles were reaching her brain but were below the threshold level so it was important that she trained herself to perceive these messages and this could only happen with more effort and training. Therefore, it was important that Charlotte developed her confidence to use her legs more and depend less on her crutches or on her mother. Following a long discussion about how Charlotte needed to retrain her muscles, setting a short-term target was brought up. What did she feel should happen next?

Mrs Banks felt that Charlotte's immediate need was to get back to school. This would help Charlotte to get out of the house and socialise with her friends. And it would be a welcome relief for Mrs Banks so that she could have some time for herself. However, she was concerned about how Charlotte would manage at school and the difficulties it might cause her in moving from class to class. Mrs Banks agreed to discuss the issue of Charlotte's return to school. The therapist agreed to liaise with school and put them in the picture about Charlotte's difficulties after Mrs Banks had made contact with school.

At the next session Mrs Banks reported that she had visited school and met with the headteacher. A number of steps were to be put in place before Charlotte returned to school. Following discussion between Charlotte and mother in a family session, it was decided that Charlotte would start attending school, starting with three half days a week and increasing attendance gradually until she achieved full attendance. Mrs Banks remained apprehensive about Charlotte's return to school. She had been to school with Charlotte on the first day and appeared satisfied with the arrangements that had been made. A peer mentor had been identified to help Charlotte in moving from class to class. Charlotte also had some classes for which she had to climb steps. It had been decided that she would be exempt from lessons in these classes and spend her time in the library.

In the next session Mrs Banks complained that the school had not taken sufficient care in looking after Charlotte's needs. For example, they had not made arrangements for someone to look after Charlotte in case the fire alarm went off. It was apparent that her catastrophic thinking was making her highly anxious about Charlotte's return to school. The therapist discussed the probability of a fire at school. Mrs Banks considered the chance of the fire alarm going off as remote and agreed to 'take a chance'.

The next hurdle for Mrs Banks arose when they were hoping to go on a family holiday to Germany. Mrs Banks had a number of relations in Germany but she was concerned about air travel and how Charlotte would manage during the holidays. She insisted on taking a wheelchair in case Charlotte had difficulties in walking when she was in Germany. Charlotte had not been keen to take the wheelchair because she felt confident that she could manage with crutches. The therapist interpreted this as a sign of her need for independence and more specifically she might not want to be seen by their relatives in Germany as an invalid. As it happened, Mrs Banks had her way and made sure that they took the wheelchair with them. Charlotte for her part had told her therapist that she was going to prove to her mother that she did not need the wheelchair while on holiday. The family holiday turned out to be a turning point. Charlotte had enjoyed the travel and the time she spent with relatives. She never used the wheelchair and, on their return home, Mrs Banks decided that it was time to stop using the wheelchair when Charlotte went out. 'If you did not need the wheelchair in Germany, you don't need it in England,' she had declared. The therapist saw this as a positive step.

Building on the need to get Charlotte to be more independent, in the next few sessions the therapist worked on trying to encourage Mrs Banks to get Charlotte off crutches, initially at home and later at school. Her anxiety was identified as a major hurdle to get Charlotte to move from one step to the next. Mrs Banks admitted that she was an anxious person, especially in matters concerning health and illness. The therapist pointed out that it was important for her to keep her anxieties to herself and not transfer them to Charlotte. Children were good at picking up anxiety signals from their parents. How could she manage her anxieties in such a way that they did not show? Over the next few sessions Mrs Banks was able to gradually distance herself from Charlotte and worry less about her. She found her man friend enormously helpful in this. As their relationship improved, Mrs Banks was able to worry less about Charlotte. During this period she made a conscious decision to make it compulsory for Charlotte not to use her crutches at home. On other occasions with the help of the therapist she 'forgot' to get the crutches into the car.

Individual sessions with Charlotte: Charlotte was seen by her therapist fortnightly for individual sessions. The therapist was keen to build a good working relationship with Charlotte and spent the first few sessions discussing topics that interested Charlotte such as her schoolwork and friends. Charlotte brought some of her schoolwork to show her therapist how good her work was. It became clear that Charlotte was worried about losing her position in class as number one student. The therapist was able to discuss Charlotte's need to be the 'top dog'. Charlotte's view was that she was only good at schoolwork and she did not want to be beaten at it too. Charlotte's self-esteem appeared to be built almost entirely on her being a good student. Over a number of sessions together with Charlotte the therapist was able to map other areas in which Charlotte was competent and reasonably good. For example, she liked children and neighbours got her to babysit. She had a flair for getting on with children and, in fact, was looking forward to her step-sister's delivery (Tanya was pregnant at this time).

Another aim of therapy was to 'sell' the rehabilitation model and gradually decrease her dependence on the wheelchair and crutches. To motivate Charlotte her therapist brought up the topic of things she missed most because of her illness at every session. The therapist set small achievable short-term targets such as walking up to the toilet without help and walking in the garden for increasing periods of time. A major part of some sessions were spent discussing what Charlotte would like to do if she was free of weakness in her legs. The objective of the exercise was to emphasise the discrepancy between what she was doing now and what she wanted to do. In the sessions she talked a great deal about how she was looking forward to Tanya's delivery. She was keen to look after the baby. This provided an incentive for the work. She was keen to be able to go to her sister whenever she wanted. Moreover, she did not want to be limping or be on crutches when she was with the baby. She wanted to be able to carry the baby and be fit to babysit for her sister. The therapist capitalised on her motivation to improve before the baby was born, setting targets of increasing difficulty.

Together with Charlotte the therapist examined the various difficulties that she might face when she returned to school. Unlike her mother, Charlotte was more concerned about dealing with questions that her peers might ask rather than the practicalities of physically getting from one lesson to another. Possible scenarios were enacted and modelled by the therapist. When she did return to school, things were not as bad as she expected. She was surprised at the sympathy and offers of help she received from her classmates. She surprised the therapist when she said that she had told them she was getting better and would be walking unaided soon. This was quite unexpected and not in the therapist's script. The therapist felt that it was a reflection of her optimism and her keenness to get back to normal life.

Liaison with school and physiotherapist: When therapy began one of the clinicians contacted school and explained Charlotte's problems to the head-teacher and the head of year. They were sympathetic and were keen to have her back. A gradual introduction to school was suggested. Contingency plans for her to remain in school if there were crises (e.g. dizzy spells) were discussed. Her mother was to meet with SENCO and the form teacher to make practical arrangements. Charlotte's physiotherapist was contacted to tell her about CAMHS involvement and the plans to get Charlotte to attend school. The physiotherapist had been visiting her at home to get her to do the prescribed exercises but had stopped seeing her because Charlotte had learnt the exercises and was able to carry them out without the physiotherapist's assistance. She was happy that Charlotte had been doing the exercises regularly. Her visits had become infrequent but she had kept a close eye on Charlotte. The physiotherapist was encouraged by the turn of events and agreed to visit school to help them to accommodate Charlotte's requirements.

Progress and outcome

Charlotte's progress in general was steady but slow. For the therapists, her return to school was an anxious time because any momentary failure had the potential to set back progress and even ruin the program. But rehabilitation to school progressed without any major problems. Some days she complained of feeling tired and missed a day or two of school. This was described by the therapists as ordinary difficulties that arise from prolonged muscular inactivity. The teachers and her classmates were supportive and encouraged her in her attendance. Contrary to her expectations, she had no difficulties in coping with schoolwork and in her own usual way she excelled.

It took Charlotte some time before she could give up her dependence on her crutches. The use of a walking stick as an interim measure was suggested by her mother. But Charlotte ruled it out as 'uncool' and 'geriatric'. The first time she was able to walk unaided was in school when she had to go from one classroom to another. Her mentor kindly agreed to carry her crutches for her. Charlotte and her peer mentor had become good friends.

One of the events that expedited progress in Charlotte was the birth of Tanya's daughter Emma. Charlotte wanted to visit her sister as often as possible and was keen to take an active part in looking after Emma. Moreover, Mrs Banks was kept fully occupied with her first granddaughter and had little time for Charlotte. Within weeks of the birth of Emma, Charlotte gave up her crutches and was walking without help.

During this period she was attending the paediatric neurologist's clinic regularly albeit infrequently. After the birth of Emma the family were reluctant to attend the clinic and complained that it took them a whole half day away from Tanya and Emma. It was negotiated with the neurologist to suspend attendance temporarily. Mrs Banks remained apprehensive about being discharged from the neurology clinic. The sessions in the CAMH clinic were reduced to once a month and Charlotte attended the last few sessions without her crutches. They were discharged a year after they were referred to the service.

Over the next few years we came to know from school that she had been attending regularly and her improvement was maintained. Her therapist ran into her in the shopping centre a few years later and found her healthy and well. Charlotte recognised the therapist and enquired after her. She never mentioned the 'weakness of her legs'.

Comments

Charlotte's case is a prime example of what CAMHS can offer to children and adolescents with somatisation problems. Admittedly, the referral to CAMHS came belatedly. Charlotte had been wheelchair-bound for some time and lost a considerable amount of schooling. Her mother was exhausted looking after her although she was reluctant to admit to it. When the referral was received the CAMH team was not very optimistic about the outcome. But Charlotte and her mother proved that they were resourceful and not as dysfunctional as perceived by the clinicians. Charlotte's desire to get better was the main motivating factor once she had got past the stage of looking for a cause for her problems. Admittedly, her mother was enmeshed with Charlotte, as any mother with a 'paraplegic' daughter would be. But once she began to realise that *her* life was being dominated by the 'illness', she was able to take risks and try new ways of managing the problem. No doubt the arrival of a baby in the family acted as a fillip and provided the impetus to her improvement, a good example of extra-therapeutic factors at work.

Other clinicians may adopt different approaches to those employed in this case. But the essential ingredients probably would have been the same: careful management of the referral from the paediatrician, a non-blaming attitude and a good working relationship with Charlotte and her mother. And, more importantly, the two clinicians learned not to underestimate the inherent potential in families to heal themselves once the barriers to recovery are addressed.

Large paediatric hospitals have well established paediatric–psychiatric liaison services that include a multidisciplinary team consisting of consultant psychiatrists, child psychologists, psychotherapists and specialist mental health nurses. Joint ward rounds or weekly liaison meetings ('psycho-social meetings') have been found to be useful ways of working where hidden psychological issues can be discussed.

Paediatric liaison services serve three groups of children and adolescence patients:

- Those with comorbid physical and mental health problems. It is well recognised that the incidence of mental health problems in those with physical illness is twice that in normal populations; for those with chronic physical problems the incidence is thrice as high.
- Those primarily with mental health problems presenting with physical problems, e.g. panic disorder presenting with hyperventilation.
- Those with somatisation disorders, the subject of this chapter.

In dealing with somatisation a major part of the work has to be with the paediatric staff. The process of referral is fraught, since many paediatricians are somatically fixated and, once investigations are normal or when their patience is exhausted, they do not see a part for them anymore and want to dispose of the case. Parents, on the other hand, may view the referral to CAMHS to mean that the child is 'not really ill' or is 'putting it on'. Many feel they are being blamed. By the time the CAMHS workers get involved in the case the tension between the two parties is palpable. It requires considerable skill to hear the paediatrician's frustration and the family's annoyance and to work with them. With the support and encouragement provided by the CAMHS workers, paediatricians can be helped to work with anxious and demanding parents. A proper paediatric/psychiatry liaison team can save a child wasteful and intrusive tests and unnecessary suffering and disability.

Another model for managing severe and unremitting adolescent somatoform disorders is through admission to an adolescent psychiatric ward. Inpatient services using a rehabilitation model involving behavioural shaping, family therapy and supportive therapies have been described (Lock and Giammona, 1999). While some specialist centres may have the resources for such programmes and find such approaches useful, for many district general hospitals even paediatric/psychiatric liaison services remain a luxury.

Box 11.1 Research on somatisation in children shows that . . .

- Disorders involving somatisation are common (about 1%) and often cause severe distress and handicap.
- Symptoms often serve several conscious and unconscious purposes such as adopting the privileges of the sick role, avoiding conflict or eliciting care.
- Useful treatment approaches include: completion of medical investigations as soon as possible; allowing the adolescent to give up the symptoms through rehabilitation, physical therapies and other face-saving strategies; family and individual therapy.
- A properly organised and resourced paediatric liaison service is effective in reducing suffering and offering better outcomes for children with somatisation.

Note

I am grateful to Marlene Vernon, Clinical Nurse Specialist, who acted as the co-therapist and undertook the individual work with Charlotte.

References

* Bass C, Benjamin S. The management of chronic somatisation. *British Journal of Psychiatry.* 1993; **162**: 472–80.
* Lask B, Fosson A. *Childhood Illness: the psychosomatic approach*. Chichester: John Wiley; 1989.
Lock J, Giammona A. Severe somatoform disorder in adolescence: a case series using a rehabilitation model for intervention. *Clinical Child Psychology and Psychiatry*. 1999; **4**(3): 341–51.
Minuchin S, Barker L, Roseman BL *et al*. A conceptual model of psychosomatic illness in children: family organisation and family therapy. *Archives of General Psychiatry*. 1975; **32**: 1031–8.

Pilowsky I. *Abnormal Illness Behaviour*. London: Wiley; 1997.

Stores G. Clinical and EEG evaluation of seizures and seizure-like disorders. *Journal of the American Academy of Child and Adolescent Psychiatry*. 1985; 24, 10–16.

Chapter 12

Conduct disorder

A worried and concerned GP telephoned the local CAMHS about a 14-year-old boy who had been violent towards his mother over the weekend. In fact, it was the mother and the grandmother, both of whom were the GP's patients, who had turned up at the surgery to complain about the unruly and violent behaviour of Sam. The GP was aware that Sam had a number of long-standing behaviour problems and had been referred to various agencies in the past, but now the situation was grave. Following an argument with his mother over the weekend he had become 'aggressive, smashed his bedroom and threatened his mother with a kitchen knife'. There had been previous complaints about his behaviour both by the mother and school. When asked about what these problems were, the GP said that Sam was known to be stealing and truanting but the GP did not have any more details. The police had been involved in the past but, as far as he was aware, there had been no charges brought against him.

The GP had known the family for some time. There was no significant medical history in Sam. His mother, who was a single parent, had been on antidepressants in the past. The GP wanted to know what medication he could prescribe to control Sam's behaviour. Of course he wanted Sam to be seen urgently and be 'sorted out' because his mother was 'at the end of her tether'. He felt under great pressure to prescribe medication to calm Sam down. It took some time to persuade the GP not to prescribe any medication. Significantly, Sam had refused to attend the surgery. Although his mother was concerned about her own safety she had not informed police because she did not want Sam to have a police record.

Soon after the telephone referral from the GP, Sam's social worker called to reiterate that the situation was getting worse and Sam was said to be in an agitated state. The situation was reaching a crisis point. The mother had been on the telephone to the social worker pleading with him to 'do something' so that she could keep Sam (and herself) safe. The social worker wanted to know what to do. Could Sam be admitted to a psychiatric unit to ensure the safety of his mother? There was also a call from the Youth Offending Team (YOT) who had been involved with Sam after he had committed a number of 'minor offences'. The YOT worker also indicated that the school had been concerned about Sam's behaviour for some time and said that he would value any input from CAMHS.

It was clear that Sam's behaviour had caused considerable concern to the family and the professional system. A number of agencies had already been involved with the family for some time and probably had lots of information on them. Everyone was now turning to CAMHS for a solution!

The issue of risk to the mother appeared real and something had to be done to ensure her safety. Of everyone involved with Sam, the social worker appeared to know Sam and his family best. In a lengthy telephone discussion with the social worker it became clear that Sam had shown considerable behaviour problems for a long time and social services had had sporadic input over a 10-year period. The immediate question, however, was how to deal with the crisis, because at the present time his mother appeared to be unable to manage him at home and she was worried about her own safety. The social worker wanted to know if Sam could be admitted to a psychiatric unit for young people. It was explained to the social worker that admission to an adolescent psychiatric unit might not be feasible and was highly unlikely because, from the available information, Sam did not appear to have a major mental disorder. The social worker had last seen Sam two weeks ago when there had been an incident in which Sam had hurt a neighbour's son. On that occasion the social worker had made two visits to the family and also talked to their neighbour. His impression of the family was that they sought help during crises but were not good at engaging with services once the crisis was resolved. He was prepared to make a home visit to assess the situation.

The social worker was hoping to visit the family. He would collect information about Sam's behaviour difficulties over the last six months or so in some detail during the home visit, in addition to other information. He agreed to gather information on the nature, frequency, severity and duration of the behaviour problems. He would be paying particular attention to the violent behaviour directed towards the mother. The pair (social worker and the CAMHS worker) had worked on previous cases and were well used to each other's method of working. The social worker was to make his own assessment and discuss it with his manager. As for immediate measures to ease the situation, a judgment would be made to remove Sam from home and place him temporarily with a relative or, as a last resort, get him placed temporarily in a children's home. Apart from dealing with the crisis, it was suggested that a network meeting be arranged as soon as possible that included all professionals involved with the family. Sam and his mother as well as any others whom she regarded as significant were to be invited.

The network meeting

The meeting was attended by the social worker, CAMHS worker from the YOT, Sam's form teacher, the special needs co-ordinator (SENCO) from school, Sam's mentor at school, his mother and grandmother. Sam had refused to attend the meeting. The meeting was chaired by the CAMHS worker. Following introductions, the aims of the meeting were outlined as follows:

1 To share information regarding Sam and his difficulties.
2 To understand the roles and relationships of the various professionals involved with Sam and share their views of the current problems.
3 To arrive at an action plan in which the task of each professional is specified so that there was agreement and clarity as to what each worker was doing.

First Sam's mother was invited to give some background information and express her concerns.

Sam's mother (Mrs Clerk): Mrs Clerk described herself as a single mother with two children, Sam aged 14, and Samantha aged 17 years. Mrs Clerk was on income support, her mother lived not far away and was her only source of support. She described the neighbourhood as rough and the family had been subject to harassment by the neighbours, partly because of Sam's antisocial behaviour.

She said that Sam's behaviour was causing her great concern. He was argumentative and rude towards her and often threatened to beat her up if he could not have his own way. He went out with friends and came back late at night in an intoxicated state. He was truanting from school and spent time with a crowd of older boys. Whenever she tried to discipline him he became angry and violent. He had punched holes in the bedroom doors, smashed a window and threatened to beat her up. He had put his hand through a window in a temper when she had refused him money. In the most recent incident, he had threatened to stab her when she refused to go to the local shop to buy cigarettes for him. She had been doing it in the past because Sam was underage but on this occasion she felt that he had been horrible to her the whole week and she was determined she was not going to buy cigarettes for him any more. He argued with his sister all the time and was rude and nasty to her. The latter had been preparing for exams and on weekends she went to the grandmother's house with her books to get away from him.

Mrs Clerk was frightened for her own safety and had been to the GP because she was convinced that 'something was wrong with him'. At this stage Sam's grandmother voiced her concerns and said that she had witnessed the violence several times and it was getting worse. He smoked and drank and came home late at night. He owed money to a number of local youth and they had been harassing him. Sam had got into fights with them on a number of occasions. She said they had sought help from various agencies over the last several years and 'no one had helped him'. Sam was not receiving the help he should and she wanted to know why he was behaving the way he did. She pointed at her daughter and said, 'You can't blame her, she has brought up one other child who is perfectly well behaved.'

Social worker: The social worker had known Sam and his family for four months on this occasion. Mrs Clerk had sought help from social services because of Sam's out of control behaviour. He had been absconding from school, shooting at the neighbours with a pellet gun and aggravating his sister by constantly arguing with her. He went out with his friends and came back late at night. He refused to get up in the mornings to go to school. Some days he would set out to go to school but go to meet his friends on the way and hang around with them. He had been smoking cannabis and drinking alcohol.

A number of different social workers had been involved with Sam and his family sporadically for the previous six years. The family had first contacted social services when Sam was 8 years of age. During the last contact (at the age of 10 years) with social services the main problems had been school-based ones. Social services remained involved with the family on this occasion for nine months and the case was closed. He was referred again two years later for aggressive behaviour and truanting from school. On this occasion the mother was referred to the local parenting group. After attending two sessions she dropped out of the group. Subsequently social services withdrew their involvement.

During his current involvement, the social worker had spoken to Sam and taken him out to the local fitness centre. Sam was interested in body building and swimming. He described Sam as a large boy who could pass for an 18-year-old. He had been polite and co-operative but refused to discuss his behaviour whenever he (the social worker) brought up the subject. He was quite disrespectful to his mother and spoke of her in derogatory terms. (At this point Sam's mother intervened and said, 'He calls me a cow and a slag.') Sam's ambition, he had said, was to join the army. On this occasion the social worker had tried to get his mother to attend a parent training group for teenagers run by the social services but the mother had not shown much enthusiasm. The best he could do was to pay occasional visits to the house and take him out bowling or to the fitness centre. He was under pressure from his team manager to close the case. But he agreed that the problems had been getting worse over the recent past. On one occasion Sam had been brought home by the police in a dishevelled state after he had got into a brawl with a group of older lads. He handed around a summary of his observations:

- Nature of behaviour: Temper outbursts, getting into arguments with mum, deliberate defiance of adults, truanting, getting into fights.
- Frequency: Temper outbursts and arguments were daily features, truanting was very frequent and he had not attended school for the last two weeks, and fighting occurred at least once a week.
- Intensity: Tempers were explosive marked by shouting, swearing, punching and kicking doors, leaving home and staying away from home overnight.
- Duration: Since the age of three or so, now getting worse.
- Context: Tempers occur whenever his requests are denied (e.g. requests for money) or when he is asked to do 'normal' things (e.g. go to school, come back home in time).
- Impact: Disrupting family life, not learning at school, police involvement, 'everyone in the family is scared of his temper', no career ambitions, delinquent peers.

As for Sam's violence towards his mother, the social worker felt that this was the first time he had threatened her with physical violence. On enquiry it had transpired that Sam had *said* that he would stab her with a knife but had not, in fact, taken a knife towards Mrs Clerk. Although he had been verbally aggressive towards her, he had not been physically violent towards her or any other family members in the past. Mrs Clerk agreed that Sam had not really threatened her with a knife, but his behaviour on that day was so unpredictable that she felt he might stab her. The social worker had spoken to Sam about the possible consequences of future violence towards his mother. His mother had been asked to call the police in event of any violence.

The teachers: His form teacher Mr Robinson described him as a 20-year-old in the body of a 14-year-old. When he did attend school he was disruptive in class and was challenging to teachers. He was particularly difficult with female teachers. He had sprayed a female teacher's car with paint. Sam responded better to him, probably because he was a man. Sam had mild learning difficulties and had rather poor verbal skills. He had been disruptive in class but this was usually preceded by situations in which Sam had been asked to do reading or written work. Sam was good at arts, crafts and design and PE. The teacher described him as a leader among his group of friends. He had been caught bullying younger children. He appeared to like the reputation he had as the 'tough guy'. Mr Robinson had witnessed him showing off to his friends how he could tolerate pain by cutting his forearm with a piece of glass and drawing blood.

He had been excluded on numerous occasions for being rude and cheeky to teachers and disrupting class. On one occasion he had openly challenged a male teacher and on another called a female teacher names.

The SENCO's view was that Sam was academically capable but his application was very poor and he was simply not interested in learning. But there was general agreement among the teachers that his reading was quite poor compared to his peers. She had attempted to provide extra help in English but Sam had not been interested. All that she could do was to keep all his teachers informed about his problems. When pulled up in class for being disruptive he would stomp away from class swearing obscenities at the teacher concerned. She had arranged for a mentor in school to befriend him and be available to him if he ever wished to discuss any of his difficulties but Sam had not shown any interest in meeting him.

Youth Offending Team worker: The CAMH worker from the Youth Offending Team reported that Sam had been involved in a number of criminal offences:

1   Two offences of shoplifting: Sam and his friends were involved in the theft of some electronic items from a supermarket. He received a caution.
2   Disturbance of the peace and drunk and disorderly behaviour: Sam and his friends had been thrown out of a pub and got into a brawl. Sam had tried to resist arrest and challenged the policeman. He pleaded guilty to the charges and was placed on a supervision order.
3   Breaking into the school laboratory and stealing chemicals: he had confessed to the offence and was on a supervision order.

As a condition of the supervision order, Sam met with the youth worker regularly. At these meetings he was cautioned about the need to keep out of trouble and warned that any future offending may result in a custodial sentence. In short, he was on the brink of being sent to jail. The YOT worker had discussed with Sam the disadvantages of having a criminal record and that his ambition of joining the army was getting rather slim. He pointed out that Sam's offences had been committed in the company of youth who were much older and many of them had criminal records. It was probable they were using him to do the thieving and while Sam got caught they had escaped punishment. The motivation for many of the thefts, in his opinion, was to buy illicit drugs although Sam had never admitted to it. The break-in at the school laboratory too was probably drug-related. He had been referred to a drug worker.

CAMHS worker

On searching the records at the clinic, it was found that the family had been seen when Sam was only three years old. This came as a surprise. But the CAMHS worker did not want to discuss this at the network meeting. The complaint at that time was that Sam did not do as he was told to do; he was aggressive and had violent temper outbursts. He had also been aggressive towards other children in the nursery. He was said to have some speech delay and was receiving speech therapy. It was recorded in the notes at this time that there were many family issues. His father had been jailed for burglary when Mrs Clerk was pregnant with Sam and there had been family violence, resulting in a number of parental separations. The notes also mentioned that the mother had been treated for depression and had had several admissions to the local psychiatric hospital for depression and overdoses and had been treated with ECT (electroconvulsive treatment) on one occasion. At the first referral Sam and the family had been seen by a member of the CAMH team and, following initial assessment, been referred to a parenting group run by social services. The family had been also asked to seek social services support. This information was not disclosed to the network meeting for two reasons: it served no useful purpose at the present time and permission had not been obtained from the mother to reveal it to the network group. It was also was likely that the other agencies may have known about some of the facts of the case and, indeed, have other pieces of information they did not want to reveal at this stage.

Network discussions: The CAMHS worker summarised the case as follows: Sam, now 14 years of age, had shown behaviour problems from a very young age. Thus the problems have been long-standing and there had been a number of stresses and difficulties in the family. He had had some speech delay. He had not had any formal educational assessment but was felt to be of average or borderline intelligence. As Sam had grown and got physically bigger, the problems too had got bigger. At the present time the mother was a single parent and was managing as best as she could with the help of Sam's maternal grandmother. The immediate concerns were:

1 violent behaviour towards his mother and
2 offending behaviour, both of which had been escalating over the past few weeks.

In addition, Sam's persistent antisocial behaviour both at home and outside was a cause for concern. It appeared that Sam's behaviour was almost completely outside the control of the adults around him. The CAMHS worker invited the participants to air their views about what could be done to bring about change.

Sam's form teacher felt that Sam had been traumatised by witnessing violence in the family when he was young and had 'identified with the aggressor'. Sam came across to him as a sad boy, despite his bravado, and needed help. He was not clear what the nature of the help should be, and wanted to know what help was available from CAMHS. The SENCO was not so sure. She thought that removal from home and placement in a secure environment was the only way to contain his behaviour. The social worker said that Sam's parents had been referred to parent training groups in the past but had not taken up the offer and wondered whether his mother would consider the new group that had been set up by social services for parents of teenagers. A number of families he had been involved with had found it very helpful. To this the grandmother and mother replied that they had been involved in such groups before and were well aware of the various techniques of child management and did not think these 'classes' were of much use. Both of them were convinced that 'something was wrong' with Sam.

When asked to elaborate on what made them think Sam had a problem *in* him, they said that from an early age he had been different from other children. He had a violent streak in him, he was uncaring and, sometimes, plainly cruel. They mentioned an instance when he had killed his goldfish by squeezing it in his hand; he was 'not like other children' and was unpredictable. For example, he had thrown his sister's school coursework out of the window on a rainy day; he had 'tried to burn the house down' by burning paper in the kitchen; he had ripped the wallpaper in his room and punched holes in the door. They had seen a television program on ADHD and received a leaflet about it. The descriptions fitted Sam perfectly. They wanted to know why he had not been assessed for ADHD. They had been made to feel that they were bad parents and asked to attend 'classes' while Sam's condition had gone undiagnosed and untreated.

The worker from YOT felt that from his point of view, Sam had to be kept away from the delinquent group he was associating with. He pointed out that Sam's offences were committed in the company of other youngsters. In his view there were push and pull factors that led to law-breaking behaviour. The push factors were his being away from school, lack of alternative interests outside home and an unsatisfactory relationship with his mother. The pull factors were his delinquent peer group, use of cannabis and drinking in their company. The YOT worker's remit was to prevent Sam from reoffending. In his work with Sam he had made it clear to Sam that the courts would take a serious view of any further law-breaking behaviour and that he was very likely to get a custodial sentence for any further infringement of the law. He was also arranging for drug counselling. But a lot depended on his co-operation and so far there had been not much evidence of it.

Following a long discussion a plan of action was drawn up:

- Arrangement for Sam to be received at school in the mornings by his form teacher. Initially he would be collected from home. His daily attendance in the morning would be checked and his mother kept informed. (Action: Form teacher and Special Educational Needs Coordinator.)
- After-school activities would be organised for Sam. (Action: Form teacher.)
- Sam would be assessed for any mental disorder including ADHD. (Action: Consultant child and adolescent psychiatrist.)
- A sessional worker would take Sam out twice a week for activities of Sam's choice. Sam would be enrolled in a local activity based group for youth. (Action: Social worker.)
- Sam's whereabouts would be supervised closely by his mother and reported to the Youth Offending Worker on a daily basis. They would impose a 'curfew' on him to make sure he returned home by 10.00 pm. A point system based on behavioural principles would be set up to enhance adherence to the curfew. (Action: Youth Offending Worker.)
- If Sam was ever violent towards his mother she was to get the police involved. In order to improve her relationship with Sam, his mother would spend one hour three times a week in activities that Sam liked. (Action: Sam's mother and grandmother.)

A date for the next network meeting was arranged in two weeks' time.

Clinical presentation and background

Individual session with mother: The consultant psychiatrist made an appointment for Sam and his family to be seen. His mother telephoned to ask to meet him on her own before he saw Sam. She wanted to discuss certain matters even before Sam was seen. She explained that she would not be free to say things in Sam's presence and he was bound to become difficult if she said anything critical of him. An appointment was made for her to be seen on her own.

Mrs Clerk was a small women and appeared older than her age. Sam was born full-term; the pregnancy and delivery had been normal. Mrs Clerk had been quite depressed following Sam's birth although she did not realise it at that time. Her husband was violent towards her, her marriage was in trouble. He drank heavily and was in trouble with the police. He was later sent to jail for robbery. Sam was a difficult baby. He cried a lot and slept very little. She did not remember much about Sam's developmental milestones. She felt that his speech was somewhat delayed but after having some speech therapy, he started talking well. After her husband came back from prison she had been subjected to domestic violence on a daily basis. She was depressed at this time and needed treatment in hospital after she took an overdose. She felt that she had been depressed for the first five years of Sam's life and had had various forms of treatments. She had left her husband several times and taken the children with her, but he had persuaded her to come back claiming that he had changed. When Sam was six years of age, one night her husband came home drunk, accused her of sleeping with other men and beat her up severely. She went to the police and was taken to a women's refuge. He was charged and she got a court order to prevent him from contacting her.

During the session she confided in the CAMHS worker that things were very bad at home and, she added hesitantly, that Sam had been violent towards her for some time but she had not mentioned it to the social worker for fear that Sam may be taken away from her. She went on to say Sam had been aggressive from the age of three years.

He had not had any unusual habits or behaviours. She felt that his problems started around the age of three. She remembered coming to see someone in CAMHS when Sam was three years of age but was disappointed with the outcome because nothing was done.

She felt guilty that she had not been available to Sam during his early years when she had been preoccupied with her own problems. She wished she had dealt with her problems more decisively and given more time to Sam. During his early years he was very demanding and she found it hard to cope. She was depressed so much that she would spend long hours in bed, leaving Sam to be looked after by his sister who was only five years old at that time. At other times she gave into him, especially when he had tantrums. When he started nursery he hit the teachers and pulled at their hair. He was excluded from the nursery at the age of four and a half!

Similar problems were reported by the primary school. The headteacher had said Sam was unprepared for school. Sam had no friends and felt rejected by his classmates. She felt that from the first day teachers did not like him and she was called to the school whenever they had problems managing him and often asked to take him back home. As her grew older his aggression had got worse and his tempers had become outbursts of rage. When he had one of his 'rages' he became red in the face, made a fist and growled at her. She was afraid that he was turning out to be like his father. He demanded money from her and, on numerous other occasions, money had gone missing from her purse. She was sure that he had taken the money but was scared to confront him. She agreed with the description of Sam provided by the social worker but she had not told him that Sam had beaten her up on several occasions. She was so scared of him that she hardly asked him to do anything and dared not say no to any of his requests. She did not want Sam to get into trouble with the police.

Sam had always found schoolwork difficult. Mrs Clerk felt that this was because he was not interested in reading or writing. He liked sports and PE. He did not get on with any of his teachers and had little regard for them. According to teachers, 'he had an attitude problem'. He had been excluded from school numerous times, later he was placed on a part-time timetable because the school could not manage him and later still, he decided to truant or not attend school.

She was convinced that 'there was something wrong with him'. Her 17-year-old daughter (by a previous partner) was compliant, intelligent and was well behaved. Sam had been tested for chromosome abnormalities because of his large stature, but no abnormalities had been found. His physical health had been remarkably good. Mrs Clerk was asked to fill in the Conners' questionnaire (Conners, 2001; *see* Chapter 9)

Individual session with Sam: Sam was brought to the assessment session by the worker from the YOT. Sam was a tall, large, rather obese boy. He was not very communicative. He said he had come only because the 'geezer from the courts' had made him attend the YOT. He said he had no particular problem and it was his mother who was making a big fuss. He denied ever having threatened or harmed his mother. He said 'Look man, I don't know who told you all these lies. I have nothing wrong with me and I don't want to see a shrink.' Asked about his court appearances, he shrugged his shoulders and said that he got into 'a spot of bother with the police'. He was more co-operative when taking about his body-building activities and about his aspiration to join the army. He was dismissive when asked about his drug use but admitted he smoked skunk to feel good. He denied feeling depressed or having thoughts of harming himself. He refused to talk of his childhood and claimed that he did not remember the past. Asked about what he wished to change, he was not sure what that meant. If it meant coming for counselling, he had had enough of it and was simply not interested.

During the interview Sam did not appear depressed, rather he was angry and annoyed that he had been asked to attend clinic. When he was told that his mother appeared rather frightened by his aggression and violence he showed very little emotional reaction. He also showed a serious lack of concern about his future and appeared to lack insight about the predicament he was in. Although he was aware that further offending may lead to a jail sentence, he remained remarkably unconcerned about it.

Case conceptualisation and formulation

Sam, 14 years of age, showed severe problems of conduct. These included extreme defiance, severe and frequent temper outbursts, threatening behaviour, truanting and getting into fights. In addition, at the time of assessment he had been offending (stealing and breaking and entering) using prohibited drugs and engaging in a number of antisocial activities. He was aggressive and violent towards others, particularly his mother, and posed a risk to her. The constellation of conduct problems he displayed has been described in the literature as conduct disorder (CD). Sam had shown behaviour problems since the age of three and has been getting worse ever since. Sam may therefore be said to show the early-onset subtype of conduct disorder that has a worse prognosis than the adolescent onset type. Detailed examination of Sam's developmental and clinical history (not mentioned in any detail here), school reports and the scores on Conners' questionnaire did not indicate that there was evidence of autism spectrum disorder (*see* Chapter 7), Hyperkinetic Disorder (*see* Chapter 9) or intellectual disability (*see* Chapter 4).

As for aetiology, in Sam's case there were a multitude of factors that may have contributed to his difficulties. Of these a number of family factors appear to have been prominent: domestic violence, criminality in the father, marital discord and his mother's mental health during Sam's early years. Because of her own difficulties Mrs Clerk appeared to have had great difficulties imposing discipline and control over Sam's behaviour from an early age. She had had a difficult childhood herself and described her own upbringing as fraught with difficulties including domestic violence and physical abuse. The cumulative effects of these family factors, in combination with Sam's temperamental difficulties seem to have produced a series of processes that had led to the current difficulties. In the light of her depression when he was young it was highly likely that there were attachment difficulties between his mother and him from infancy. Sam appeared to hold her in contempt and Mrs Clerk had had little control over him since childhood.

Theoretical perspectives

The term 'conduct disorder' (CD) refers to aggressive, destructive and disruptive behaviours in childhood that are serious and likely to impair the child's development. Examples of these behaviours include excessive levels of fighting or bullying, often causing injury, breaking household objects and frequent refusal to obey commands and keep to house or school rules. In DSM-IV, the distinction is made between oppositional defiant disorder, which is characterised by recurrent negativistic, defiant, disobedient and hostile behaviours, and conduct disorder, characterised by the presence of repetitive and persistent violations of societal norms and other people's basic rights. In ICD-10, oppositional and conduct problems are both included under the heading of conduct disorder.

The central feature of CD is repetitive and persistent violations of age-appropriate social norms and rules or violation of other peoples' rights. It is the presence of many antisocial behaviours and their persistence that is the hallmark of conduct disorder. In younger children this typically this includes severe temper outbursts, hitting and kicking people, destruction of property, disobeying of rules, lying, stealing and spitefulness. In older children and adolescents it may include behaviours such as frequent fighting, severe aggression, cruelty to people and animals, serious theft, truancy, intimidation of others, running away from home, drug misuse and arson. The various behaviours that come under the umbrella term 'conduct disorder' fall into four overlapping classes: aggression and defiance (fighting, physical violence); deceitfulness (stealing, breaking and entering); destruction to property (fire setting); and serious rule violations (truancy, running away). Table 12.1 summarises the main features of conduct disorder as described in DSM-IV.

It should be emphasised that the use of the term 'disorder' does not imply dysfunction *in* the young person or child. Although classified in psychiatric practice as a disorder according to DSM-IV and ICD-10, it is a *description* of a constellation of behaviours and a convenient shorthand for the purposes of study and communication. Behaviour problems in children and youth have been the subject of intense studies over the last three decades and we now possess a vast

Table 12.1 Behaviours included in DSM-IV Conduct Disorder

Aggression to people (and cruelty to animals)	Deceitfulness and theft	Destruction of property	Serious rule violations
Bullying, threatening, intimidating	Breaking into a house or car	Destroying others' property	Staying out at nights
Initiating physical fights	Cheating or conning others	Intentional fire setting	Running away from home
Using a weapon to cause damage to others	Stealing without confrontation		Truancy
Physically cruel to people			
Physically cruel to animals			
Stealing with confrontation			
Forced sexual activity			
Using a weapon			

knowledge base about the causal influences, developmental processes and the course of these difficulties. A number of excellent research studies, some spanning a period of three decades, have added to our knowledge on the subject. Many of the studies have focused on the processes involved in the development of the problem while others have addressed issues of management and development of services. This section provides a very brief outline of what is known on the subject that is relevant to our discussion about Sam.

Variously termed as antisocial behaviour in childhood, aggressive conduct of childhood and, most commonly as behaviour problems, conduct disorder is one of the commonest problems in children and youth. Early studies by Rutter and colleagues showed a prevalence rate of 4% in the rural population and 9% in an urban area (Rutter *et al.*, 1975). It is thrice as common in boys as in girls. These findings have been confirmed by numerous epidemiological studies. The more recent national morbidity survey in England and Wales of over 12 500 children aged 5–15 found that 5% of children exhibited clinically significant conduct disorder (Meltzer *et al.*, 2000). More worryingly, its prevalence is rising. There is accumulating research evidence to show that, in general, antisocial behaviour in childhood is persistent in more than 45 percent of the children, leading to delinquency and antisocial behaviour in adulthood (Robins, 1978). Follow back studies of young delinquents have shown that 90% had had childhood-onset conduct disorder (Farrington, 1995). The number, frequency and intensity of the various behaviour difficulties are directly proportional to their eventual outcome.

Early onset and adolescent forms of conduct disorder: Two pathways in the development and progression of conduct disorders from childhood through adolescence into adulthood have been described (Moffit, 1993):

1 Early-onset, life-course-persistent: In this group severe problems of behaviour are encountered in early childhood and are associated with temperamental difficulties and these tend to persist into adolescence and adulthood.
2 Adolescence-limited: Here the problems begin in adolescence and are thought to be more due to deviant peer influences. Often they improve in early adulthood.

There is strong evidence that the earlier the onset of antisocial behaviour, the worse is the prognosis. Sam may be said to belong to the first group, as his problems appear to have started early, as early as 3 years of age, with serious disobedience, authority conflict and rule-breaking behaviour. His mother appears to have lost control of him early in the course of the development of problems and, partly because of her mental health problems and partly because of lack of support, she had not taken up the offer of enrolling in parent training. It was evident that she neither had the competence nor the resolve to change her behaviour now. Her desire to have him diagnosed reflected her sense of hopelessness and feeling of defeat. She was vainly hoping for a magic solution to the problem.

Aetiology/risk factors: Both genetic and environmental factors contribute to the development of conduct disorder. Environmental causes include family factors such as parenting style, attachment, parental mental illness, harsh and erratic discipline, and parental rejection of the child, to name a few. Child factors associated with conduct disorder involve temperament, poor verbal skills, low IQ and hyperactivity. The main child, family and environmental risk factors are listed in Table 12.2. Readers may note that Sam had almost all the risk factors associated with conduct disorder.

Table 12.2 Summary of risk factors associated with early onset aggression and conduct problems in children. Sam had been subject to most risk factors except those marked with an asterisk

Child risk factors	Family risk factors	School and contextual risk factors
Below average intelligence*	Parental psychopathology (e.g. depression), criminality	Rejection by prosocial peers
Difficult infant temperament	Parent–child attachment problems	Harmful school responses
Specific Reading Retardation	Coercive parenting	Low socio-economic status/ poverty
Attention deficit (ADHD)*	Marital problems, family violence, family instability	Association with aggressive/ antisocial peers
Other developmental problems	Lax and ineffective discipline, lack of monitoring	School exclusions

Patterson's 'coercive cycle' hypothesis proposes that parents inadvertently behave in ways that promote oppositional behaviours (*see* Chapter 1). There is some evidence to support this hypothesis, although the failure of the child to reinforce effective parenting may also contribute to such sequences, and parental behaviours may be influenced by genetic factors similar to those that influence the child's conduct problems. Most of the recent evidence suggests that the combination of inherited vulnerability plus negative parenting, especially early negative affect and intrusive control, contribute to the development and the persistence of conduct problems.

The role of the environment in which the child grows up is pivotal to the development of antisocial behaviour. A useful idea is the concept of Environmental Status Examination (ESE, Munger, 1998). This refers to the exploratory process involved in identifying the person's fit with his or her environment. The main assumption here is that behaviour problems stem not from any brain or personality dysfunction in the chid, but from inadequate environmental supports including improper 'fit' between a particular child and a particular setting. Understanding the behaviour of the child requires first the understanding the context within which the behaviour occurs. This necessarily involves the child, the family, school, the peer group, the community and other networks. In conducting an ESE a detailed description of how the child's time is spent, with whom and where is obtained. The evaluation involves an assessment of the pattern of time use at home, school, with peers and other activities so that a clear picture of the child's environment is obtained. This involves studying and intervening with the family, school and the community. From the information that is gathered, an environmental support plan (ESP) may be devised, specifying what supports are required to enable the child to make reasonable progress towards behaviour changes.

Prognosis: Conduct disorder is strongly associated with social and educational disadvantage. Many children with conduct disorder leave school without qualifications or are permanently excluded. Drug and alcohol misuse are common. In adulthood they continue with their antisocial and offending behaviour. Health, social and law enforcement services spend vast resources 'servicing' this group. The economic cost to society arising from conduct disorder is very high indeed. The financial cost incurred by antisocial behaviour from childhood to adulthood has shown to be 10 times greater that for those with no disorder. At 1998 prices for public services the mean individual total cost was £70 019 for conduct disorder compared with £7423 for the no problem group. The main part of the expenditure was by law enforcement agencies (prison and justice system) followed by extra educational provision, foster and residential care and state benefits (Scott *et al.*, 2001).

The outlook for children with conduct disorder is poor. Numerous long-term follow-up studies show that early childhood conduct disorder continues into later childhood, adolescence and ultimately into adulthood (as antisocial behaviour). The folk notion that children 'grow out' of behaviour problems is unfounded and is not true of severe, clinically significant conduct difficulties. As a rule, conduct disorder comes to the attention of health and social services late in the course of its development when the problems are already severe and the possibility of reversing the trend are long past. It should be noted that in oppositional defiant behaviour, parent training is effective only in children under the age of 10 years. Poor prognostic signs include the following: early onset (before the age of 10 years), male sex, severity of conduct problems, multiple behaviour problems, and presence of aggression.

The pioneering studies of Lee Robins (1978) were amongst the first to demonstrate the stability of conduct disorders in children. In this study, follow-up into adulthood of a large sample of child patients with conduct disorder who attended child guidance clinics showed that:

1 adult antisocial behaviour virtually required childhood antisocial behaviour
2 most antisocial children did not become antisocial adults; only 40–50% became antisocial adults
3 the variety and number of antisocial behaviour in childhood was a better predictor of adult antisocial behaviour than any particular behaviour
4 adult antisocial behaviour is better predicted by childhood behaviour than by family background or social class.

Numerous studies, too many to mention here, have subsequently confirmed these findings.

Studies on delinquents have produced similar results. The Farrington study (see below) showed that 40% of 7- and 8-year-olds with conduct disorder became recidivist delinquents as teenagers and over 90% of recidivist juvenile delinquents had conduct disorder as children. Thus conduct disorder severe enough to come to the attention of professionals shows continuity over time and carries a poor prognosis.

Undoubtedly, problems of conduct fall along a continuum from benign infringement of discipline to serious law-breaking behaviours. A diagnosis of conduct disorder represents one extreme end of the continuum of antisocial behaviour. By definition conduct disorder implies persistent rule-breaking behaviour that is of sufficient severity to cause social, educational or relational impairment. When rule-breaking behaviour becomes infringement on the law it is called delinquency.

Delinquency: Offending behaviour, i.e. breaking the law, is considered to be part of the spectrum of conduct problems. Delinquency is a legal term applied to persons between the ages of 10 and 17 who have committed an offence that would be regarded as criminal in an adult. Delinquency is a societal problem and has been the subject of several studies. One such study worthy of mention is the Cambridge study of delinquent development, a remarkable piece of research that prospectively followed up a population of boys aged 8 years for a period of 32 years. Data collected from a variety of sources showed that (Farrington, 1995):

- One third the population between 10 and 17 years was convicted of offences.
- Offending behaviour increased up to the age of 17 and showed a decrease thereafter.
- 75% of those convicted as juveniles reconvicted between 17 and 24.
- On average, criminal careers began at 17, lasted 6 years and ended at 23 and included 4.5 offences leading to convictions.
- Between 18 and 32 years there was a 75% decrease in offending.
- At 32 a small minority (6%) were still offending and were chronic offenders responsible for 50% of all crime.

Progress and outcome

At the second network meeting the findings of the mental health assessment were fed back to the group. It was made clear that Sam did not show evidence of ADHD or any other mental disorder (apart from conduct disorder). Other members of the network reported that most of the decisions of the first meeting could not be implemented, mainly because of Sam's intransigent attitude. He had continued to truant, keep out late and been engaged in criminal activities. The YOT worker reported that Sam had been involved in a break-in into an elderly couple's house and stolen money. He had been arrested and released on bail awaiting trial.

In the days that passed by he offended again while on bail. He had got into a vicious fight with a group of youths and beat up one of them and was charged for grievous bodily harm. He received custodial sentences for both offences and was sentenced to jail for 18 months. After release from jail he lived with his mother for a short time. Soon after, however, she refused to have him because of his aggressive behaviour towards her and social services were involved again. He was placed in independent living in a hostel for young people. He continued to be involved in various offences.

Comments

Sam typifies the problems posed by a child/youth with severe conduct disorder. Unfortunately there were few protective factors in Sam, his family and his immediate environment that might have provided a different trajectory of development. Opportunities for early intervention were missed partly because his mother was under considerable personal stress arising from the marital situation and her depression. It would be intriguing to know if the outcome would have been any different if she had taken up the offer of parent training and implemented it in all earnestness.

Sam's case raises a number of issues. What services are available for children and young people with behaviour problems and which services are responsible for delivering such services? What is clear with this group of children is that interventions need to be intensive and prolonged if they are to achieve good outcomes. Given that standard management of conduct disorder by all services is not effective, there is a need to rethink about what services should be offered.

Are problems of conduct mental health problems? There is much controversy about the inclusion of conduct disorder within mental health classificatory systems. Some notable authorities have persuasively argued against its inclusion under metal health disorders. For example, Robert Goodman (1997) has argued for the exclusion of conduct disorder from child mental health services, the same way medical services do not take responsibility for dangerous driving, homelessness or unemployment. He contends that conduct disorder is a social and educational problem that has no identifiable health component. He points out that antisocial behaviour in adults is usually considered a social problem; similar behaviour in children is often categorised as a mental health problem. They require social and educational solutions and not mental health interventions. There is much to be said for avoiding medicalisation of social problems and confining CAMHS involvement in CD to those subgroups where there are comorbid and treatable conditions such as HKD.

Wakefield, a reputed American scholar, approaching the subject from a theoretical perspective, has put forward the powerful argument that in conduct disorder, thus far, there has been no demonstration of internal dysfunction in the child in order to qualify for a diagnosis under DSM-IV (Wakefield *et al.*, 2002). He points out that the text of DSM-IV states that a diagnosis of conduct disorder should be made only if symptoms are caused by internal pathological dysfunction and not if the symptoms are a reaction to a negative environment. He has produced evidence to show that clinicians' judgements about the presence of conduct disorder are based on the presence of presumed internal dysfunction. For example, when a child experiencing repeated sexual abuse ran away from home, lied repeatedly and stayed out late, clinicians were unlikely to make a diagnosis of conduct disorder. Currently there is no evidence of internal dysfunction (such as failure of mechanisms involved in empathy, impulse control, guilt and moral conscience) in children with conduct disorder.

Many authorities have pointed out that a psychosocial model is more appropriate for conduct problems in children and youth rather than a mental health model. Unfortunately psychiatric literature and government strategy documents refer to all maladjusted children as having mental health problems. There is no doubt that children with conduct disorder are a major problem for parents, teachers and society as a whole and they need help and support. The question though is whether it is useful to view these problems as mental health problems and, consequently, expect CAMHS to take responsibility for delivering such services.

Given that the development and maintenance of conduct problems involve multiple risk factors it is only to be expected that no single intervention would be sufficient to produce appreciable change. If interventions are to be successful they should target the multiple systems at the level of the child, family, school and the community. It is worth noting that individual child centred therapy is singularly unhelpful in conduct disorder. Many who work with children, especially those involved in primary care, often naively believe that treating these children and adolescents with various types of counselling, anger management and other forms of individual psychotherapy is effective. Research has repeatedly shown that, on their own, various forms of individual psychotherapy are of little value with the conduct disordered population. In oppositional defiant behaviour and mild forms of conduct disorder parent training is the treatment of choice, especially in younger children (*see* Chapter 1).

In the case of severe conduct disorder, research studies over the last 20 years have unequivocally demonstrated that a combination of multimodal and multi-level interventions that are skilfully co-ordinated hold the best opportunities for success. A recent innovation in the treatment of children and young people with severe behaviour and emotional problems is the *system of care approach*. The central theme of such approaches is that children with severe antisocial behaviour need services that are well co-ordinated, comprehensive and delivered in natural environments. It involves comprehensive, interagency, community-based systems of care in which professionals and parents work together collaboratively to serve the needs of the child with severe conduct difficulties and their families. One such model that has been studied extensively and proven to be effective with antisocial youth is Multisystemic Therapy (MST). (Another example of the systems of care approach is the Multidimensional Therapeutic Foster Care model; *see* Chapter 6.)

MST is an intensive family and community-based treatment for adolescents who engage in severe antisocial behaviour including delinquency and substance misuse (Henggeler *et al.*, 1998). MST is provided through a home-based model of service delivery with the primary goal of bringing about change through 'intervening comprehensively at the individual, family, peer, school and possibly even neighbourhood levels' (Henggeler *et al.*, 1998, p8). Some of the main features of MST are:

- It incorporates empirically validated procedures (typically behavioural and family interventions).
- It is delivered mostly through home-based family sessions.
- School, neighbourhood and community interventions are employed as needed.
- The therapist provides direct service and acts as case manager in accessing other community-based services.
- The therapist provides intensive input with daily contact and services are made available 24 hours, 7 days a week
- The therapist carries a low caseload (3–6 families) and provides time-limited (3–5 month) interventions; therapists work in teams of 3–4 practitioners and receive weekly clinical supervision.

The application of MST to youth with severe conduct problems has been studied in a number of trials and the results have been promising. These studies have demonstrated reduction in re-offending rates, decrease in antisocial behaviour symptoms in the adolescent and a decline in the overt levels of conflict. It is unfortunate that the potential of the MST, developed in the US in the 1980s, has not been fully utilised in the UK (it is just beginning to be piloted in some areas). Unfortunately setting up MST and other systems of care are not within the gift of individual clinicians or CMHS teams.

Given the high cost to society of antisocial behaviour in children, it is surprising that policymakers and the government have not paid sufficient attention to preventing conduct disorder. The case for preventative interventions in conduct disorder, as opposed to therapeutic strategies, is overwhelming. There is already evidence from early community interventions during the preschool and early school years that targeting the most behaviourally disturbed children (the top 10% who score high on a screening measure) through parent training groups and academic training has a significant impact on children with behaviour problems. Several early (preschool) intervention projects are being carried out in the UK, US and Canada at the moment and preliminary reports show promising results. At the same time research findings caution us against approaches that simply address conduct problems without addressing the social, family and individual factors that are associated with these problems. There is a need to position programmes aimed at the amelioration of conduct problems in a broad policy context, aimed at reducing socio-economic inequalities, reducing family adversity and addressing a wider range of social and economic problems.

Box 12.1 Research on conduct disorder shows that . . .

- CD is common and is seen in 4–9% of children; it is three times more common in boys.
- Aetiological/risk factors for development of CD are well documented (*see* Table 12.2).
- In general, CD tends to persist over time and carries a poor prognosis; early-onset CD has a worse outcome than adolescent-onset CD.
- Individual and group therapies are remarkably ineffective.
- At the present time the only proven method of treatment for moderate to severe CD including delinquency is Multisystemic Therapy.
- Targeted prevention of early-onset CD appears to hold the best promise.

References

Conners CK. *Conners' Rating Scales – Revised, Technical Manual*. New York: Multi-Health Systems; 2001.

*Farrington DP. The development of offending and antisocial behaviour from childhood: Key findings from the Cambridge Study in Delinquent Development. *Journal of Child Psychology and Psychiatry*. 1995; **36**: 929–64.

Goodman R. Child mental health: who is responsible? *BMJ*. 1997; **314**: 813–17.

*Henggeler SW, Schoenwald SK, Borduin CM *et al*. *Multisystemic Treatment of Antisocial Behaviour in Children and Adolescents*. New York: Guilford Press; 1998.

Meltzer H, Gatward R, Goodman R *et al*. *The Mental Health of Children and Adolescents in Great Britain*. London: Office of National Statistics; 2000.

Moffit TE. Adolescent-limited and life-course persistent antisocial behaviour: a developmental taxonomy. *Psychological Review*. 1993; **100**: 647–701.

*Munger RL. *The Ecology of Troubled Children: changing children's behaviour by changing the places, activities and people in their lives*. Cambridge: Brookline Press; 1998.

Robins LN. Sturdy childhood predictors of adult antisocial behaviour: replication from longitudinal studies. *Psychological Medicine*. 1978; **8**: 611–22.

Rutter M, Cox A, Tupling C. Attainment and adjustment in two geographical areas. *British Journal Of Psychiatry*. 1975; **126**: 493–509.

Scott S, Knapp M, Henderson J *et al*. Financial cost of social exclusion: follow up study of antisocial children into adulthood. *BMJ*. 2001; **323**: 1–5.

Wakefield JC, Pottick KJ, Kirk SA. Should the DSM IV diagnostic criteria for conduct disorder consider social context. *American Journal of Psychiatry*. 2002; **159**: 380–86.

Chapter 13

Post-traumatic stress disorder

The referral letter came from the GP and was soon followed by a telephone call. The GP had seen a 6-year-old boy called Charles with his parents. His parents had reported that his behaviour had deteriorated over the last few months and that he was unusually aggressive and difficult to manage. He behaviour was worse when travelling by car and he was frightened of the dark. The family had been involved in a bad road traffic accident (RTA) about a year ago in which his grandmother died. The GP wondered whether the change in behaviour was related to the RTA. She had considered the possibility of an occult head injury, but Charles had not had any overt injuries or any loss of consciousness that might have suggested any brain injury. She was not sure whether his behaviour change was the result of post-traumatic stress disorder. She wanted to know whether she was doing the right thing by referring Charles to CAMHS. The member of staff who took the telephone call agreed for him to be seen in the outpatient's clinic.

Clinical presentation and background

An appointment was offered for the family and in the first assessment interview Charles was seen together with his parents, Mr and Mrs Hunt, and his 10-year-old sister, Molly. The family had been involved in a road traffic accident about 13 months ago. The family had visited Charles's grandmother and were on their way back home when the accident happened. Charles and his grandmother were in the back seat. His mother was seated in front and his father was driving the car. It had been a rainy day and visibility was poor. They were driving on a country lane when a truck had hit their car, causing the car to roll over and land on its side. Charles, his grandmother and his father were trapped in the car. His mother managed to get out of the car and ask for help from cars passing by. When the police arrived on the scene they found that they could not open the car doors. They smashed the windows and got Charles out of the car. But they had to wait for assistance to cut open the car to get his grandmother and father out. His father sustained a broken arm and his grandmother was badly hurt. Charles received a number of bruises on his head and body and was in a state of shock when he was rescued from the car. They were taken to the local hospital, X-rays were done and Charles and his parents were allowed to go home. His grandmother was admitted to hospital for treatment of her injuries, which included a fractured hip. She remained in hospital for a few weeks and was transferred to a rehabilitation hospital but her condition deteriorated and she died 3 months later.

The accident had had a severe impact on the family. Mr Hunt could not return to work for 3 months and Mrs Hunt had to give up her part time job. In addition she had also to cope with the death of her mother. Following the accident there had been a significant change in Charles's behaviour. From being outgoing and pleasant, he had become clingy, fearful and insecure. Initially he had refused to sleep alone and although he shared the room with his sister he wanted his mother to sleep with him. Over time his sleep difficulties had got better but he experienced nightmares and woke up screaming. He was frightened of the dark and insisted on having the nightlight on in his room. His sister, Molly, who had not been involved in the accident, objected to this and complained that it disturbed her sleep. Charles was also scared of dark rooms and corridors in the house. He would refuse to go to the kitchen unless he was accompanied by his parents or sister. Soon after the accident he had refused to get into the car but was now able to travel by car. However, he found it difficult to be in a car if he felt it was being driven fast and would shout, 'Slow down, slow down.' One particular problem for the family was that he became very anxious and panicky when travelling at night. The parents made sure that they did not cause him distress by undertaking night journeys. However, on one occasion, unexpectedly, there was some delay in getting back home from a visit to a family friend in Wales. As it got dark, Charles had become anxious and started shouting and crying in the car and 'gone into his panic mode'. They had to break the journey and spend the night at a hotel. But he was a 'nervous wreck' that evening and had hardly slept that night.

The parents had also noticed other changes in him. They had found him to be losing his temper easily and having tantrums. He was noticed to be shouting back at his mother and being rude to her. On one occasion he threatened to run out of the house. These behaviours, the parents said, were uncharacteristic of Charles, who had previously been a compliant and pleasant boy. Another important change that had overcome Charles was his fear of being sick. Soon after the accident he had started complaining about feeling sick and insisted on having a bowl by his side while at home. He carried this bowl around wherever he went because he was scared that he might be sick at any time. However, he had never been sick. No amount of reassurance by his parents and the GP had made him give up the bowl. Soon they had realised that it was a fear of sickness, rather than actually feeling sick that made Charles worried and upset. His fear of sickness was causing other problems too. He refused to eat when they went out to friends and relations or to restaurants. He also refused to eat anything after 5 pm in the evening for fear of being sick. In spite of these difficulties, Charles was attending school and there had been no adverse reports from there.

In the evenings there were times when Charles would become agitated and frightened for no reason. He usually clung to his mother for comfort and said in a frightened voice, 'It's coming, it's coming.' This behaviour had been happening two to three times a day but lately had got less frequent. The parents had also noticed that any loud noise made Charles jump. For example, while they were at a restaurant there had been a big bang outside and Charles was startled and went into a panic. Soon after the accident he had started to wet the bed and suck his thumb, but these had got better with time. The family attributed the change in his behaviour to the accident and its aftermath.

Developmental history: Charles's birth was normal and he had been a healthy and active baby. Apart from occasional attacks of asthma, there was no significant medical history. His developmental milestones had been normal and he had been early to walk and toilet train. He had never been to a hospital until the day of the accident. He had attended the local playgroup and later the nursery. He had socialised well with the children and had not shown any difficulty with separation from his parents. He was good at reading and drawing. He had been an energetic and vibrant boy until the accident.

Family history: The family consisted of Mr and Mrs Hunt and two children, Charles, aged 6, and Molly, aged 10 years. Mr Hunt worked for a local company and Mrs hunt had been a part time secretary. There was no significant history of psychiatric or nervous problems in the family. The death of the maternal grandmother in the accident had been a difficult issue for the family to come to terms with. Mrs Hunt blamed herself for having offered to bring her mother home for the weekend and Mr Hunt felt more could have been done by the hospital to help her recover from the fractured hip. He felt that she had been allowed to get depressed while in the rehabilitation hospital and she had refused to eat or drink and gradually 'withered away'. He felt they should have recognised the depression and treated it more aggressively.

Individual assessment of Charles: At the end of the family session, the therapist focused on Charles. Given his young age, he was seen with his mother. Charles was a short, chubby boy with short hair. Initially he was wary and appeared to be not sure as to what he was expected to do. He was given paper and felt pens and asked to draw whatever came to his mind. Charles busied himself drawing a picture of a house with a garden. He said that it was their house and indicated to the therapist where his room was in the house. This gave the opportunity of asking about his room and the difficulties he had at night. At this point in the interview Charles became chatty and appeared to be eager to talk. The therapist was careful not to bring up the issue of the accident prematurely and decided to allow Charles to take the lead.

Charles said he was scared to go to bed and did not know why he felt that way. He said he was scared at nights by the dreams he had. He described the dreams as scary but was not able to give any more details about them. When asked about what sort of thoughts came into his mind when he was trying to get sleep, he said he remembered the accident especially the 'big noise' he heard at the time of the accident. He was worried that it could happen again. Travelling by car at night was difficult because it was dark in the back seat and he felt something terrible could happen. He said that he remembered the accident every day, especially when he was on his own. The worst time was bedtime, when he kept remembering the accident in great detail. He said he remembered the 'scene' of the accident, the 'bang' and how the car rolled over. He remembered the flashing lights of the police car and the ambulance. These thoughts and 'pictures' came into his mind every day and were worse at night.

Charles talked about his grandmother and how he found her bleeding when she was pulled out of the car. He remembered being taken by ambulance to hospital and being checked out by the doctor. He had screamed when he was separated from his mother because each of them was examined separately. He talked about the sadness that engulfed him when he heard about the death of his grandmother. He had attended the funeral and he vividly remembered his mother crying at the funeral. Charles was particularly worried that another accident could happen and that all of them could get killed. When asked about his fear of being sick, Charles said that in the evenings he felt that he might be sick. Therefore, he kept the bowl with him and in case he became sick he could vomit into it. But this had never happened and he agreed what he had was a fear of sickness, rather than being sick. He said that it usually started as a funny sensation in his tummy and then he would feel that he was going to be sick and got frightened. He was reluctant to eat in the evenings out of fear of being sick. One way he had managed to do this was to have his evening meal as early as possible. He knew that his parents were worried that he was not eating enough. He had been taken to the doctor, who had commented about his being thin and having lost weight. He had encouraged him to eat more and have more milk.

Charles's ambition was to become a fireman so that he could rescue people from burning houses and vehicles. He had a number of friends at school and got on well with them and the teachers. He said he avoided the 'rowdies' in class and there were many in his class. He said he was fond of his mother and father and was worried that something might happen to them.

School report: A school report obtained later confirmed Charles's description of himself. He was described as a boy of above average ability, who was good at drawing and storytelling. The report commended his behaviour and said that he was a delightful boy. The teachers were aware of the accident but had not observed much difference in Charles's behaviour at school. He liked sports and was said to be good at swimming.

Case conceptualisation and formulation

Charles had been a well behaved and well functioning boy prior to the accident. There had been a remarkable change in him following the accident. He exhibited the typical features of post-traumatic stress disorder (PTSD) 13 months after the RTA. Re-experiencing phenomena were prominent with frequent recollections of images, thoughts and affects associated with the accident. These occurred spontaneously, especially at night and at bedtime and made him fearful and anxious. Trauma reminders such as loud noises, darkness and being driven fast triggered traumatic memories, resulting in high levels of anxiety and fear. There were prominent avoidance behaviours, including not travelling at night. Avoid-ance was also evident in the drawings he did during the initial session. Hyper-arousal was evident by the exaggerated startled response and hyper-alertness to dangers, especially when travelling by car and at night. In addition to the symptoms of PTSD described above, he also showed incident specific new behaviours, such as anger, irritability and separation anxiety, which were probably unrelated to the trauma. Regressive behaviours such as enuresis and thumb-sucking, which were evident soon after the accident, had got better at the time of assessment. Obviously Charles had been saddened by the death of his grandmother and missed her a great deal. But at the time of assessment, grief was not considered to be a significant factor in Charles's presentation.

Overall, Charles presented with the typical features of PTSD that could be expected for a child of his age. Some of the symptoms had shown improvement but he had been traumatised severely by the accident and 13 months after the accident was showing a significant degree of distress and impairment in terms of symptoms of PTSD. There was one symptom that eluded explanation at this stage, namely his fear of sickness. The therapist made a mental note to explore it in some detail in future.

A number of factors appear to have made the experience of the trauma difficult for Charles. Apart from the suddenness and the severity of the incident, the reaction of his family members was a significant contributor to Charles's distress.

His father had been injured in the accident and probably suffered with post-traumatic features as well. Neither his mother nor father had been assessed for post-traumatic features, let alone receiving any help. In a later session with the parents it became clear that in the first six months they had suffered from intrusive thoughts about the accident and fear of going too far from home but had eventually recovered from them. Their difficulties in coping with the symptoms of PTSD, litigation issues, and physical ill health no doubt interfered with their ability to support and help Charles. His grandmother's injuries, the prolonged illness and the subsequent death no doubt contributed to difficulties experienced by the family as well as Charles. Mrs Hunt in particular had been grieving the death of her mother and over the previous year the family had been under considerable stress because of the direct and indirect effects of the accident.

Theoretical perspectives

Anxiety and fear are normal responses to threatening events. Following extreme trauma intense fear, disorientation and increased arousal are common (acute traumatic reaction). These usually abate over a period of days or weeks. However, in a significant proportion of those exposed to trauma, the symptoms may last longer and show little reduction in intensity. In those instances where the psychological effects of trauma last longer than four weeks and caused significant distress and disability, it has been called postraumatic stress disorder (PTSD). The subject of PTSD has received considerable attention in the recent past because of the many manmade (bombings, war) and natural disasters (hurricanes, tsunami). The plight of children exposed to such disasters has been a particular concern. In PTSD three main groups of symptom are seen as characteristic both in adults and children:

- Re-experiencing symptoms: Recurrent and intrusive recollection of the event, recurrent dreams, intense distress on exposure to cues that symbolise or remind of the event.
- Avoidance and emotional numbing: Efforts to avoid thoughts, feelings and cues related to the event, avoidance of activities, places and people associated with the event, inability to recall important details around the events, feeling of detachment, estrangement or alienation from other people.
- Increased arousal: Hypervigilence, exaggerated startle response, sleep difficulties, irritability and anger outbursts, difficulty concentrating.

In general, older children and adolescents are more likely to exhibit adult-like PTSD symptoms. Some children with PTSD, especially those who have been exposed to multiple and chronic trauma (e.g. sexual abuse), may have prominent dissociative symptoms. Dissociation is a mental process, which produces a lack of connection in a person's thoughts, memories, feelings, actions or sense of identity. During these periods the person feels 'switched off' from reality. Dissociation may sometimes take the form of hallucinations, de-realisation, de-personalisation or disorganised thinking and behaviour. These symptoms may be difficult to distinguish from psychotic states and should be understood as manifestations of PTSD rather than a form of psychosis. In one study about 40% of severely maltreated children were found to meet the full PTSD criteria soon after being removed from their parent's care; 2 years later this figure had been shown to decrease to 33%.

While the older adolescent may manifest most of the features of PTSD mentioned above, younger children may show a somewhat different picture. Attention has been drawn to the lack of visual flashbacks, numbing symptoms and amnesia in young children. Primary school children may show frequent post-traumatic re-enactment of trauma in play, drawings or verbalisations. Sleep disturbance is particularly common in pre-pubertal children. Studies show that post-traumatic reactions are common in infants, toddlers and young children, although the presentation may vary.

Scheeringa *et al.* (1995) have proposed an alternative checklist to DSM-IV criteria for detecting PTSD in young children (under 4 years) on the basis of analysis of 25 previous studies (*see* Table 13.1). These authors differentiate between post-traumatic play (which is compulsively repetitive, represents part of the trauma and fails to relieve anxiety) and play re-enactment (which also represents part of the trauma but is less repetitive and more like the child's pre-trauma play). Either of these may fulfil the re-experiencing criteria, as can non-play recollections of trauma (which are not necessarily distressing) or nightmares. They also suggest that in the avoidance/numbing category, only one of the following is required: constriction of play (with or without post-traumatic play), social withdrawal, restriction of range of affect or loss of acquired temperamental skills. They also propose that a new category of symptoms, new fears and/or aggression be considered a part of post-traumatic stress response.

Table 13.1 Key features of post-traumatic disorder in young children (under 4 years of age) (Scheeringa *et al.*, 1995)

Re-experiencing	Avoidance	Increased arousal	New behaviours
Post-traumatic play	Constriction of play	Night terrors	New aggression
Play re-enactment	Social withdrawal	Difficulty going to sleep	New separation anxiety
Recurrent recollections of the traumatic events	Restricted range of affect	Night walking	New fear of the dark
Nightmares	Loss of acquired developmental skills	Decreased concentration	Fear of toileting alone
Flashbacks or dissociation		Hypervigilance/ exaggerated startle response	New fears not related to trauma

One of the earliest and best known studies on PTSD in children is Lenore Terr's 'Chowchilla Study' (Terr, 1979). She followed up 26 school-aged (age 5–14 years) children who were kidnapped from their school bus by three armed men in 1976. The kidnappers drove the children for 11 hours in a van with blackened windows. They were then buried in an underground truck trailer. After spending 16–17 hours underground they managed to escape. All of the children developed PTSD symptoms. This prospective study with controls demonstrated that children could suffer from devastating psychic trauma if the trauma was extreme enough and was directly experienced. In this study incidence of PTSD was 100%. Numerous other studies with children and adolescent survivors of traumatic experiences have been carried out since. Notable amongst these studies are those carried out by Yule and colleagues (2000) following the sinking of the cruise ship, *Jupiter*, in 1988. They assessed 200 child and adolescent survivors of the disaster and demonstrated that the children displayed many of the typical post-traumatic reactions shown by adult survivors. Child symptoms included re-experiencing the event with repetitive intrusive thoughts and flashbacks, avoidance reactions and increased arousal. Half the survivors had symptoms that met the criteria for PTSD. Many had depression and anxiety as well as a range of other symptoms, including separation difficulties. In many cases the debilitating effects of the disaster resulted in adjustment difficulties at school, home and with peers. About one third recovered within 1 year, but one quarter still suffered from the disorder after 5 years (Yule *et al.* 2000). This study illustrates three features of the response to a single event disaster:

1 not all children experiencing a traumatic event develop PTSD
2 of those with PTSD many recover over time and
3 the rates of PTSD are high and in a high proportion of them the symptoms persist.

Precipitants of PTSD: PTSD can follow any frightening event that is perceived by the child as being threatening. Defining the stresses that lead to PTSD in children has been problematic. There has been a growing recognition that subjective evaluation of the threat by the child or adolescent is directly related to processing trauma related information.

What constitutes a traumatic event? The list is long. In general, exposure to violence, witnessing murder, rape and suicidal behaviour, experiencing sexual or physical abuse, severe accidental injury, road traffic accidents and natural disasters are considered to be traumatic events. A number of authors have made a distinction between single event PTSD and multiple events or chronic stressors that lead to PTSD. Terr (1991) conceptualised two types of PTSD determined by the type of trauma experienced. She suggests that Type I traumas (one sudden blow traumas, such as a motor vehicle accident or sniper attack) result in classic DSM symptoms of re-experiencing, avoidance and increased arousal, whereas experiencing Type II traumas (variable, multiple, long-standing traumas, such as ongoing child physical and sexual abuse) result in denial, numbing, dissociation and rage. Other authors have drawn attention to the differences between witnessing traumatic events (e.g. seeing a murder) and experiencing trauma (e.g. being shot).

There are important differences between children who experience child sexual abuse and one off traumatic events. Abuse occurs in the context of severe parental dysfunction, parental conflicts, psychiatric disorders and poor parenting. Typically, abuse occurs on many occasions over a period of time and the relationship of the abuser to the child is crucial in determining the effect on the child. Investigating the cause–effect relationship in chronic sexual abuse has been fraught with difficulties because of the confounding variables that impact on the child. For example, a child placed with foster parents following child sexual abuse may have experienced many of the following adverse experiences:

dysfunctional parenting, parental conflict and violence, exposure to protracted investigations, removal from home, separation from parents and repeated placements outside home.

Mediating factors: A number of studies have examined mediating factors in the development of PTSD in children. A review of 25 studies (Foy *et al.*, 1996) indicates that three factors have been found to consistently mediate the development of PTSD in children:

- the severity of the traumatic exposure
- trauma related parental distress
- temporal proximity to traumatic events.

There is universal acknowledgement that every person will experience psychological distress if the stressor is severe enough. There is a direct dose–response relationship between the perceived severity of trauma and the post-traumatic response. Although the objective severity of trauma is directly proportional to the stress reaction, subjective factors are important in mediating the effects. The implications of these findings are that both subjective and objective factors must be taken into account in making a full assessment of the child. The clinician should not only try to get a clear account of the traumatic event in detail but also attempt to gather as much information as possible about the child's perception and experience of what occurred. It is, therefore, important to ask the child what they expected to happen to them and to others during the event and whom they hold responsible for them.

In addition to the severity and degree of threat to the child, an important factor that influences the development of PTSD symptoms is the reaction of the parent/ parents to the event. Children who see their parents in an overwhelming state of distress react to traumatic events more adversely than when parents cope with the trauma better. It is particularly important where the trauma involves both the child and the parent. The child who witnesses a mother who is injured and hospitalised experiences separation anxiety and panic in addition to the initial trauma experience. Often the picture is complicated by the fact that in instances where parents too suffer from PTSD this can impede the recovery of children from the effects of trauma. The third factor shown to be of importance is the period of time that has lapsed after the event. In a 7-year follow-up study of adolescent survivors of the *Jupiter* sinking, Yule *et al.* (1990) found that overall 50% of survivors had presented with PTSD at some point, mainly in the first few months. At 7-year follow-up around 15% still met the criteria for PTSD, with many others showing signs of stress reaction that were not sufficient to meet diagnostic criteria. A high proportion was depressed and although the numbers are small, the rate of suicide attempts was threefold that of a group of matched controls (Yule *et al.* 2000). The longest follow-up study so far is the study of children involved in the Aberfan landslide. Thirty three years after the event almost 30% of those interviewed met the criteria for PTSD (Morgan *et al.*, 2003). Thus PTSD in children and adolescents must be considered as a seriously disabling disorder that can lead to interference in development and adjustment over many years.

Several studies have documented significant comorbidity of childhood PTSD with other psychiatric disorders. Clinical depression is the commonest disorder that is associated with PTSD. There is debate as to whether the depressive symptoms are part of PTSD or whether PTSD precipitates or leads to depressive symptomology. A number of reports record comorbidity between PTSD and other anxiety disorders such as panic disorder, as well as substance misuse. The relationship between PTSD and externalising behaviour problems seems obscure. Many case studies have implicated an association between chronic PTSD and borderline personality disorder, particularly in sexually abused children. Studies show that most adult females with a diagnosis of borderline personality disorder report sexual abuse during their childhood. It has been suggested that borderline personality disorder represents very severe and chronic manifestation of PTSD and has been termed 'complex PTSD' by some authors.

Psychological models of PTSD: At present a variety of psychological models have been put forward that addresses the different features of the disorder. All of the models account for some aspects of the disorder but no one single theory has captured the entirety of the manifestations or has the power to explain all the features seen in PTSD. Ehlers and Clark (2000) have put forward a cognitive model of PTSD that attempts to explain several PTSD phenomena and provide a framework for treatment. They suggest that PTSD becomes persistent when individuals process the trauma in a way which produces a sense of serious current threat. They hypothesise that this state of affairs is thought to arise from three sources:

1 Disturbance of autobiographical memory: Traumatic memories are different from normal autobiographical memories in that they are poorly elaborated and contexualised.
2 Negative appraisals of trauma and/or its consequences: Self-blame, guilt, over-responsibility regarding the traumatic event are common in PTSD.
3 Maintaining behaviours: These include behavioural and cognitive strategies such as avoidance, dissociation and thought suppression, which may lead to temporary relief from negative affect but, in the long term, help maintain the symptoms.

The cognitive neuroscience view of memory suggests that memory is composed of multiple systems (autobiographical, episodic, declarative and so on). It has now been proposed that memories of personally experienced traumatic events can be of two distinct types (Brewin, 2001):

• Verbally accessible memories (VAM): These are ordinary autobiographical memories that are narrative-based, coherent, easily retrieved and have a 'there and then' quality.
• Situationally accessible memory (SAM): These are specific trauma-related memories that are triggered automatically, are vivid and detailed yet fragmentary and incoherent. They are difficult to express in words and have a 'here and now' quality.

Flashbacks, trauma-related dreams and intense emotions associated with the trauma are features of SAM. SAM memories are difficult to control and the emotions that accompany them are restricted to those that were experienced during the trauma such as fear and helplessness. Different parts of the brain are thought to be associated with the two systems of memory. The treatment implications of the model are that for one to 'work through' the trauma memories change is required in three areas (Ehler and Clark, 2000):

- The trauma memory needs to be elaborated and integrated into the person's existing 'normal' autobiographical memory.
- Distorted appraisals of the trauma and/or its consequences need to be modified.
- Dysfunctional behavioural and cognitive strategies that prevent elaboration or deter reassessment of appraisal should be abolished.

Effective interventions are those that achieve change in these three areas. Recent studies have provided preliminary support for several aspects of the model.

Rating scales to measure PTSD symptoms: There are several rating scales that assess the effect of trauma in children and adolescents. One such scale suitable for children above 8 years is the 8-item Impact of Events Scale-Revised (IES-R; Yule, 1997). Subsequently this was expanded to a 13-item version (CRIES 13) that measures the various symptoms of PTSD. Scores can be calculated for three subscales: intrusion, avoidance and hyperarousal. It has been used in children in Kosovo and Bosnia since the war. It is considered to be a sound screening instrument and is available online at www.childrenandwar.org/CRIES-13.doc.

Choice of treatment and management

Despite the high prevalence of childhood trauma, studies regarding psychotherapy for children suffering from PTSD are scarce, especially regarding the treatment for paediatric PTSD following single-incident trauma. Treatment practices for this population rely mainly on the paradigms of therapy for adult PTSD and paediatric PTSD following sexual abuse. No evidence exists that a particular treatment approach (e.g. individual, group or family) of delivery of the therapeutic treatment is superior. The best available evidence supports outpatient *trauma-focused* psychotherapy containing cognitive-behavioural components, including exposure strategies, stress management, cognitive/narrative re-structuring and parental treatment components. While psychotropic medication has been found to be helpful in reducing symptoms of PTSD in adults, in children and adolescents, their use has little to add to psychological management. The National Institute for Health and Clinical Excellence (NICE) has recently reviewed the evidence base for the treatment of PTSD in adults and children and recommends trauma-focused cognitive behavioural therapy (TFCBT) and eye movement desensitisation and reprocessing (EMDR) as the two first-line treatments for PTSD (NICE, 2005).

Individual trauma-focused therapy: There is general consensus that the cornerstone of treatment involves helping the individual re-experience the trauma and its meaning in affectively tolerable doses in the context of a safe environment (Pynoos, 1990). Only in this way, it seems, can the overwhelming traumatic experiences be mastered and integrated into the person's personality and emotional life. The essence of most effective treatments for PTSD involves the reconstruction and repetition of a detailed oral or written trauma narrative. How this principle is applied to children and adolescents depends on their developmental level.

There is now general consensus that psychotherapy in children with PTSD should be *trauma-focused*. Non-directive forms of therapy including non-directive play therapy, individual child psychotherapy and counselling have little place in the treatment of children with PTSD. Such techniques avoid directly discussing the traumatic event and reinforce the child's own avoidance of talking about the trauma. The reluctance on the part of many therapists to directly discuss trauma-related issues with the child is often related to their own anxieties about the need not to upset the child. Parental emotional reaction to the traumatic event and parental support of the child are powerful mediators of the child's PTSD symptoms. Most authors describing treatment for children with PTSD recommend including one or more parent directed components. Others have used parents as cotherapists.

Clinical consensus among experts in the field suggests that the essential components of any form of treatment for children with PTSD include the following:

- direct exploration of the traumatic event and its impact with the child
- exposure techniques
- exploration and correction of inaccurate attributions and cognitive assumptions regarding the traumatic event
- use of specific stress management techniques
- inclusion of parents in treatment.

EMDR: Francine Shapiro, an American psychologist, first described EMDR in 1989 as a psychological treatment to alleviate the distress associated with traumatic memories. During EMDR, the patient is asked to attend to emotionally disturbing material, e.g. a distressing traumatic image in brief sequential doses whilst simultaneously focusing on an external stimulus such as eye movements, hand taps or bilateral audio stimulation. Therapists usually encourage patients to focus on traumatic material for around 25 eye movements over a 1–2 minute period. Brief feedback is then obtained about any noticeable cognitive, emotional or physical changes. Further eye movements are then made with the patient focusing on this new material. This process continues until the individual reports a subjective reduction in levels of distress related to the traumatic experience. An individual treatment session normally lasts around 90 minutes and several sessions might be required to process an individual memory or image (Shapiro, 2000). Research into its effectiveness shows that EMDR performed as well as exposure-based therapies (Davidson and Parker, 2001). The meta-analysis on which the NICE recommendations are based also resulted in similar conclusions.

Management plan for Charles

The main objectives of treatment for Charles were to:

1 reduce Charles's intrusive thoughts
2 restore sleep and reduce nightmares and
3 reduce fears associated with trauma reminders.

Charles was seen weekly (initially with parents) and parents-only sessions were held fortnightly.

Individual sessions with Charles: In the first treatment session Charles was seen in the presence of his mother. The therapist told Charles that he had seen a number of children who had experienced the same sort of problems that he had been through and that the purpose of the sessions was to help him understand what happened in the accident and try to overcome his various fears. He was told that the sessions would involve drawing, playing and talking. A box with paper, felt-tip pens, crayons, some string, scissors, human figures and plasticine was provided. He was told that the box and its contents were for his exclusive use during the therapy period. They would be discussing the accident and what happened thereafter. The therapist told him it was only natural that Charles felt upset and frightened whenever he was reminded about the accident. Most children who have been through bad accidents, he was told, had bad dreams and all sorts of fears and worries. But these things got less and less with time. The purpose of the sessions was to help Charles get over the frightening dreams and thoughts that he experienced as soon as possible.

Next he was asked to draw some scenes from the accident as he saw and remembered it. (Some therapists might have begun with free drawing; in Charles's case the therapist's judgement was that Charles would not be too upset by drawing the trauma scene.) Charles hesitated for a while and wanted to know whether he should use the pencils or felt-tips. The therapist asked Charles to make the choice. Charles chose felt-tip pens saying that with felt-tips he could use various colours in the drawing. Unprompted by the therapist, Charles then proceeded to draw an upturned car and the vehicle that hit it. He drew himself lying down by their side. The therapist encouraged him to put more details into the picture and asked him to describe the scene in some detail. He drew bodies by the roadside and said one of them was his grandmother, the other was his father. At every step the therapist asked for more details and vivid descriptions including the colour, smell and sounds, as well as Charles's feelings at various moments during the accident. He was requested to describe the events in the present tense 'as if it was happening now'.

He said that he was seated in the back seat, together with his grandmother. Both of them were wearing seatbelts and his grandmother had given him a sandwich to eat. It was dark in the car and it was raining outside. His grandmother had been talking to him about taking him on holiday with her. Suddenly there was a big crash, he heard a big noise and he was jolted from the seat. He realised that the car was turning around and that everybody was shouting. He remembered his grandmother falling on him and he was squeezed underneath. He was sure he saw some sparks. He had pains in his chest and thought he was going to die. He heard his parents trying to open the car door and then scream that the door had got locked. He could not remember what he said but he knew he was shouting and crying. He was quite sure that every one of them was going to die. He did not remember how he was pulled out of the car but felt it was a long time before he was rescued. He said that during the time that he was in the car, he felt trapped and suffocated. He felt sick and dizzy and wished it would end soon.

The therapist wanted him to tell the story in 'slow motion' paying attention to how he felt and what he experienced. Charles described the sound of metal crashing, the smell of something burning and the screams that followed. He described the sight of blood on his body but was not sure whose blood it was. He had pain in his right knee but it was not severe. He remembered that he kept rubbing his knee. He said when he was in the car his heart was beating so fast that he could hear it. He felt the heaviness of his grandmother on him and could not move his limbs. Strangely he did not feel much pain until they arrived in hospital. He could not remember what injuries he had. He was sure he was not bleeding.

He said that when he was trapped in the car it was hot and he was sweating. He remembered that when he came out it was very cold and he started shivering and a policeman gave him a blanket. He remembered his grandmother being carried in a stretcher to the ambulance and he was able to describe the trip to the hospital. He had been clinging to his mother and had vomited all over her while in the ambulance. He said everything looked as if it was happening in a dream and he thought, 'this is not true; it was not really happening'. He felt he would wake up from the dream and everything would be alright.

While at the hospital his mother was taken for examination, leaving him on his own, and he had screamed so much that they allowed him to accompany her. He described the smell of antiseptic in the hospital and remembered a doctor examining him and cleaning his wounds. He had had a few cuts on his body and arms. He drew his shirt over his head to show the therapist the scars in his arms and abdomen. It was late at night that they got back home and he cried on his way back home because his grandmother had been left at the hospital. He kept asking his parents, 'Is she going to die?' He said that nobody in the family slept that night. They huddled together in one bed. He remembered that his father had his arm in a plaster. He did not go to school for the next few days. They went to see his grandmother in hospital. He was relieved that she was alive and she had told him that she was getting better.

Throughout the account of the incident, Charles was alert and stiff. His voice trembled at times and sometimes his drawings became untidy because his hand was shaking, especially when he was describing the heat and stuffiness while he was trapped inside the car. He was introduced to the concept of the fear thermometer and asked about what his 'temperature' was when he was talking about the incident. He said when he started talking about the accident it was at 6 (out of 10) but then later it came down to 4. The therapist said that in future the therapist would check with him to see where the temperature was at any given moment when they discussed the accident. Before the end of the session he was asked what he found most difficult to talk about. Charles felt that describing how he felt while he was trapped in the car was about the most difficult thing to discuss because he had never thought about before. He said the 'temperature' was close to 8 and he was sweating for a short time. Before ending the session he was praised for the courage that he had displayed in describing the accident and the therapist acknowledged how difficult it was for him to re-experience it. It was agreed that he would bring a toy car and a toy truck to one of the subsequent sessions to demonstrate how the accident happened.

It was noted that Charles had been eating during the accident and been sick following the accident. It was hypothesised that his fear of sickness arose from this experience. He seemed to have linked the accident with the feeling of sickness and hence it could be conceptualised as re-experiencing phenomenon. In one of the sessions the issue of feeling sick was discussed. Charles was able to talk about 'normal sickness' as he experienced it when he had been ill with bronchitis and asthma in the past before the accident had occurred. The therapist wondered whether the feeling of sickness reminded him of the accident. Charles was not very sure of it.

Drawing and narration: In later sessions a technique was used with Charles which involved drawing the worst two moments of the accident. The worst moment for Charles was when he felt trapped in the car and felt the weight of his grandmother on him together with the screaming and the hotness he experienced. This was named scene 1. The second worst scene was that of his grandmother being lifted out of the car and there being blood all over her (named scene 2). In the initial exposure sessions, Charles was required to give detailed verbal descriptions of scene 2 while drawing a picture of it to aid visualisation. He was encouraged to give a very detailed verbal account of the scene. Charles was asked to draw a large picture of the scene when he saw his grandmother pulled out of the car (*see* Figure 13.1). Entire sessions were spent on drawing scene 2 and describing it in great detail. He was asked to describe the bodily sensations he experienced, the sweating, feeling sick, pounding of the heart and the sight of his grandmother, the blood and what he thought would happen next. He was instructed to describe the event in the first person and in the present tense. In addition, details of responses in terms of sight, sound, touch, taste and smell were evoked. Charles was guided through the description with questions evoking details of thoughts and feelings. He was also instructed to 'rewind' to particularly distressing images and to visualise and hold images until his distress diminished. With each session, exposure continued for approximately 20 minutes and his fear temperature ratings were recorded.

Following each subsequent exposure session his fear levels came down progressively and he was able to recollect the scene with relative ease. In later sessions similar exposure was carried out for scene 1 and repeated several times. At this point his parents were encouraged to undertake the exposure programme at home for his fear of travelling by car at night using systemic desensitisation techniques. Initially he was to be driven for not more than 10 minutes at night as he sat in the back seat of the car with his mother. Later the time period was to be increased by 10 minutes and later he was to sit on his own in the back seat for longer and longer distances. He was taught deep breathing to relax himself during the exercise.

Subsequent sessions were devoted to exposure to combined scenes 1 and 2. In a later session Charles felt he was ready to bring a toy car and truck to enact the accident in the session. Most of the session was spent describing how the accident happened. Although Charles did not see the truck coming towards them, he had an idea about the truck coming from a side road and hitting the car. He replayed how the car had turned over. He remembered some new details, like when the glass window was smashed, and said that some of the cuts he had sustained were probably from the glass. He described the loud noise and the shock that it gave him.

Imaginal exposure: Another technique that was used with Charles was exposure in imagination. In this session first he was asked to do regular deep breathing and undergo progressive muscle relaxation. Then he was asked to imagine scene 2 with his grandmother being lifted out of the car. The therapist took him through the various sensations and emotions he experienced and asked him to think about various details of the scene, including the sight of blood, the smells and the shouting that accompanied the scene. To help him stay with the memory, he was repeatedly asked questions such as 'What do you see?', 'How does that feel?' and Where do you feel that?' Charles found the first imaginal exposure exercise, which took more than 30 minutes, easy and said initially his fear temperature had risen to 6 but later he felt more comfortable and at the end

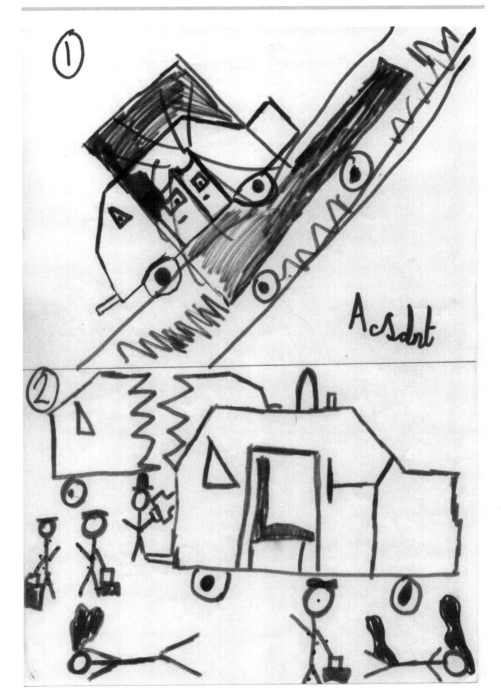

Figure 13.1

of the session in fact he felt relieved. This exercise was repeated twice over the next sessions.

During another session imaginal exposure to scene 1 was carried out. On this occasion, following preparation (deep breathing and relaxation), he was asked to imagine scene 1 and put himself in the trapped car and the therapist took him through the various sensations and emotions he experienced and asked him to think about various details of the scene, including the weight of his grandmother, the sense of suffocation and the shouting. Unexpectedly, Charles became tense and agitated during the *in vivo* exposure to scene 1 and reported feeling sick. He wanted to know if he could have a bowl to vomit into. The therapist talked him through a relaxation session and controlled breathing. It took 10 minutes or so for his anxiety levels to return to normal. This session proved to the therapist that his fear of vomiting was indeed associated with the trauma. For Charles it also was proof that he could control the fear of vomiting. Charles did well during the relaxation exercise, which took more than 30 minutes, and said initially his fear temperature had risen to 8 but later he felt more comfortable and at the end of the session in fact he felt relieved. The exposure exercise was repeated in subsequent sessions.

Charles blamed the driver of the truck for causing the accident. He said the driver had been drunk. He was weepy when he talked about the death of his grandmother and how she had hoped to take him on holiday. When asked whether he could have done anything to prevent the accident or the death of his grandmother, he said he was not very sure anything could have been done but he said that the doctors could have done more to save his grandmother from dying after she went into the rehabilitation hospital. Clearly he was echoing the family's opinion of blame for grandmother's death. In some of the sessions the focus was on bereavement issues associated with his grandmother's death to aid him through the bereavement process. During this period the family visited grandmother's grave and laid flowers.

Externalising intrusive thoughts: Charles was also taught techniques to help gain control over intrusive re-experiencing symptoms. This was through a process of externalisation where Charles was helped to think about thoughts as something from outside the body that got into his head and occupied it and got him worried. He was to learn methods of keeping these thoughts away the way a goalkeeper kept a football away from the goal (Charles was very interested in football and was a good football player). He was to hold the thought and throw it way or, if it was too strong, he was to deflect it over the goalpost. In effect this included postponement of the thought and distraction. He was also to set aside some time to practice goalkeeping of thoughts. This involved periods of about 10 minutes during which he would sit in a chair comfortably and try to get the thoughts into his mind. Charles found these techniques intriguing and very quickly mastered the principle behind them. The parents had been prepared to help him practice his behaviours and use progressive relaxation techniques when appropriate.

During the course of therapy, Charles reported that the nightmares were getting less and that he was getting better at sleeping in his own bed without calling for his mother. He was encouraged to try to overcome his fear of the dark and take chances to walk to the kitchen from the drawing room. The therapist made a link between the experience of feeling trapped in a dark car and his difficulties in travelling by car at night and wondered whether it triggered off memories of the accident. Charles was not sure, but agreed to think about it when he was next travelling by car at night. By now, Charles had stopped carrying the bowl around. But he continued to feel nauseous in the evenings. A discussion about how the brain got messages from the stomach was discussed. The therapist said it was likely that he was getting false messages and that the best way of coping with them was to be able to relax at times like that. He was taught deep breathing and muscle relaxation and encouraged to use such techniques whenever he felt sick.

Parent sessions: The aim of parent sessions was to explain Charles's difficulties on the basis of his traumatic stress symptoms. During the discussion it became clear that father too had flashbacks and re-experiencing phenomena. He was very bitter that the compensation claim had not been properly dealt with by the insurance company. He continued to have dizzy spells and headaches because of a whiplash injury. He was asked to contact his GP to get help with both his physical and post-traumatic problems. The family was surprised that the nausea that Charles complained about might be linked to the accident. This made them feel sympathetic towards Charles because in the past the family, especially his sister, had blamed Charles for being a 'sissy' and carrying about a bowl like 'a beggar'. The therapist impressed upon the family how trauma reminders could bring on anxiety. Charles's difficulty in travelling in the car at night was discussed and it was agreed that after some preparation in individual sessions, they would take him on car rides at night, starting with a 5–10 minute ride and gradually increasing the time to an hour and more.

Progress and outcome

In all, individual work with Charles involved 16 weekly treatment sessions. The first symptom to improve was his sleep problems. There was dramatic improvement in nighttime sleep as he reported fewer nightmares. He was also able to sleep without asking to be comforted by his mother at night. At this time he said he was getting less frightened by the intrusive thoughts of the accident. He was getting better at ignoring them. Later he reported that the intrusive thoughts were getting less and that he was able to fight them back using the goalkeeper metaphor. In parallel with these improvements, his anger outbursts and irritability got progressively better.

The family organised the exposure exercises for travelling by car at night, starting with 10-minute rides and increasing them to 30 minutes. Charles gradually got better at managing his fear and anxiety although he did not use the relaxation exercises. He said he found the exercises a 'bore'. The fear of sickness took longer to overcome. Although he was able to stop using the bowl, on questioning he said that he still experienced nausea by nighttime but he was eating normally and was able to eat at normal hours and when the family went out. Overall there was very good improvement by the 16th session.

Before he was discharged a final session was held which involved imaginal exposure to scenes 1 and 2 combined. Charles reported that his fear temperature was 3 during the exposure session, confirming that Charles had, to a large extent, overcome the PTSD symptoms. His father had received some help from local psychiatric services for his PTSD symptoms and had also been seen by a neurologist for his dizzy spells and whiplash injuries. Before termination of sessions, the family was asked to visit the site of the accident and spent some time inspecting the place and talking about what had happened. The exercise was a success and none of the family members including Charles reported much anxiety or fear.

Three months after discharge the therapist telephoned the family and spoke to the parents and Charles to find out how they were progressing. They reported that Charles had been on a trip to Wales and he had been able to sit in the car on a night trip which had lasted more than 2 hours and had, in fact, fallen asleep.

Comments

The treatment of Charles was considered to be relatively easy. The family was co-operative and understood the problems associated with PTSD, which made them treat Charles with more sympathy and consideration. The traumatic event was a single event and the degree of trauma was relatively mild judging by the severity of symptoms. Fortunately, for Charles it was not complicated by bereavement issues. Charles proved to be resilient and resourceful and undertook the exposure exercises without much reluctance. The main concern for the therapist was to provide sufficient exposure to bring about habituation without overstepping the mark. The sessions were prolonged and sometimes took 90 minutes before Charles's anxiety hit baseline. This happened particularly during the first few sessions. Imaginal exposure was hard going compared to exposure through drawings and play.

Treatment of PTSD, especially single event PTSD, produces good outcomes and is gratifying to treat as long as it is well planned and properly executed. The techniques of exposure need to be adapted to the developmental level of the child and his or her inclinations. Some adolescents are good at writing about their experience while others may 'think in pictures' and have good iconic imagination. Using the strengths of children to achieve exposure to the traumatic memories requires flexibility and adaptability on the part of the therapist. Technique matters little as long as the aim of treatment – 'helping the individual re-experience the trauma and its meaning in affectively tolerable doses in the context of a safe environment' is achieved (Pynos, 1995).

Unfortunately PTSD is common in children seen in CAMHS but often remains undetected. Many minor aversive experiences like bullying and mugging sometimes produce post-traumatic reactions which may not fulfil the diagnostic criteria for PTSD but can be equally as disabling as the full syndrome. Well-placed screening questions may help identify post-traumatic symptoms. At the other extreme, some children who have been subjected to chronic and unremitting trauma present a 'mixed' clinical picture in which other behaviours might overshadow PTSD features. This is especially true of children who have been physically or sexually abused. Child sexual abuse is a particularly malignant form of abuse and may present with various symptoms including those of PTSD. The treatment of PTSD in child sexual abuse is discussed here because often the PTSD features go undetected and untreated in this population of children.

Treatment of PTSD in child sexual abuse: Research on child sexual abuse shows that the impact of child sexual abuse is highly variable. Although no specific syndrome of post-sexual abuse has been identified, studies suggest that more than 50% of sexually abused children meet partial or full criteria for post-traumatic stress disorder. As with any potentially traumatic experience, the effects depend not only on the characteristics of the incident but also on the child's vulnerability and resilience. Two thirds to one half of sexually abused children appear to improve over time but many either do not improve or deteriorate. Post-traumatic symptoms may be triggered in traumatised children by

1 trauma reminders
2 loss reminders and
3 change reminders.

Many of the problematic behaviours of sexually abused children are often related to one or more of these reminders and it behoves the clinician to make the links so that it makes sense to the carers.

There has been a recent increase in the number of empirical studies evaluating treatment outcome for sexually abused children (Saywitz *et al.*, 2000). All studies consistently favour *abuse-specific* CBT over other forms of treatment. As Saywitz *et al.* say, 'It bears repeating, however, that there is little empirical support for generic therapies applied indiscriminately to all cases regardless of the referral question. Hence, as with referrals for traditional psychiatric disorders or other potentially traumatic events, clinicians who work with sexually abused children need to think strategically. Specific symptoms need to be targeted with specific strategies.'

Specific elements of the TF-CBT model typically include the following:

- **Exposure/direct discussion of the traumatic event:** Exposure, whether intense and prolonged (such as imaginal flooding) or graduated (such as gradual exposure) involves ongoing exposure to specific stimuli that are associated with the traumatic event.
- **Cognitive interventions:** Cognitive distortions may occur as a part of the attempt to understand or explain why the traumatic event occurred. Self-blame, survivor guilt, overestimation of danger and a view of the world as unsafe are common. Correcting cognitive errors by identifying, evaluating and eventually correcting them is a part of the CBT approach.
- **Stress management:** Relaxation and thought stopping or thought replacement are typically used to reduce arousal.
- **Parental treatment:** The parental treatment component is an important element of TF-CBT and consists of the following:
  - exploring their own thoughts and feelings about the child's experience and resolving their personal trauma related distress
  - learning effective parenting skills
  - providing optimal support for their children.

Recently there has been a deluge of publications that attest to the effectiveness of TF-CBT in children who have been sexually abused. One such study was a multisite randomised controlled trial for children with sexual abuse-related PTSD symptoms conducted by Cohen *et al.* (2004) that examined the differential efficacy of trauma focused cognitive behaviour therapy and child centred therapy for treating PTSD and related emotional and behaviour problems in children who had suffered sexual abuse. This was a large study consisting of 229 children aged 8–14 years and their primary caretakers. The children had significant symptoms of PTSD with 89% meeting the full DSM for PTSD criteria. A total of 90% of the children had experienced traumatic events in addition to sexual abuse, such as sudden unexpected death or life-threatening illness of a loved one, witnessed domestic violence or other PTSD-level traumatic events such as medical trauma or traumatic custody situations. Analysis of the results indicated that children assigned to TF-CBT compared to those assigned to child-centred therapy demonstrated significantly more improvement with regard to PTSD, depression, behaviour problems, shame and abuse related attributions.

Box 13.1 Research on PTSD in children and adults says that . . .

- About half the children exposed to single incident trauma exhibit features of PTSD.
- In a high proportion of such children symptoms persist for more than 5 years.
- For treatment to be effective, interventions need to be trauma-specific.
- The basic requirement of effective treatments is 'emotional reliving' of the trauma in tolerable doses in a supportive therapeutic environment.
- Two methods of treatment have been shown to be effective: trauma-focused CBT (TF-CBT) and eye movement desensitisation and reprocessing (EMDR).
- PTSD is common in child abuse but often goes undetected.

References

Brewin CR. A cognitive neuroscience account of posttraumatic stress disorder and its treatment and behaviour. *Research and Therapy*. 2001; **39**: 373–93.

Cohen JA, Deblinger E, Mannarino AP. A multisite, randomized controlled trial of children with sexual abuse-related symptoms. *Journal of American Academy of Child and Adolescent Psychiatry*. 2004; **43**(4): 393–402.

Davidson PR, Parker KCH. Eye Movement Desensitisation and Reprocessing (EMDR): a meta analysis. *Journal of Consulting Clinical Psychology*. 2001; **69**: 305–16.

Ehlers A, Clark DM. A cognitive model of post-traumatic stress disorder. *Behaviour Research and Therapy*. 2000; **38**: 319–45.

Foy DW, Madvig BT, Pynoos RS *et al*. Etilogical factors in the development of post-traumatic stress disorder in children and adolescents. *Journal of School Psychology*. 1996; **34**: 133–45.

Morgan L, Scourfield J, Williams D *et al*. The Aberfan disaster: A thirty three year follow up of survivors. *British Journal of Psychiatry*. 2003; **182**: 532–6.

NICE (National Institute for Health and Clinical Excellence). *The Management of PTSD in Adults and Children in Primary Care and Secondary Care*. Clinical Practice Guideline Number 26. London: Department of Health; 2005. Available at www.nice.org.uk/page.aspx?o= CG026.

*Pynoos RS, Eth S. Witness to violence: The child interview. *Journal of the American Academy of Child and Adolescent Psychiatry*. 1986; **25**: 306–19.

*Saywitz K, Mannarino AP, Berliner L. Treatment of sexually abused children and adolescents. *American Psychologist*. 2000; **55**(9): 1040–49.

*Scheeringa MS, Zeanah CH, Drell MJ *et al*. Two approaches to diagnosing post-traumatic stress disorder in infancy and early childhood. *Journal of the American Academy of Child and Adolescent Psychiatry*. 1995; **34**: 191–200.

Shapiro F. *Eye Movement Desensitisation and Reprocessing: Basic principles, protocols and procedures*. 2nd edn. New York: Guildford Press; 2000.

Terr LC. Childhood trauma: an outline and overview. *American Journal of Psychiatry*. 1991; **148**: 10–20.

Terr LC. Children of Chowchilla: a study of psychic terror. *The Psychoanalytic Study of the Child.* 1979; **34**: 1543–50.

Yule W, Bolton D, Udwin O *et al.* The long term psychological effects of a disaster experienced in adolescence – I: the incidence and course of PTSD. *Journal of Child Psychology and Psychiatry.* 2000; **4**: 503–11.

Yule W, Udwin O, Murdoch K. The 'Jupiter' sinking: effects on children's fears, depression and anxiety. *Journal of Child Psychology and Psychiatry.* 1990; **31**: 279–95.

Yule W. *Anxiety, Stress and Post-traumatic Stress in Childhood. Child psychology portfolio.* London: NFER-Nelson; 1997.

Chapter 14

Deliberate self-harm I: overdose

The referral arrived by fax from the paediatric ward. It was a routine referral for assessment of deliberate self-harm (DSH) and was in keeping with the protocol agreed between the hospital paediatric services and the local CAMHS. The patient had been admitted the previous evening. The referral form had been completed but was cryptic and short in detail:

> Name: Amrit Dhaliwal
> Age: 15 years 6 months (Date of birth given)
> Arrival at A & E: 9.40 pm Friday (date given)
> Seen in A & E: 10.05 p. m. Friday
> Admitted to (name of ward): 10.10 p. m.
> Parents: Mr & Mrs Dhaliwal
> Complaint: Taken 30 tablets of paracetamol around 9.00 p. m.
> Reason for OD unclear. ?family problems. No past history of OD.
> Examination: Conscious, reluctant to give history.
> To be seen by CAMHS. Patient fit to be interviewed.

On receiving the referral the CAMHS worker telephoned the ward to make two clarifications: Who had parental responsibility and had the social services been involved with her or her family? Did the parents speak English and was there a need for an interpreter when seeing the family? The reply was straightforward. Amrit lived with her parents and social services have not been involved. In short, the parents had legal responsibility for her. On the second question, both parents spoke English and there was no need for an interpreter. A time was arranged for Amrit and her family to be seen in the ward.

Clinical presentation and background

On going through the clinical notes in the ward it was found that Amrit had told the ward doctor that she took 30 tablets of paracetamol around 9.00 p.m. 'because she had been under pressure from school'. She had been treated at A&E. Medical investigations showed that she had paracetamol in her blood but the levels were not high enough to warrant active treatment. She had been kept in the ward overnight until she could be seen by CAMHS on 'the next working day'.

The nurse looking after her said that she had found Amrit to be a polite and 'nice' girl. Amrit had been quite chatty to other patients and the nurse did not feel she was depressed. Amrit had not volunteered information about the overdose and said that it was silly of her to have taken the tablets. The nurse had not asked for any more details. The parents appeared to be quite caring. From the ward's point of view she was fit for discharge.

Individual interview: Initially Amrit was seen on her own in a side room. She was a slim girl in a dressing gown. She appeared quite tense and anxious and had a serious look on her face, as if she did not know what to expect. The clinician introduced himself and told her that it was usual for anyone who had taken an overdose to be seen by a member of the CAMHS team and it did not necessarily mean that there was anything wrong with her mind. The clinician assured her that he was not there to 'tick her off' for what had happened. He was there to find out about the circumstances of the overdose and see if he or a member of his team could be of help to her and her family. He told her he would treat the information she gave him with utmost confidentiality so that she could feel free to discuss things with him. Confidentiality would only be broken on issues that concerned her safety. When it came to keeping her safe, obviously, her parents would have to be involved. And he would not talk to her parents about other things she had said without her permission. He wanted to make sure that she understood what he said.

She was asked first about her experience in A&E. She said she was brought to the hospital by her mother. She was seen by a nurse first and then by a doctor. She was given something to drink that tasted horrible and she had been sick. She described her experience in the ward overnight as frightening because initially she had been admitted to an adult ward where the patients were quite seriously ill. She was later transferred to the children's ward. This place was much better, but the kids in the ward were babies and young children. She had been quite bored and could not wait to go home.

Amrit was in year 10 at a local school. She said she liked school, particularly her friends. She had a mixed group of friends that consisted of boys and girls, Whites, and Asians and Afro-Caribbeans. She got on better with boys than girls. She described herself as an average student. She was good in English and wanted to be a primary school teacher. There had been no bullying or other problems at school. She got on well with her father, but did not get on with her mother that well. Amrit identified several reasons for the strained relationship with her mother. Her mother, she said, expected her to help with the family business and housework at the expense of Amrit's social life. The family ran a newsagent's shop. Her mother helped her father in the business and Amrit and her brother joined them in the shop after school. She would work at the counter when time permitted. She and her brother did most of their schoolwork while at the shop. She denied any particular problems at home.

The conversation then moved to the overdose. The clinician told her that he had seen quite a number of young people of her age after they had taken overdoses and wanted to go through with her the circumstances of the overdose in some detail.

> *Clinician:* Can you describe to me what happened?

> *Amrit:* Mum and I had been to the careers evening at school. On the way back she said things to me that were hurtful. She said that I was not trying hard enough or something like that and that she was disappointed with me. She is never happy with me. She does not like my friends. She does not like the way I am.

Clinician: So, you felt irritated and upset with your mother. How did you decide to take the take the tablets?

Amrit: I am not sure. After we got back I did not want to have dinner, but mum said that she'll tell dad when he got back. He really gets angry if I go to bed without dinner. So I pretended to eat my dinner and went back to my room. I was fed up. It had been going on for some time and I could not see things any getting better. It was the same thing every day over and over, again and again. I felt I could not go on like this. I could not stop crying; I could not sleep either. It was like torture. I went to mum's room and took the packet of tablets from the drawer. I sat down on the bed and took them with a glass of water.

Clinician: How many tablets were there and how many did you take?

Amrit: I took all that was there. I think there were 30 tablets.

Clinician: How long had you been thinking about taking the tablets?

Amrit: Just that night.

Clinician: On the Friday night how long had you been thinking of taking the tablets, hours, minutes?

Amrit: May be ten minutes or so; when I was in the room and I could not stop crying.

Clinician: Did you do anything to prevent being found out, like locking the room or things like that?

Amrit: No I just went to bed as usual; I did not tell anybody, if that is what you mean.

Clinician: Did you let any body know about it, telephone anyone or write a note or letter to anyone?

Amrit: No. Everything happened so quickly.

Clinician: What happened after you took the tablets?

Amrit: I went to bed.

Clinician: What happened next?

Amrit: When dad came home that night, he came to my room to talk to me. Mum must have told him about the argument we had had. He found the empty packet on the bedside table. He put me up and asked me whether I had taken the tablets. They brought me to the hospital.

Clinician: What sort of thoughts were you having just before you had taken the tablets?

Amrit: I am not sure. I was sort of fed up. Mum is never happy with me. She does not like the way I dress, the way I look, does not like my friends. She does not like me going out with friends. We have arguments all the time, day in day out.

Clinician: Let me get it right. You had been unhappy for some time and on this occasion, after an argument with your mother, you felt fed up; you thought things will not get any better.

Amrit: I felt that things will be the same . . . nothing will get better . . .

Clinician: When you took the tablets what did you expect to happen?

Amrit: I was not sure. Maybe that all my problems would be gone. I would not have to worry or face another day.

Clinician: You mean once you are dead you will not have to face another day? Did you really want to die?

Amrit: (shakes her head with tears in her eyes)

Clinician: Is it a 'no'?

Amrit: Yes; I mean it's a no (smiles).

Clinician: People take overdoses for lots of different reasons. I'll give you a list of such reasons. Sometimes they are a bit mixed up and are not very sure as to why they took the overdose. Please tell me which of those are true or not true in your case. (Clinician went through the list in Box 14.1, making sure she understood them.)

Amrit's main motivation for taking the overdose was to escape from an unbearable situation and to show her parents how unhappy she was. Amrit did not know the seriousness of paracetamol overdose or its toxicity and had not really thought about it. The clinician took this opportunity to tell her about the dangers of paracetamol overdose (e.g. liver toxicity).

Box 14.1 Motivation for deliberate self-harm (Hawton and van Heeringen, 2000)

1 To die.
2 To escape from unbearable anguish.
3 To get relief.
4 To escape from a situation.
5 To show desperation to others.
6 To change the behaviour of others.
7 To get back at other people/make them feel guilty.
8 To get help.

Mental state examination: Amrit appeared to be an intelligent and articulate teenager. After some initial reluctance she was able to talk about the difficulties in the relationship with her mother and the extended family clearly and convincingly. She held good eye contact and appeared to be at ease with the clinician in describing the difficulties. When speaking of friends and school she brightened up but broke down when discussing issues concerning her grandmother and the extended family. She denied experiencing feelings of sustained depression in the previous weeks and months. She said she felt sad and unhappy at times and these were usually related to what happened between her and her mother. She enjoyed going out with friends and 'having a laugh'.

When asked about the reason for taking the overdose, Amrit said that there had been some bullying, mainly name calling, at school. She had fallen out with the group of girls she used to hang around with. She smiled at this point and said that it had been silly of her to have taken the overdose and wanted to know whether she could go home. The clinician felt that she was trivialising the reason for the overdose and wanted to probe a little further.

At this point the clinician wondered whether there were things about which she was unhappy. Amrit said that her mother wanted her to be at the shop late into the evenings while she preferred to spend time with friends, especially on Fridays and weekends. This was a source of tension between the two of them and often led to arguments. On a number of occasions she had defied her mother and gone out with her friends.

Another reason for conflict between the mother and daughter was over schoolwork. Although Amrit was reasonably good in her schoolwork and always completed her homework in time, her mother appeared dissatisfied with her school performance and felt that she should be doing better. The clinician wanted to know what the disagreement was about. Amrit felt that her mother compared her to her cousins who were high achievers. Amrit had a number of maternal aunts and uncles and numerous cousins. Most of her cousins went to private schools and were 'high flyers'. One of the cousins was doing law and another was doing medicine. It was clear that it was no coincidence that Amrit took the overdose soon after the careers evening at school which she and her mother had attended.

Developing the theme further, the therapist explored with her the relationship of her family with the extended family. Her mother had three brothers and one sister and all of them were married and had children. Amrit's mother was not on talking terms with the rest of the family because she had married against the wishes of her family. Her maternal grandparents lived with their son and his family in a big house in a nearby town. Amrit visited her grandmother regularly but she had always felt that her grandmother favoured the other grandchildren. Amrit became tearful when spoke about how she felt about her grandmother. She was most upset when she spoke about how, for their grandparent's 30th wedding anniversary, all the grandchildren had got together and given a trophy with all their names inscribed on it but her name was not included.

When asked about her friends and how her family felt about them, she said she knew that her mother was not happy with some of her friends, especially the boys. Amrit felt that her mother was somewhat distrustful about her relationship with boys and it was one reason that she kept her from going out with her friends. She felt that her mother was overprotective and wanted to choose her friends for her. Amrit described her social life in some detail. She enjoyed being out with her friends but spoke little about her friends at home because she knew that her mother did not like her going out with them.

Family interview: By now it was clear that there were a number of areas of conflict that were directly associated with the overdose. Next, the parents were asked to join the session. Following introductions and a brief social chat, each was asked to describe Amrit and what they liked about her. Her father, Mr Dhaliwal, described her as a loving and likeable girl who was good in her schoolwork and was helpful to the family. He could find no fault with her. He has always been proud of her. Her mother agreed but said that she was showing the usual teenage behaviour. They were asked how they were dealing with the 'teenage behaviour'. 'Not very well,' said the mother. Mr Dhaliwal said he left these matters to his wife to deal with. They had their usual quota of arguments as any mother and teenage daughter would.

Mr Dhaliwal said the overdose had come as a big shock to him. He described how he saw the empty packets in her bedroom and could not believe that Amrit could have done such a thing. He had always thought of her as a sensible and level-headed girl. He was not sure what they were not doing right as a family. All during this time he remained calm but seemed concerned. Amrit was gazing at the floor with tears in her eyes. When it came to Mrs Dhaliwal's turn, the tone of the conversation was different. Her mother described her as a nice girl, but Amrit wanted to have her own way. She was too keen on her friends and less keen on helping her or her husband. She said that Amrit was an intelligent girl and used to be top of the class. Over the last two years her schoolwork had suffered and she was getting to be like her friends, interested only in going out and having a good time. Amrit intervened at this point and said that she helped her mother with her work at home and at the shop. This lead to an exchange of words between them and resulted in a minor argument. Her father looked at them in a detached way and glanced at the clinician as if to say, 'Look, this is what happens at home.'

The clinician defused the situation by asking about the stresses they may be experiencing as a family. The father said they had to work hard as a family because his previous business had gone under and now he had taken over a newsagency. It involved long hours of work and he was pleased that all the members of the family helped him with the business. The finances were not excellent but they had settled the debts. Her mother said that Amrit had been a delightful baby and, apart from infantile eczema, she had always been healthy. Her developmental milestones were normal. She had liked school since she started nursery. She always had lots of friends and been a popular girl at school. She was asked about a time when she felt particularly close to Amrit. About a year ago Mrs Dhaliwal was admitted to hospital and underwent keyhole surgery for gallstones. Unfortunately, there were complications and she had another operation. She was in hospital for about four weeks and when she got back home it took her a long time to get back into a routine. She was particularly touched by the care and concern Amrit had shown for her soon after her discharge from hospital. During this period Amrit had been very helpful in taking care of her and in looking after the home.

When asked to identify what the main problems were in the relationship between them, Mrs Dhaliwal said that Amrit wanted to be 'like the white girls' and was bent on going out and having a nice time rather than concentrating on her studies. She agreed that Amrit needed her independence and autonomy but was worried about her safety and did not want her to get into trouble. Mr Dhaliwal thought that his wife was 'overworried about Amrit and was too strict with her'.

Case conceptualisation and formulation

From the assessment it was evident that Amrit had been unhappy for quite some time. Discussions about her career appeared to have brought to the surface underlying difficulties that are typical of families with adolescents: issues of autonomy and independence for the young person. Amrit's drive for independence was at odds with her mother's expectations of a dutiful daughter of her age. Although her father appeared to understand Amrit better, he was seen to be taking a peripheral role in the matter, leaving it all to the mother to deal with the problems. Obviously the family was experiencing difficulties in negotiating acceptable levels age appropriate autonomy for the young person. These difficulties had put a lot of strain on the mother–daughter relationship and Amrit was beginning to get alienated from the family. There were indications of more deep-seated problems involving the extended family that needed exploration. On mental state examination, there was no evidence of depression or other psychiatric disorder.

Risk assessment: The overdose was an impulsive act and Amrit had not planned it. The immediate precipitant was the disagreement with her mother over issues of career choice, socialisation and application to schoolwork. There were no serious family issues such as abuse, there was no evidence of psychiatric disorder such as depression, conduct problems or substance misuse. This was her first overdose. The family appeared to be a caring one and there was no indication of serious dysfunction in the family. However, there were two factors that caused some concern:

1 The overdose was a lethal one. Thirty tablets of paracetamol could have caused serious liver damage and even death, if it had not been detected and treated early. On the other hand, Amrit had little knowledge of the dangerousness of paracetamol. Because her perception of the dangers of taking the tablets was inaccurate, this factor could be disregarded to some extent. More worrying was the availability of and accessibility to large quantities of non-prescription drugs in the home and shop. This was taken up with the family later.
2 Amrit had made no attempt to disclose the overdose to anyone. She had gone to sleep and not told anyone of the overdose. Although she had not actively taken precautions to avoid discovery, this was a more serious situation and was an indication of the difficulties in communication within the family, principally between Amrit and her mother. The significance of non-disclosure of the overdose to anyone within or outside the family and her failure to seek help was brought up for discussion with the parents later.

On balance, in Amrit's case the risk was considered to be low. Even though the immediate purpose of the overdose had been to escape from an unbearable state of mind, it had served the purpose of highlighting Amrit's predicament and had made the family take serious notice of her mental anguish and, if possible, do something to make it better. At the end of the assessment the clinician was left with a number of questions: What underlying family belief systems were preventing the family from successfully negotiating Amrit's need for a degree of autonomy acceptable to the family and her? What was the part the extended family played in creating the context for the current problems? How could the clinician assist in opening a dialogue between Amrit and her parents in a way that allowed Amrit to reconnect with the family? How could Amrit manage future problems within and outside the family without resorting to risky behaviours such as self-harm?

Treatment choice and management

Immediate management: The main objectives in the immediate management of an adolescent presenting with deliberate self-harm are:

- minimising the immediate risk of repetition or suicide completion (risk management)
- establishing rapport with the young person (and family) so that follow-up appointments are taken up and further work made possible
- mobilisation of family support (or other support systems, if the family is unavailable, unwilling or is unhelpful)
- recognising and treating, where indicated, coexisting psychopathology (particularly depression).

The first priority in the management of adolescents who take overdoses is to ensure the safety of the young person. The immediate aim is to minimise the immediate danger of repetition. The main factors that are associated with risk of repetition of deliberate self-harm are given in Table 14.1. When the risk is considered to be high, a decision has to be made about how the young person's safety could be ensured. This may involve keeping the young person in the current hospital for a longer period of time, work with the family and the adolescent and reassessment of risk, or admission to an adolescent psychiatric inpatient unit. Admission may be necessary when the risk is high or in the presence of a serious psychiatric disorder such as severe depression. Social services involvement may be necessary when parents are found to be negligent or unreliable in protecting the young person.

Table 14.1 Factors associated with risk of repetition of attempted suicide

For non-fatal repetition	For suicide
- High suicidal intent in current episode	- Older age
- High suicidal intent at the time of examination	- Male gender
- Lethality of attempt as perceived by the adolescent (may be inaccurate)	- Leaving a suicide note
- Intensity of precipitating factors	- Previous attempt(s)
- Previous suicidal behaviour	- Psychiatric history: depression, anti-social personality
- Current psychiatric disorder (depression, conduct disorder) or substance abuse	- Living alone (away from home)
- Chronic psychosocial problems (e.g. severe parenting problems, abuse, social services involvement, alternative and unstable care histories)	

Amrit was not actively suicidal and the risk of taking another overdose was judged to be low. She had a supportive family that acknowledged the seriousness of the situation and was keen to accommodate her needs. The responsibility of keeping her safe was entrusted to the family. They were to:

1 keep her under supervision at home so that for the next few days an adult was with her all the time when at home and
2 take away all medications, sharp objects, and so on.

The parents were told about the importance of keeping medications under lock and key both at home and in the shop.

In order to mobilise parental support the parents were seen as a couple. The purpose of this part of the session was to:

1 highlight seriousness of the problem and engage them in future work in addressing family issues and
2 help them understand the meaning of the act of deliberate self-harm.

It is usually necessary to increase parental anxiety in order to mobilise parental support. The clinician stressed the seriousness of the overdose, pointing out that Amrit had not disclosed the overdose to anyone. Had it not been discovered in time she might have succeeded in killing herself. It was therefore important that they took action to both keep her safe and address the underlying problems. They were reassured that Amrit did not show any mental health problems. Although they were a close family and all of them cared for one another dearly, as a family they were facing problems in the negotiation of the needs of an adolescent for independence and autonomy. Following this discussion dates for family sessions were arranged.

When Amrit was seen on her own at the end of the session, she was happy that she could go home. This part of the session focused on two issues: Amrit's 'reason for living' and on coping strategies. She was asked to name the things she would miss most if she had succeeded in her suicide attempt. Amrit was surprised by the question and, after some thought, she said she would miss her parents most. She went on to talk of her best friend who had been very close to her. She spoke of her hopes of wanting to be a primary school teacher; she wanted to show her grandmother that she and her mother were not 'losers'.

Next, the importance of thinking about how she dealt with stresses was emphasised. Taking overdoses and engaging in self-harming behaviours, it was said, are indications that people were not dealing with their problems in a healthy and adaptive way. She agreed that the method she had used to convey her distress to the family was a dangerous one. While the clinician understood some of the difficulties she was experiencing with the family, it was important that she learned better and more useful ways of coping with stresses. Following a brief discussion about how she would cope if in the following days she encountered similar problems, it was agreed that she would talk to a friend over the telephone or go out for a walk. She also agreed to telephone the clinician if things did not get better. The clinician's name and work telephone number were given. Appointments were made for the family and her to be seen the next week. The clinician felt Amrit (and the family) understood and that she was sufficiently engaged with the clinician to want to attend follow-up appointments.

Subsequent management and aftercare

Despite the frequency of DSH in adolescents and the important place it occupies in CAMHS, there is not a single empirically validated method of psychotherapy developed for suicidal and self-destructive behaviours in adolescents. In a systemic review of 20 randomised controlled trials on interventions in deliberate self-harm in adults, Keith Hawton, one of the foremost researchers on the subject, concluded: 'There is insufficient evidence on which to make firm recommendations about the most effective forms of treatment for patients who have deliberately harmed themselves. This is a serious situation given the size of the problem of Deliberate Self Harm throughout the world and the importance of dealing with the problem to prevent suicide' (Hawton, 2000).

There is consensus that, barring young people who exhibit psychiatric disorders, brief time-limited interventions are the treatments of choice for the majority in this group. A problem specific to adolescents who self-harm is the high rates of clinic non-attendance and non-compliance. Hence the clinician has to pay particular attention to increasing compliance. This includes giving a definite appoint for follow-up at the time of assessment, scheduling the appointment to within a week or, at most, two, and involving family members and, where there is involvement of other significant adults (e.g. social worker, the mentor), involving them in the treatment.

A number of psychotherapeutic methods of intervention are available for this group of adolescents. For example, problem-solving therapy, family therapy and cognitive therapy have been employed. A meta-analysis of six randomised controlled trials in adult DSH patients has reported that problem therapy improved depression, hopelessness and personal problems (Townsend *et al.*, 2001). In light of the overall paucity of empirical studies of treatment of adolescent suicidal behaviour, the following principles, based on the extant literature and clinical experience, seem reasonable and appropriate:

- addressing the contextual crisis that had precipitated the suicidal attempt
- addressing any mental health problems in the adolescent (and parents)
- focusing on problem-solving strategies.

Since the working hypothesis with the Dhaliwal family was that the family were experiencing difficulties in negotiating adolescent developmental tasks, family meetings were arranged to address these issues. Concurrently Amrit was to be seen for individual work. The proposed interventions were to be brief and time-limited. A particular issue was the cultural context to the problems that involved the relationship between Amrit's family and her grandparents. This was to be brought up in family sessions. Amrit and her family were seen in family sessions and couple sessions that ran concurrently with individual sessions for Amrit. The following is a condensed account of the sessions.

Family sessions: The main aims of the family sessions were:

1   to help open up a dialogue between the parents and Amrit, paying special attention to issues concerning autonomy and independence
2   to help the parents provide nurturance without necessarily infantilising or depriving autonomy for the young person.

Early in the family sessions there was disagreement between the parents about how Amrit should be managed. The mother was more concerned about Amrit's choice of friends and the amount of time she spent with them. She felt Amrit should spend her free time on her schoolwork and helping with housework. Her husband felt that Amrit's behaviour was no different from those of girls of her age and his wife's way of dealing with it only made it worse. Amrit's mother said that Amrit was an intelligent girl who could become a doctor or a lawyer if only she applied herself to her schoolwork better. She was particularly concerned about some of Amrit's girlfriends, who she felt had a bad influence on her. When asked to expand on this she said, in a rather reluctant voice, that the girls she went out with had boyfriends and they slept with them. She did not want Amrit to follow in their footsteps. At this point Amrit intervened and said that her mother wanted her to be like her cousins who were high flyers. This brought up the issue of the role of the extended family.

The therapist enquired about the reaction of the grandparents to the overdose. There was a pause in the conversation as the parents glanced at each other. Amrit broke the silence and said that the grandparents had not been told about it. Her mother said, 'I did not want them to know about it because it would be another reason for them to have a go at me.' This led on to a discussion about her relationship with her parents. She said she was not on talking terms with her mother. The difficulties between the two of them dated back to her marriage to Amrit's father. Her parents had been opposed to it and, after the marriage, had severed all relationships with her. She had been considered the black sheep of the family for marrying someone they did not approve of. Her two sisters had married husbands chosen by their parents. She had met her husband at the local shop and they had fallen in love. Her family considered him to be beneath their standing. They were Kenyan Asians and came to the UK when all Asians were made to leave Kenya. The family had settled down in Birmingham and started a business. Over the years the family had done well and were proud of their achievements. All her sisters married into well-off families.

Although she did not visit or speak to her mother, she had wanted Amrit to keep in touch with her side of the family, especially her cousins. Amrit visited them regularly but was becoming more and more reluctant to go. Amrit said that her grandmother treated her differently to her cousins. One of the things she did not like was the way she was treated like a poor relative. The grandmother would make sarcastic comments like, 'Are you going to find a man of your own?' and her cousins would laugh at this. At other times her grandmother was patronising and would give her pocket money. Amrit was particularly hurt about receiving money from her grandmother for her birthday instead of presents. Her mother agreed with Amrit and said that she too was annoyed at the way her mother treated Amrit. But she did not want Amrit to lose contact with her family.

Amrit's father appeared to take a back seat during the sessions and allowed the daughter and mother to tell their stories. When asked for his views, he said that Amrit had always been a mature girl, he could trust her to make the right choices and he did not see any problems with the way she chose her friends. He did not consider her behaviour to be any different from someone else of her age. But he had left it to the 'women' to sort their problems out. He said he had a good relationship with Amrit. But he had been busy with establishing his business and found little time to spend with the children. However, he had taken Amrit, as well as her brother, to football matches. All three of them enjoyed football matches and supported the same football team. There was some light-hearted discussion about how their mother would shout at them when the three of them watched football matches on television. He felt that Amrit was entitled to her freedom and independence, as long as she did not misuse them. He had enough confidence in her to allow her to learn for herself by making her own mistakes, if necessary.

There appeared to be a striking difference between the way in which each parent approached the issue of adolescent autonomy. The therapist wondered aloud how that difference could have come about. Amrit said that her father was more 'modern' than her mother. At this point her mother objected to it and said that she was not as old-fashioned as Amrit thought. It struck the therapist that there might be a cultural difference between Amrit's father and her mother. The discussion moved to Amrit's father's background. Her father had been born and brought up in Birmingham. His parents had come to the UK in the 1960s. He had gone to the local comprehensive school but had not been interested in studies. He had a sister who was married to a local 'white' man. Amrit called him fondly 'Uncle Peter'. Amrit wished that Peter had children so that she could have cousins from her father's side of the family as well. It struck the therapist that there was a generational difference between the parents. Amrit's father was a second generation Asian living in the UK, whilst Amrit's mother belonged to the first generation of migrants, having come to this country with her family when she was about 10 years of age. Moreover, her family structure appeared somewhat rigid and had a powerful influence on her. The therapist was intrigued by the fact that Amrit's mother had separated from her parents and left home in what appeared to be a highly conflictual situation. She had felt ostracised by the family for marrying Amrit's father, who the family considered to be an outsider. It was interesting to note that her main anxieties centred around Amrit's growing up and leaving home. It was also clear that she was guilty about the way she had left her family of origin and had not yet come to terms with it. She appeared to have a highly ambivalent relationship with her own mother.

In one of the family sessions, issues of acculturation were discussed. It transpired that Amrit's father was more acculturalised to the host culture than his wife. For example, he preferred to eat fish and chips and pizza rather than chapattis. He had a mixed group of friends, many of whom were British-born Asians and whites. He was an ardent supporter of one of the football clubs and took every opportunity to go to football matches. Although a Sikh by religion, he hardly went to the gurdwara. Amrit's mother, on the other hand, had a more traditional lifestyle. Most of the time she wore a shalwar kameez, she preferred traditional Indian food and, although she spoke good English, she had an Indian accent.

The therapist asked both of the parents what their aspirations and hopes were for Amrit. Her father said that ultimately it was up to Amrit to make the necessary choices in life and he would be glad to go along with whatever her preferences were. When asked to expand further he said that as far as careers were concerned he was quite happy for Amrit to choose whatever career she felt suitable for her; and as for choice of future partners, he felt that it was up to her to decide on whom she wanted to marry and he would have no problems in adapting to whoever his son-in-law was, whether he was white, black or brown. He added that it was unfair for them to expect Amrit to behave like a 'typical Asian woman'. She had been born and brought up in this country and, therefore, thought and behaved like people here. Amrit's mother had a very different view. She felt that Amrit should keep to Asian values and be careful not to be drawn into the 'false family values' of the host country. She was particularly concerned about Amrit having white boyfriends and getting pregnant before being married.

At this point the therapist disclosed his hypothesis that each of them thought differently about Amrit and her future because they belonged to different generations of immigrants. Her father was more acculturalised into the UK culture than her mother and, therefore, thought and acted more like the British, while his wife, not being a second generation immigrant, took a more traditional view of the role of women in society in general, and Amrit in particular.

Another complicating factor was Amrit's mother's relationship with her own family and the therapist wondered whether she wanted Amrit to be 'a high flyer' and marry someone of Asian origin in order to compensate for the disappointment she had caused her family when she got married to Amrit's father against their wishes. At this point Amrit's mother broke down and said that she had been labouring under intense guilt for having broken up with her mother over her marriage to Amrit's father. Ever since the marriage she said she had been treated by her family as an outcast. She had never been invited for family occasions and whenever she met with members of her extended family, they had treated her as an embarrassment or not spoken to her. She felt that her parents and some other family members looked down upon their family because they were not as well to do as them.

At this point the therapist asked her, 'Are you hoping, then, that Amrit would live up to the expectations of your parents so that you would feel equal to them and be accepted by them?' She acknowledged that there was some truth in the statement. She would want to show her mother that she was capable of bringing up a daughter who was successful and well behaved. The therapist pointed out that probably she thought that she herself was not 'successful and well behaved'. There appeared to be a number of personal issues for Amrit's mother to come to terms with. Her wish for Amrit to have a more traditional lifestyle was mixed with the unresolved conflict of separation from her mother and her perception that she had been a disappointment to her parents.

At this juncture the therapist asked Amrit her ideas about what she wanted to be and what sort of woman she wanted to grow up to be. Amrit said that she wanted to be a professional working woman. She was more likely to become a teacher because she liked children and teaching. She said she was particularly good at listening to children and young people and felt that she would be a good teacher. As for getting married, she said she would like to get married some day and would probably marry a man of Asian origin. Both her parents were surprised by this statement. She said that Asian men were more reliable and more committed to relationships. There were white boys who were as good but she would not take a chance. She said that she would like to have a traditional Indian wedding but would not want to be 'just a housewife'. This provided enough material for a long discussion with the family. Her mother was very surprised and said, 'I thought you would choose a white boy and have a church wedding.' In the rest of the session the therapist continued to amplify the differences between Amrit's hopes, expectations and desires on one hand, and her mother's perception of Amrit's choices and preferences.

The therapist observed that there was a lot for the family to discuss and suggested that they set aside some time to have a family discussion around issues that were brought up in the family sessions. They agreed to discuss these issues at home as a family after each family session. In later family sessions, they reported having made progress in understanding each other's viewpoints. They said they were spending more time with each other and that the relationships had improved.

Individual sessions: The main aims of individual sessions with Amrit were:

1 to identify the main problems for *her* and set about how she would solve them
2 to help deal with future disappointments and crises in a more appropriate way without resorting to maladaptive behaviours like deliberate self-harm.

A problem-solving approach was adopted in the individual sessions with Amrit. Problem-solving therapy is described in greater detail in Chapter 15. A brief account of the application of it is given here. Amrit was asked to identify the main problems for her, and encouraged to generate as many solutions for each of them. Following some discussion, Amrit identified two problems that she felt were important:

1 her difficulty in getting her mother to understand that she was a responsible and trustworthy young person and
2 she wanted to be able to deal with her grandparents, especially her grand-mother and some of her cousins in an assertive and dignified way.

After a long brainstorming session it was decided that she would be frank with her mother about her relationship with her friends. She was aware that her mother was unhappy about the relationship with some of the boys (and girls) whom the mother considered not very well behaved. She said, 'Whenever she sees boys and girls together, she thinks that they are going to have sex.' Amrit felt the best way to win her mother's trust would be to tell her that she was not 'sleeping around' and that she had high moral standards for herself. She went out with friends because she enjoyed their company and it made her feel good. She said she learned a lot from her friends about life in general and how they coped with their problems. She said that she would assure her mother that she would keep to agreed times regarding her return home. There had been a few occasions when Amrit returned home late and her mother had been ringing around to find out her whereabouts.

As for her relationship with her grandmother, she said that she was always left with a disquieting feeling whenever she met her grandmother. Her reluctance to go to her grandmother's was something that she wanted to work on. She felt that she should visit her grandmother, albeit infrequently. She felt the best way of dealing with her grandmother was to tell her directly how she felt about the treatment she received from her. This would be a difficult task; she agreed she would choose the right time when she was alone with her grandmother to tell her how she made her feel small. She said that of the many cousins she had, there were two who had been quite friendly towards her and treated her as an equal. She felt that she should develop a good relationship with these two cousins by visiting them at their homes. She would begin by telephoning them and having some 'small talk' and test out to see if she would be welcome in their homes.

The therapist brought up the subject of how she coped with stress. The discussion centered around how to recognise the signs of stress early and the various strategies she could use to cope with it. She was able to construct a list of the actions she could take when she felt under pressure. These included the following: going out for a walk, telephoning her best friend and asking her dad for a special time to discuss the problem. (*See* Chapter 15 for a discussion of problem-solving strategies.)

Theoretical perspectives

Deliberate self-harm is common among adolescents. Statistics show that 19 000 to 20 000 young people between 10 and 19 years of age are seen annually in general hospitals in England and Wales following an attempted overdose (Hawton and Fagg, 1992). But hospital data are gross underestimates of the true prevalence of deliberate self-harm in young people in the community. Most adolescents who deliberately harm themselves do not attend hospital. Hawton *et al.* (2002) surveyed more than 6000 pupils aged 15 and 16 years in 41 schools in England and found almost 400 participants (6.9%) reported an act of deliberate self-harm in the previous year. Of these only 12.6% of episodes resulted in presentation to a hospital. DSH was almost four times more common in females than in males. The study found that the main methods of self-harm were cutting (67%) and poisoning (31%); more than 55% of these had repeated self-harm. Suicidal ideation (without self-harm) was even more common with 15% reporting thoughts of self-harm in the previous year. These findings are in keeping with the findings from other studies that find that 7–10% of adolescents in the community attempt suicide (Safer, 1997).

In stark contrast to rates of attempted suicides, *completed suicides* are rare in this age group. In 1998 the rate of suicide for males aged 15–19 years was 52 *per million* and the corresponding figure for females was 13 in England and Wales (McClure 2001) (when deaths deemed to be due to undetermined and accidental causes were included the total number of suicides was 135 and 43 per million for males and females respectively). Thus when contrasted with attempted suicide rates in this age group, it emerges that the ratio of those who engage in self-harm to suicide victims is almost one thousand to one (6.8% vs. 65 per million).

Several conclusions may be drawn from the above studies:

- The rates of DSH are very high in young people (about 7%).
- But (fortunately) rates for completed suicide are very low (about 65 per million), a ratio of 1000:1,
- Self-injury (self-cutting) is more common than overdoses (2:1).
- Suicidal thoughts are very common among adolescents (15%).

The implication of these findings is that the prediction of suicide, a rare event in this age group, in the context of high frequency behaviour that may lead to it (i.e. attempted suicide), is an extremely difficult task. It is important to remember that in risk assessment one is attempting to make two types of predictions: risk of repetition of self-harm and risk of death by suicide. The risk factors associated with each of these overlap but are also different (*see* Table 14.1). A number of attempts have been made to develop ratings scales to predict suicide but most have been shown to have poor predictive power. What this means is that existing methods of risk assessment are insufficient and inaccurate to make predictions.

Despite the fact that suicide is the third most common cause of death in young people aged 15 to 24 (the first and second being accidents and cancers) and that every teenage suicide is an extremely tragic event, prediction of suicide risk is 'a risky business'. A fundamental problem is predicting a rarer event because false positive rates would be too high for predictions to be useful. It has been argued that using deliberate self-harm as a marker for suicide risk is misleading from a public health point of view. Professionals, particularly those in primary care, often respond with disproportionate panic when an adolescent discloses self-harm or suicidal ideation.

Assessment of adolescents who harm themselves is one of the most common and demanding emergencies in CAMHS. Young people who harm themselves are not a homogeneous group; rather they differ widely according to their backgrounds, problems and in their outcomes. A clinically useful classification has been produced by Richard Harrington (2001). He divided those deliberately self-harming adolescents into four clinical groups:

1 Family dysfunction group: This group is formed of young people with poor intra-familial relationships, low levels of nurturance in the context of disturbed family relationships characterised by low warmth and communication problems. The majority of adolescents who take overdoses, about 60%, fall in to this group. They and their families require interventions designed to promote communication and problem solving.
2 Acute crisis group: Young people experiencing transient problems or acute crises constitute about 20% of cases of DSH. They usually do not require more than one follow-up appointment.
3 Psychiatric disorder/high risk group: The most common disorder is depression; this group also includes those who are at high risk irrespective of psychiatric symptomatology. They account for about 10% of all overdoses and require psychiatric assessment and follow-up. Some may need inpatient care.
4 Chronic psychosocial problem group: Adolescents with a history of chronic problems and a history of social services involvement, chaotic parenting, abuse or experience of foster care. They constitute about 10% of adolescents who take overdoses. Repetition of deliberate self-harm is common in this subgroup. This group often needs social work input and multidisciplinary management.

On the basis of the above classification of DSH Amrit's case was considered to come under the family dysfunction group. The main issues were related to communication within the family, balancing the adolescent's quest for independence with the parent's concern for safety within the cultural context and expectations of the family.

The literature on adolescent DSH is voluminous and although we know a great deal about the risk factors for adolescent suicidal behaviour, little is known about how best it is treated or prevented. DSH is not a diagnosis but a description of behaviour. Assessment of a young person who had taken an overdose involves paying attention to the following five factors:

1 Motive
2 Circumstances of attempt
3 Presence of a psychiatric disorder
4 Precipitating and maintaining problems
5 Coping skills and support.

Motivation or the reasons for the attempt has been addressed in many studies. Based on extant research Hawton and van Heeringen (2000) have developed a useful list of eight reasons given by adolescents for taking overdoses (*see* Box 14.1). The risk factors associated with repetition of DSH have been well documented in literature. Box 14.2 summarises the various factors to be considered in assessment of suicidal intent.

Box 14.2 Factors that suggest high suicidal intent (Hawton, 2000)

- Act carried out in isolation.
- Act so timed that intervention is unlikely.
- Precautions taken to avoid discovery.
- Extensive premeditation.
- Preparations made for the act (e.g. purchasing tablets, saving up tablets).
- Communicating intent to others beforehand.
- Not alerting potential helpers after the act.
- Admission of suicidal intent.

Self-injury: It is important to make a distinction between those taking over-doses and those involved in self-injury (e.g. self-cutting). In the vast majority of cases self-injury suicidal intent is low and the main motivation is to get relief from a heightened emotional state such as anger, frustration or misery (*see* Chapter 15).

Multiple repeaters of self-harm: Adolescents who frequently repeat self-harm constitute a distinct subgroup that is associated with a number of significant problems in other areas of functioning.

Case example: Repeated attempter

Naomi, age 15, was admitted to the children's ward after ingesting a number of tablets belonging to her mother. Her overdose followed an argument with her mother over where she should be living. The overdose occurred in the back-ground of chronic and ongoing relationship problems with her mother, who had severe personality problems. There was predictable pattern to the events. Naomi would go to live with her aunt when the conflict with her mother became unbearable for her. After a few weeks with her aunt she would come back to her mother in the hope things would have changed, but within a few months she and her mother would begin quarrelling again and Naomi would move out. Her mother admitted to having a volatile temperament and having taken several overdoses herself, some of them in the presence of Naomi. Naomi's older brother had been in trouble with the police; her two younger siblings had been taken into care and placed for adoption on account of inadequate parental care. This was Naomi's fifth overdose within a period of two years. In the past Naomi had cut herself on the forearms. At various times she had truanted, shoplifted and had got into fights with her peers at school. She and her family were seen in the CAMHS but little progress was made mainly because of her mother's demand for a diagnosis rather than seeking solutions. The situation continued unchanged over the next three years during which time she took several overdoses. When she was 18 years she was seen by adult psychiatric services and a diagnosis of borderline personality disorder was made. However, she refused to adhere to any treatment plan.

Three overlapping categories of frequent repeat DSH can be delineated:

1 **Those with poor impulse control:** This group of adolescents has mainly conduct and antisocial behaviour problems. They have difficulties in managing

anger and for them taking overdoses is seen as one way of coping with difficult situations. Many of them are predelinquents or delinquents and represent a major therapeutic challenge.

2 **Those with chaotic past histories:** Adolescents placed in local authority care and those with past histories of physical and sexual abuse constitute another subgroup of frequent repeaters. In those children living with families, severe family dysfunction and instability is common; parental mental health problems including self-harming behaviours are common are frequent this group.

3 **Those with substance misuse or alcohol abuse:** Substance misuse and alcohol abuse are strongly associated with DSH and requires that both behaviours be addressed.

These special groups are more at risk of completed suicide and need different approaches to treatment. A form of treatment that combines group therapy with individual work called Dialectical Behaviour Therapy (DBT) has been developed in the US by Marsha Linehan (1993). DBT is an intensive form of manualised cognitive behavioural therapy shown to be effective in chronically suicidal adults including those with a diagnosis of borderline personality disorder. DBT conceptualises suicidal and self-destructive behaviours as having important affect regulating properties as well as serving to elicit helping behaviours from an otherwise invalidating environment. From this perspective, suicidal behaviours are considered maladaptive solutions to overwhelming, intensely painful negative emotions.

Progress and outcome

During the period of treatment Amrit was enthusiastic in carrying through the various ideas that were generated. On several occasions she had opened the discussion about her friends with her mother, making sure that her father was present during these conversations to support her. She said that she could see a distinct change in her mother's attitude towards her. She was pleased that her mother was more flexible about her going out with friends. For her part, she had tried to keep to agreed times about coming back in the evenings. She had invited two of her friends, both boys, to visit her at the shop so that her mother could get to know them better. Her mother had commented that they were responsible young men.

The 'generation gap' between the parents had been a hot topic of discussion in the family. In the beginning her mother had been reluctant to accept that her level of Anglicisation was less than that of her husband, but over time she had tended to agree with it. Nevertheless, she would repeatedly say that one should forget one's roots. She had also tried to influence Amrit and her husband to take more interest in cultural events.

Amrit did not confront her grandmother about the stepmotherly treatment she meted out to her. She said she needed more time. But she had returned the money her grandmother sent her for her birthday (by post). At the time of discharge the relationship between Amrit and her grandmother was frosty. Amrit was seen fortnightly for a period of six and a half months. The therapist felt she had made good progress and become better at problem solving. Over the next three years she did not come to the attention of the services through taking an overdose or otherwise.

Comments

Assessing DSH is a core task for most CAMHS practitioners. It involves an element of unpredictability in that the case may be relatively simple (as in the instance of a situational crisis) or incredibly complex (as in a case of one with prolonged social service involvement or severe depression). Most services now have guidelines, protocols and 'risk assessment strategies' in place; some of these documents go for the overkill and detail what should be done and by whom.

As in all clinical work, a sound assessment forms the basis of management. The clinician is best served by using a well thought-out framework for assessment taking into account the various risk factors detailed above. In thinking about management the four groups of self-harming adolescents described by Harrington mentioned above may be useful. Many adolescents with mental health and other serious problems, who may not otherwise seek help from health or social services come to the attention of CAMHS through self-harming behaviours. Clinicians involved in assessment of adolescents who take overdoses need to be adept at identification of conditions like clinical depression.

Many adolescents are skilful at minimising problems and often tend to trivialise the significance of the overdose. This is especially so when they want to be discharged from the hospital. They tend to give simplistic reasons for the DSH episode (e.g. bullying, falling out with friends, minor arguments with parents). It is important not to take these explanations at face value and look for discrepancies such as lethality of the DSH and in the professed explanation. In Amrit's case the initial explanation that was offered was school bullying and the clinician had to gently probe into other likely problem areas to enable her to talk about her difficulties in the family.

Adolescents who deliberately harm themselves are notorious for not keeping follow-up appointments. Studies show that up to two thirds drop out of treatment. It is therefore important to try to build a relationship with the young person during the time of assessment. The aim is to make the assessment interview a good enough and useful enough experience for the young person that they feel understood and listened to. Giving an appointment date and time then and there for follow-up appointments within the next week or two have been found to increase adherence. Some CAMHS teams have 'liaison teams' or a small number of team members dedicated exclusively for servicing this group of clients.

Cultural issues were important in Amrit's case. The issue of acculturation and the role of the extended family proved to be vital in understanding the context of the overdose as well as in the management. Acculturation is the process of cultural change resulting from contact with another (usually dominant) culture, whereby an individual selectively adopts cultural values of the latter. Acculturation occurs both at an individual and broader group levels. An awareness of issues related to this is important when dealing with ethnic minorities and refugees. A useful discussion of acculturation and its relevance to mental health may be found in Bhugra and Bhui (2001).

> ## Box 14.3 Research into deliberate self-harm (DSH) says that . . .
>
> * DSH is common; about 7% of adolescents in the community deliberately harm themselves.
> * But completed suicide is rare compared to the rates of DSH (about 1 in 1000).
> * Deliberate self-injury is twice as common as overdoses.
> * Prediction of suicide is fraught with dangers; risk assessment hardly assesses risk.
> * High risk is indicated by: high suicidal intent, depression, chronic psychosocial problems, comorbid conduct and substance misuse.
> * There is little research evidence to support specific forms of intervention; problem-solving approaches are commonly used in a majority of cases.

References

Bhugra D, Bhui K. *Cross-cultural Psychiatry: a practical guide*. London: Arnold; 2001.

Harrington R. Depression, suicide and deliberate self-harm in adolescence. *British Medical Bulletin*. 2001; **57**: 47–60.

Hawton K. General hospital management of suicide attempters. In: Hawton K, van Heeringen K, editors. *The International Handbook of Suicide and Attempted Suicide*. Chichester: John Wiley; 2000.

Hawton K, Rodham K, Evans E *et al*. Deliberate self-harm in adolescents: self-report survey in schools in England. *BMJ*. 2002; **325**: 1207–11.

*Hawton K, van Heeringen K, editors. *The International Handbook of Suicide and Attempted Suicide*. Chichester: John Wiley; 2000.

Hawton K, Fagg J. Deliberate self-poisoning and self-injury in adolescents: a study of characteristics and trends in Oxford, 1976–1989. *British Journal of Psychiatry*. 1992; **16**: 116–23.

Linehan MM. *Cognitive Behaviour Therapy for Borderline Personality Disorder*. New York: Guilford Press; 1993.

McClure GMG. Suicide in children and adolescents in England and Wales 1970–1998. *British Journal of Psychiatry*. 2001; **178**: 469–74.

Safer D. Self-reported rates of suicide attempts by adolescents. *Annals of Clinical Psychiatry*. 1997; **9**: 263–9.

Townsend E, Hawton K, Altman DG *et al*. The efficacy of problem-solving treatments after deliberate self-harm: meta-analysis of randomized controlled trials with respect to depression, hopelessness and improvement in problems. *Psychological Medicine*. 2001; **31**: 979–88.

Chapter 15

Deliberate self-harm II: self-injury

The form teacher of a local school telephoned the CAMHS in a state of high anxiety and wanted to discuss an urgent problem that had arisen at school. She was directed to a member of staff who had been assigned the task of taking emergencies for the day. The teacher was very worried and concerned about Emma, a 15-year-old girl in her form. It had been brought to her attention by other pupils in the class that Emma had cut herself with a Stanley knife that she had brought to school. Alarmed at hearing it, the teacher had summoned Emma and was shocked to see fresh cuts in her forearm. She had taken her to the emergency room and got the wounds dressed. She had discovered that Emma had a number of old scars in both her forearms. On enquiring about it, Emma had told her that she had been cutting herself for some time. The teacher did not know what she should do and wanted some advice.

She described Emma as a girl who was 'invisible' in class. She had had no problems in the past. She was an average student and had a small group of friends. As far as the teacher was aware there were no particular family problems. She described Emma as a somewhat shy girl with poor self-esteem. She was somewhat overweight and had been reluctant to participate in physical education. On this occasion Emma had cut herself while in the toilet. A fellow pupil had seen it and reported it to her. The teacher was puzzled about Emma's behaviour and wanted to know how best to help her. The CAMHS worker told her that as an immediate measure it would be sensible to inform her parents because of issues of safety and also to get the injuries attended to at the accident and emergency department at the hospital. The CAMHS worker agreed that Emma needed help but since the service did not take referrals direct from schools, could the teacher ask her parents to get her referred to CAMHS through the school nurse or her GP? However, if she was being referred to the hospital they (the hospital) would, as a matter of routine, refer her to CAMHS.

The teacher had been shocked by what she saw. She said she had never seen so many cuts in anyone's arms. Emma had told her that she had been cutting herself for a number of months. She was most surprised that Emma had not been able to tell her why she had been injuring herself. She had known Emma and her family for some time and, as far as she knew, there were no particular problems. Emma had been well behaved in school and the family appeared caring. The teacher wanted to know if Emma was mentally ill and whether she would need 'psychiatric treatment'. Emma's classmates had been clearly shocked by 'the attempted suicide' by Emma. She wondered if, at a later date, someone from CAMHS could talk to her class about self-harm. 'The entire staff at school had been somewhat shaken by her "attempted suicide" in school,' she said 'and we would value some advice on how to deal with such pupils who are suicidal.'

Later that day the GP telephoned and requested an urgent appointment for

Emma. Apparently the school had informed her parents and she had been taken to see the GP. The GP said that the self-inflicted injuries were superficial and were not serious. Emma had admitted to him that she had been cutting herself for more than two years but was unable to give sufficient reasons for her behaviour. He was somewhat concerned that although she did not appear depressed she was remarkably unconcerned about her self-harming behaviour. He wanted her seen as soon as possible and was faxing the referral letter. The referral was discussed in the team meeting and an early appointment was made for Emma and her family. There was also the general issue of talking to schools about self-harm in adolescents and this was to be brought up as an agenda item in the team meeting.

Clinical presentation and background

Emma and her parents, Mr and Mrs Day, attended the first session. They informed the therapist that Sean, their 18-year-old son, had started college recently and was unable to attend the session. Mr and Mrs Day had not known about Emma's self-harm until the school had brought it to their attention. They were surprised that Emma was engaged in such behaviour. They felt that Emma was a 'mature' girl who could look after herself. She had not been a cause for concern and they felt she was self-sufficient and independent. They did not know what was going on in her mind. They described Emma as a bright girl who had never been a bother to them from an early age. From the time she started at school they had been amazed that she had been able to take care of herself and needed very little help. She would get herself ready for school without much help and at the age of eight or so was making herself a packed lunch. They were surprised that Emma was cutting herself. In the past she had told them that she had been subjected to bullying at school but they had not taken it seriously. The school was one of the best in the area and the headteacher was excellent. They were sure that she would take care of it. Emma, they observed, tended to exaggerate things.

One of their concerns was that Emma was somewhat overweight and this obviously invited some name calling in school. But Emma had done little about dieting although she knew what a healthy diet was. Her mother had spoken several times to her about going on a diet, but Emma had not been interested. Mrs Day was on a diet herself and was proud that she had lost weight. She had joined WeightWatchers and found it helpful. She had tried to persuade Emma to join her in attending WeightWatchers groups, but Emma had adamantly refused. She had taken Emma to the GP and got her referred to a dietician but Emma had not been keen on it.

'Now that she has started cutting herself it is time that she took the matter of losing weight seriously and did something about it,' said Mrs Day. Her father felt that she should talk to someone about her problems. He was not sure what those problems might be. During the interview Emma spoke very little and glanced several times at the therapist with a helpless look on her face. Her mother took notice of Emma's interactions and observed, 'You feel guilty about what you have done, don't you? You are a good girl, you won't do it again.'

When asked about Emma's development, her mother said that she remembered very little of her as a baby because 'she was no trouble at all'. 'She was a nice baby, she never caused me any trouble at all,' she said. The pregnancy and delivery had been normal and Emma had had no medical problems. Her developmental milestones had been normal. The parents had experienced lots of problems with Sean, who was 3 years older than Emma. He had had infantile eczema and required a lot of attention. He had temper tantrums and was 'always on the go'. They described a number of instances when he had had various accidents or upset relatives by being rude to them. One incident Mr Day remembered in particular was when Sean got lost when they were on a family holiday when he was 7 years of age. They described the event in great detail, taking turns to remind each other of details of the incident, apparently enjoying recalling it. Emma appeared annoyed by this but said nothing.

The parents had been together for two years and got married before Sean was born. Soon after, they had moved into the area because of Mr Day's work. He worked as middle manager in a local firm and Mrs Day worked in the clerical service. They did not report any particular problems. Certainly there were no mental health problems in the family. They described themselves as sociable people with many friends. Sean had started at the local college recently.

Individual session: When seen on her own Emma was rather reluctant to talk about herself. She was somewhat overweight and had many spots on her face. She said that she liked school but was having difficulties with friends. The girls in her year did not like her and she had only one friend called Sarah, but she too had become indifferent towards her. She felt that Sarah had been influenced by the other girls. She liked the teachers; she was good at her schoolwork. 'It's the only thing I am good at, nothing else.' She spent a lot of time on her homework. She did not like PE or anything related to sports. She occasionally went out with Sarah.

She had been cutting herself for the last two years. She was asked to remember the first time she had cut herself. Initially Emma said she could not remember when it was. But with persuasion she recollected that it happened when she was in year 8. She had been pushed from behind when she stood in a queue in class and had fallen down. Everyone had laughed and she remembered someone calling her 'a fat blob'. She had felt stupid and foolish. When she came home that day her mother had noticed the dirt on the school uniform and asked her about it. She had told her mother what had happened. Her mother had looked at her incredulously and said, 'What did you do? People don't push you for no reason!'. She had gone to her room and started crying. 'I felt that I was a nobody and that no one liked me. Not even my mother,' she said, 'I cried for a long time and later took a pair of scissors and cut my forearm. It hurt first, but later it was OK. I wiped the blood with tissues and flushed it in the toilet'.

Following this incident, Emma had been cutting herself one or two times a week. She had kept it a secret from everyone for some time. Her friend Sarah had seen the scars in her forearms one day and asked her about it. She had confided in her and asked her to keep it to herself. It typically occurred when something made her upset. She would come to her room and take the pair of scissors, go to the toilet and cut herself. She wiped the blood with toilet tissues and flushed them down the toilet. At times she had used the set of dividers from her geometry set or pieces of glass to hurt herself. Most of the self-cutting occurred at home but more recently she had started carrying something sharp with her in her school bag all the time so that she could use it if there was a need. It gave her a sense of security. On the last occasion there had been the usual name calling and a girl had kicked her under the desk. Emma had excused herself from class, gone to the toilet and cut herself with the Stanley knife.

Not every incident of self-cutting was related to school problems. In fact, most instances of self-injury were unrelated to school bullying and occurred mostly at home. Emma was asked to think of a time when it happened at home. The following conversation ensued:

> *Clinician:* Can you think about what feelings overcome you just before you start cutting yourself?
>
> *Emma:* I am not sure . . . (Thinks) Some anger . . . some irritation . . . some frustration . . . maybe . . . It is difficult to describe . . .
>
> *Clinician:* It is difficult to pinpoint, is it?
>
> *Emma:* That's right, difficult to name it.
>
> *Clinician:* Why do you think you harm yourself? Can you think of the reasons for it?
>
> *Emma:* I don't know . . . I am not sure . . .
>
> *Clinician:* Do you think 'I have had enough; I want to kill myself?'
>
> *Emma:* No. It's not that . . . I am not thinking of doing away with myself. No, no. Definitely not.
>
> *Clinician:* What is it then? What purpose does it serve? In what way does it 'help' you?
>
> *Emma:* (Pause) I feel better after it. It may sound strange (smiles uneasily). It makes me feel better, as if all the hurt is gone.
>
> *Clinician:* It looks as if it helps you to cope with all the unmanageable and intolerable feelings. Am I right about it?
>
> *Emma:* That's about right.
>
> *Clinician:* Would you do it on days you are not upset? Suppose there was a week when things were OK, would you do it then?
>
> *Emma:* Not likely. It happens only when I am upset, not otherwise.
>
> *Clinician:* Is it possible, just possible, that you are punishing yourself by cutting yourself?
>
> *Emma:* I don't think so. I feel guilty about it now that you ask me.

During the discussion it became clear that the motivation for the behaviour was not to kill herself but to achieve relief from an unbearable state of mind. Although she did not understand what lead to the rising tension in her mind, she was sure that self-cutting provided relief from intense negative feelings. She denied thinking about other ways of killing herself such as by taking an overdose.

In the latter part of the interview she was talkative and came across as intelligent and witty. She said that she had been feeling unhappy with 'everything' in her life, but was unable to identify anything in particular. She said she had got used to the bullying at school. Asked about what she wished most to see happen, she felt she needed more friends at school and to be accepted within the group. Would all her problems disappear if she had more friends tomorrow? Emma became solemn and serious at this point. She started crying and said in a faint voice, 'It's mum and dad . . . They are never there . . . We never do things together . . . They are always away.' She described her loneliness and feeling of emptiness when at home. Her brother was out with friends and her parents were away at their favourite pub. They had an active social life. Her father went to the pub every evening and was known as a good snooker player. She spent most evenings at home on her own doing her homework or watching television. She had been going out with friends, especially Sarah. But that did not make her feel any better. She said it was as if something was missing; she was not sure what it was. She denied any past or present abuse.

There were other times when she felt hopeful and even happy. She wanted to be a veterinary nurse. She liked animals, but her parents had refused to let her have pets. They had argued that it was too much work and responsibility. She liked drawing and art. She was good at sketching animals. But nobody took any notice of her drawings except her art teacher.

Emma came across as unhappy and sad rather than depressed. She felt unloved and uncared for. Her accomplishments and achievements were met with silence and disregard by her parents. School bullying added to her sense of worthlessness and irrelevance. A second individual assessment session was arranged. During the second session held the next week, the therapist took up the issue of her relationship with her parents. Emma was intensely loyal to her parents and described them as dutiful parents who looked after her every need. She felt that she was not close to either of them but was inclined to blame herself for it. Unlike her brother, she did not have a good social life, and this was again her fault. She was not good at making or keeping friends. She belonged to the group of kids in school who were 'discards' and no one cared about them. They were not included in activities, social events or invited to parties.

The therapist asked about relationships within the family. Emma said that there had been some marital problems between her parents a few years ago. She was not sure of the details but was aware of a time when her father was about to leave the family for someone else. Her mother had begged him to stay and, after a period of being separated, they had decided to stay together. She felt that her mother did not leave her dad's side because she did not trust him. She felt that they were quite happy now. Her brother was an outgoing person and had lots of friends. He did not depend on his parents as much as she did. She was neither happy at school nor home. Asked about when this sense of unhappiness began, she said things had never been good as far back as she could remember. She was particularly concerned about the way she was treated by her mother. She said that she could not discuss any of her problems with her mother because 'she did not listen'. For example, if she complained of a headache, her mother would say 'It's not a headache, it is just your imagination' or 'I have a bigger headache'. When she had complained of bullying at school the response was that Emma 'asked for it' and that she should be able to deal with it rather than moan about it. Emma had stopped telling her parents about her difficulties for fear of being blamed and ridiculed. 'It is bad enough that I have to put up with the name calling at school; I don't want to her to make me feel small.'

With encouragement from the therapist she explained that whenever she tried to talk to her mother about her experiences, she felt that she was not being heard. She said that they did not take what she said seriously and often turned it around and made her feel it was all her fault. If she tried to tell her how hurt she was at being betrayed by her friend, her mother's reaction was: 'You don't really mean it, Emma; you kids fall out and get back together, wait and see.' If she complained of not having many friends, her mother would say, 'Cheer up, snap out of it. You will get over it.' Emma felt that her mother trivialised her feelings. She remembered that when she was a child she had often said, 'You say no but you mean yes, I know.' Emma had found all this confusing and was not sure whom to believe. She was now convinced that she was not as good as the other girls. None of them liked her and it was all her fault.

When discussing the self-harm instances Emma was asked to describe them in detail. Most of the incidents occurred at home when she came back from school. On such occasions, she was alone at home; she was bored and felt angry. At such times she remembered some of the incidents of bullying at school or the remarks made by other girls and the humiliation she had felt. She would also think about the good times other girls might be having and feel left out. This would make her feel angry, sad and frustrated; the feelings would build inside her and she would reach for any sharp object and cut herself. The pain and the sight of blood gave her a sense of release and relief. She had hoarded a number of sharp objects in her room such as scissors, pieces of glass and small knives. She had now got used to carrying a knife or a piece of broken glass with her in her school bag for 'emergencies'. Both her forearms were covered in numerous linear scars resulting from self-cutting; she explained that the cuts were superficial and had never required suturing.

Case conceptualisation and formulation

Based on the information derived from the assessment sessions, it was felt that Emma was using self-cutting a way of coping with her intense feelings of sadness, anger and frustration. She experienced a sense of relief after cutting herself and was using it as a means of coping. She was not intending to kill herself or harm herself. Rather it could be argued that the self-cutting behaviour was an alternative to attempting to kill herself or harm herself in any other way. As maladaptive it was, it served the purpose of keeping her safe. Although the immediate and more visible problem was school bullying and lack of friends, the underlying difficulty was the invalidation of her private experiences by her parents, especially her mother. Whenever she expressed her difficulties, her parents appeared to trivialise, disregard or dismiss them and make her feel that it was all her fault. Growing up in such an invalidating environment made her angry, sad and miserable. In addition she was experiencing problems with peers. She was keen to have friends but had not been successful in making and keeping friends in spite of all her efforts.

Although she was unhappy and miserable, there was no evidence of clinical depression. There was no pervasive depression in her mood or anhedonia (loss of enjoyment). In fact, she wanted to be out with her peers enjoying life. It was her inability to find the right friends that made her sad and angry. In psychiatric literature, the feeling of chronic, low grade depression has been described as dysthymia (see later). One of the important factors that contributed to the self-harming behaviour was the unavailability of the parents both physically and emotionally. They appeared to be spending little time with Emma or at home for that matter. For reasons of their own they had an active social life that excluded

Emma. The reasons for this were unclear. It was likely that, following the marital problems, they had organised their lives in such a way to enhance their relationship that did not factor Emma into the relationship equation. Perhaps they felt that now that Emma was grown up she did not need them. The net result was that Emma felt rejected and isolated by both the family and her peer group. The various factors that contributed to Emma's self-injurious behaviour are shown in Figure 15.1.

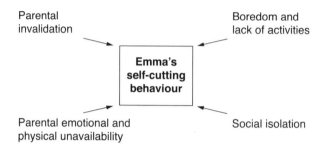

Figure 15.1 Hypothesised factors contributing to Emma's self-cutting behaviour.

Theoretical perspectives

In the literature a number of terms have been used describe self-injurious behaviour. Terms such as deliberate self-harm (DSH), parasuicide and attempted suicide have been used to describe a variety of behaviours ranging from taking overdoses, attempted hanging, self-cutting and other forms of self-injury. At the very outset it is important to make a distinction between attempted suicide and self-injury. All major reviews and studies uphold this distinction. Most workers in the field of study agree that that the self-injurer does not intend to die as a result of his/her actions. In the overwhelming majority of adults and adolescents who engage in self-injury the main intention is not one of suicide. Indeed it has been argued that self-injury is a form of anti-suicidal behaviour that represents the person's coping method to *prevent* committing suicide. The correlates of self-injury including motivation, associated problems, aetiology and outcome are vastly different from those who engage in other forms of DSH such as overdose. Undoubtedly self-injury is a maladaptive form of coping.

A comparison of psychiatric diagnoses in adult self-injurers and those who attempt suicide supports this distinction (Ferreira de Castro *et al.*, 1998). In contrast to those who attempted suicide, less self-injurers were diagnosed with major depression (56% vs 14%). On the other hand the self-injury group was more likely to be dysthymic (12% vs 7%) or have adjustment disorder with depressed mood (24% vs 6%). The main conclusion from the study was that the psychiatric profile of those who self-harm in order to die and those who self-injure to cope are very different.

Self-cutting is relatively common in the general population. A US study showed that 4% of the general population (all ages) and 21% of clinical samples report self-cutting behaviour (Briere and Gill, 1998). The peak incidence of self-cutting occurs between 16 and 25 years. In adults, self-cutting behaviour is known to be a prominent feature of patients with borderline personality disorder.

One of the few studies in children and adolescents to compare self-cutters and self-poisoners was carried out in the study of English school children by Keith Hawton and colleagues. In the study involving more than 6000 pupils aged 15 and 16 years they found that self-cutting was almost three times more common than self-poisoning. This study also showed that there were significant differences in motivation between the two groups. Less than 1% of self-cutters spontaneously mentioned that they wanted to die (compared to 10% of self poisoners). Self-cutters were significantly more likely to have carried out the act impulsively (having thought about it for less than one hour) than self-poisoners. The most common motivations for self-cutting were to get relief from an unbearable state of mind and punish oneself. The most frequently endorsed reason given by self-cutters suggested that many used deliberate self-injury as a form of coping (Rodham, Hawton and Evans, 2004).

Self-injury, i.e. physical injury to oneself, has been divided into three types (Favazza, 1998):

1 **Self-mutilation**: rare forms of major mutilation such as castration, amputation of limbs occurring in psychotic states.
2 **Stereotyped self-injury**: repetitive forms of self-injury, biting, head banging seen in those with severely intellectual disability and autism.
3 **Superficial or moderate self-injury**: the common form of self-injurious behaviour, the subject of this chapter. This includes self-cutting, scratching, skin picking and interference with wound healing.

The commonest form of self-injury in adolescents is superficial self-cutting of the arms, and less commonly the thighs. The mode of cutting is usually light superficial cutting without harming the arteries. Some adolescents make superficial scratches or carve words. Witnessing the multiple parallel scars in the forearms of a habitual self-cutter can be an alarming sight. A variety of sharp objects are used to inflict injuries ranging from razor blades to pieces of glass and other sharp instruments. Superficial/moderate self-injury often begins as episodic self-harm to relieve tension but soon becomes repetitive and even addictive. Some adolescents have been known to cut themselves over 100 times. Self-injury results in release of beta-endorphins, morphine-like substances, in the brain that lead to a feeling of euphoria and well-being. This is thought to be responsible for the habitual pattern of self-injury. Some have argued for it to be included under impulse-control disorders because of the relatively automatic nature of the act. Approximately 50% of self-cutters report that they do not feel the pain during the act of self-injury.

Pragmatic and theoretical descriptions of the various motivations in self-injurious behaviour may be broadly grouped under three headings:

• **Affect regulation:** When intense feelings build, the person is overwhelmed and unable to cope. By causing pain, self-injury reduces the level of emotional and physiological arousal to a bearable level. Self-injury eases tension and relieves anger. It is also a way of escaping from numbness and the subjects injure themselves to feel *something*. In states of dissociation and depersonalisation, it helps the person to be grounded in reality. For many it is a way of expressing emotional pain that they cannot bear.
• **Communication:** Communicating to others the extent of their turmoil,

expressing feelings that they cannot convey to others through speech and conveying their need for support

- **Control/punishment:** Continuing abusive patterns from the past by re-enacting them, punishing oneself for being 'bad', exerting a sense of control over one's body when one cannot control other things in life.

Those who self-injure report more use of problem avoidance as a coping strategy and perceive themselves to have less control over problem-solving options. This feeling of disempowerment is related to the chronic invalidation many of them have experienced.

Linehan (1993) talks about people who self-injure having grown up in an invalidating environment as follows:

> An invalidating environment is one in which communication of private experiences is met by erratic, inappropriate, or extreme responses. In other words, the expression of private experiences is not validated; instead it is often punished and/or trivialised; the experience of painful emotions [is] disregarded. The individual's interpretation of her own behaviour, including the intents and motivations of behaviour, are dismissed . . . Invalidation has two primary characteristics. First, it tells the individual that she is wrong in both her description and her analysis of her own experiences, particularly in her views of what is causing her own emotions, beliefs and actions. Second, it attributes her experiences to socially unacceptable characteristics or personality traits.

Everyone experiences invalidations like these at some time or another, but for people brought up in invalidating environments, these messages are constantly received. Parents may mean well but be too uncomfortable with negative emotions to allow children to express them, and the result is unintentional invalidation. Chronic invalidation can lead to self-invalidation and self-distrust, and the 'I never matter' feeling.

A feature common to many self-injurers is the feeling of chronic low grade depression. This condition has been called dysthymic disorder. The key feature of dysthymic disorder is the occurrence of a sustained depressed mood for more than one year accompanied by other depressive features such as altered appetite and sleep, low energy and lack of enjoyment. Low self-esteem and feelings of hopelessness are common. The condition differs from clinical depression (major depression) in that it is not episodic or acute although a depressive episode may be superimposed on pre-existing dysthymia (double depression).

Self-injurious behaviour may occasionally be a feature of other conditions. Although self-injury may not be the salient feature of such presentations, it is important to exclude the possibility of such conditions when faced with an adolescent who is repeatedly self-injuring.

Child abuse: Child sexual abuse may occasionally present as repetitive self-injurious behaviour. Many children and adolescents who have been sexually abused or have been subjected to neglect are known to exhibit self-cutting behaviour. In such children dissociative experiences are common. Dissociation is a mental process, which produces a lack of connection in a person's thoughts, memories, feelings, actions or sense of identity. During the period of time when a person is dissociated, certain information is not associated with other information as it normally would be. For example, during a traumatic experience, a person may dissociate the memory of the place and circumstances of the trauma from his or her ongoing memory, resulting in temporary mental escape from the fear and pain of the trauma and in some cases a memory gap surrounding the experience.

'Emergent' personality disorder: This is a controversial group. Usually personality disorders are not diagnosed in children and adolescents under the age of 18 years. In adults the term personality disorder is used to describe an enduring and inflexible pattern of behaviour and experiences involving affective expression, ways of relating and poor impulse control. The category of borderline personality disorder (BPD) is particularly relevant to our discussion of self-injurious behaviour. The hallmarks of BPD are enduring patterns of unstable and intense interpersonal relationships, impulsivity (substance misuse, recklessness, binge eating), affective instability (intense irritability, anger, depression) lasting hours, feelings of emptiness and fear of abandonment. Repeated suicidal behaviours such as taking overdoses and self-mutilation are common. Although there is agreement among clinicians that BPD or emerging BPD is evident in some adolescents, the current international classificatory systems prohibit the diagnosis of personality disorder in children and adolescents.

Occasionally older adolescents may qualify for a diagnosis of BPD usually in the context of chaotic family histories of abuse, neglect and parental psychopathology. DSH is often a prominent feature as illustrated by the following case.

Harry was a 16-year-old boy when he came to the attention of CAMHS. He was adopted at the age of 3, having suffered severe neglect and abuse as a child. He had been hospitalised as a baby for failure to thrive and, later, with several fractures. He was deemed to have learning disability but had managed reasonably well at the local school until the age of 15. His adoptive parents were used to 'his ways'. He had been known to talk of killing children, stealing from old people and letting them burn. His parents attributed his attitude to 'immaturity' and 'lack of understanding'. He had no friends because of his unpredictable and aggressive outbursts. He would make friends with one or two boys and go all out to please them but soon fall out with them and never contact them again. His friends were afraid of him because of his unpredictable behaviour and avoided him. He had taken several overdoses but could not explain why he took them. He had been admitted to hospital with repeated deep self-cutting that required surgical intervention. On different occasions he had swallowed fishhooks, put objects into his nose and pierced his tongue with a screwdriver. He wanted his parents by his side all the time and was afraid of being left alone.

Choice of treatment and management

Of the various forms of treatment that have been studied in the management of DSH (uncomplicated by the presence of other disorders) brief problem-solving therapy is regarded as the one with the most evidence to support its application. In an extensive literature review of randomised controlled trials of treatments for patients with DSH, Townsend *et al.* (2001) examined six trials in which problem-solving treatment was compared with control treatments. Meta-analysis of the results showed that those offered problem solving therapy had significantly improved scores for depression, hopelessness and improvement in their problems compared to control groups.

Problem-solving therapy (PST) is a brief treatment aimed at helping the young person to acquire basic problem-solving skills, by taking him/her through a series of steps: identifying personal problems, constructing a problem list that clarifies and prioritises them, selecting a target list of problems that the person wants to solve, generating possible solutions for the problems; implementing the solutions and reappraising them. This usually involves about 6 one hour sessions and includes work to be undertaken between sessions. It can be delivered by any experienced mental health professional, with suitable training and supervision.

PST teaches clients a systematic strategy for approaching problems. Problem-solving therapy serves the dual purpose of treating clients' immediate problems and preparing them to deal with future problems on their own. Problem solving is taught to clients by using cognitive modelling, prompting, self-instructions and reinforcement. The distinguishing feature of PST is that it links the current psychological difficulties or symptoms the person is experiencing with their current problems (as opposed to CBT which associates thoughts with emotions and behaviour). In Emma's case a decision was made to adopt the PST approach to address her difficulties in prioritising and analysing her problems while recognising that some of the problems she encountered were not within her control. For example, her parents played an important part in the way Emma felt about herself by disconfirming her feelings, motives and behaviours. This invalidating environment was thought to be a major factor in creating Emma's difficulties. Her parents were to be included in the treatment process to the extent they were considered important in carrying out the problem solving activities for Emma. The aim was to promote Emma's autonomy and self-efficacy with the help of her parents. A number of problem solving treatment sessions were arranged for Emma and her parents were included in some of the sessions. The format of the sessions are described below under the seven steps of the PST model (D'Zurilla,1986; Maynors-Wallis, 2005).

Step 1: Adopting a problem-solving orientation: The therapist explained to Emma that the purpose of the treatment was to identify the main problems that were associated with her symptoms. Rather than tell Emma what her problems and symptoms were, the therapist was interested in finding out from her what she considered her main concerns were. After all, she was the one who wanted things to change and she knew her problems better than anyone else including the therapist. After some discussion about what the symptoms and problems meant, Emma identified her main 'symptom' as self-injury. She had not attempted to stop harming herself previously, because she felt it was automatic and made her feel better.

Next the therapist encouraged her to examine what her main problems were. Although the therapist had his own ideas about the factors that contributed to her self-injurious behaviour, it was important that she was encouraged to talk freely about her problems. Together with the therapist she drew up a list of problems that she considered important. Emma's problem list consisted of the following:

1 lack of friends
2 bullying at school and
3 unhappiness at home.

After talking about each of these difficulties she came to the conclusion that it was mainly the three problems that made her unhappy and miserable. She acknowledged that if she did not have 'the three problems' she would not be self-harming. This was a turning point in the treatment: Emma was making a link between her 'problems' and her symptoms. The therapist spent some time trying to amplify the connection between her problems and the self-injurious behaviour and proceeded to outline the task before them: 'The next step is for the two of us to work through each one of the problems so that your "symptom" will get better and also look at ways of how you can enjoy life better and feel more fulfilled.' She was told that it would involve her active participation, maintaining records and doing regular homework tasks.

Step 2: Identifying and defining the problems: The next stage was to choose a problem on the list and apply problem-solving methods. It was important to be realistic and address a problem where some progress could be made rather than opt for one that was complex. Emma chose the task of making friends. She was helped with defining the problem accurately and objectively. Her difficulty was to get some of her classmates to do things with her or for her to be able to join in their activities. She had felt that she was always in the periphery of her peer group. The problem was thought to be complex and it was important to break it down into manageable tasks. First she had to identify the girls with whom she wanted to be friends and then think about how she could engage them (conversation, activities, hobbies). One of Emma's problems was that she prejudged the outcome even before trying. She needed encouragement to suspend her judgement and carry out the agreed tasks.

Step 3: Setting achievable goals for problem resolution: The first task was to set some achievable goals that would help her make friends with the identified girls. The therapist explored with Emma various ways of getting two of her ex-friends to talk to her. Her ultimate goal was to be able to join them in going out. She was reminded that it was important that she started on a new footing without dwelling on what might have happened in the past. She had to forgive their past mistakes and make a fresh start. She had also to be prepared to try again and again if the initial overtures were not successful.

Step 4: Generating solutions: At this stage she was encouraged to produce as many solutions as possible. Through brainstorming a list of possible steps were identified. These included approaching each of them individually, saying sorry for any past mistakes, and discussing common topics of interest. Emma wanted to invite them home and get permission from her parents for them to cook a meal because one of the friends was interested in cookery. She also wanted to ask them whether she could join them in going to the cinema or a concert. The list was long reflecting her long-felt desire to make friends and belong to a group.

Step 5: Weighing up and selecting solution/s: Emma was helped to make a list of pros and cons of each of the solutions, their feasibility, pitfalls and disadvantages. It was clear that she was being overambitious. She agreed on three solutions that had a good chance of succeeding. One task was to get talking to each of them separately to make a fresh start. This needed a lot of courage to overcome her reluctance and shyness. She had to think of the subjects they were interested in for discussion. She was also coached in complementing her friends and asking about how they got on with various activities that they liked such as cooking and sports. Another aim was to invite them to go to the cinema next week. She was aware that the offer may be turned down and she had to accomplish the first task before proceeding with the next. The third objective was to invite them home. For this she needed permission from her parents and also be ready with a number of activities that they may be interested in.

Step 6: Implementing the preferred solution: She was aware that each of the tasks needed lot of planning. If they did not turn out to be as successful as she hoped them to be, she would, with the help of the therapist, try other ways of overcoming the problem. A detailed discussion of how each of the tasks would be accomplished helped Emma to think about the details involved in implementing the solution. A number of alternative ways in which she would respond if it did not go according to plan were rehearsed. She was helped to make contingency plans if things did not turn out the way she hoped they would. For example if, on starting a conversation, her friend did not respond positively, she would say, 'Perhaps we will talk about these some other time,' and leave the place gracefully. She was encouraged not to give up the attempt and to persevere with approaching the friend. Emma proved to be resourceful in foreseeing possible barriers to implementation of the plan and devising countermoves to make it a success. To tempt her friends to visit her at home, she planned to rent a film that they liked. She agreed to make a note of the outcomes.

Step 7: Evaluating the outcome: At the next session a week later, she had managed to hold a conversation with the two friends. Initially they had been surprised that Emma had come to them and initiated the conversation. They believed that Emma was angry with them and would not speak to them again. The invitation home had not gone well. They had given one excuse or other and refused to visit her at home. Emma had invited herself to their place and was surprised that they agreed to it. The therapist commented that he was impressed with her creative thinking and ingenuity. She had postponed the idea of inviting them to the cinema to a later date. The therapist was keen to know what she had learned from the exercise. Emma said that she had overestimated the problems with her friends and commented, 'After all I am not too bad when it comes to making friends.' She added, 'And they too are not as bad as I thought.'

The problem solving experiment with her friends was a prelude to the more important task of getting her parents to be emotionally available to her and take her concerns seriously without disqualifying her. Although family interventions including formal family therapy would have been the natural choice of treatment for such problems, the therapist decided to use the problem-solving approach to deal with the issues. Since Emma had little control over her parents' behaviour, for this part of the treatment the therapist was to act as her advocate. Accordingly, family sessions were arranged to explore the possibility of working with them on a problem solving approach.

For this part of the PST, Emma identified the main problems as lack of parental involvement with her. More specifically, she described the problem as their lack of availability. 'They are too busy with their lives and I feel neglected,' she said. She had tried to talk to them in the past and it had not worked. Her mother had argued that Emma was going out with her friends anyway and was not at home. While this had been true on one occasion, Emma felt that her mother was using this as an excuse. Having described the problem the next step was to set achievable and measurable goals. Emma wanted her father to take an interest in her activities and her mother to listen to her. On further exploration, it was decided that one of the gaols would be get her father to come to school to discuss the issue of bullying. The name calling and pushing had been continuing at school, although Emma had learned to ignore them. She felt getting her father involved with the school would achieve two things: get him involved in protecting her and help stop the bullying. Another possibility was for them to spend time with her at home. This would improve the relationship between Emma and her parents and open channels of communication between them. Another solution was for Emma and her mother to go shopping together.

Implementing the plan required careful planning. The therapist agreed to bring up the issues during the family session but also wanted to know what she would give back to the parents in return. During the individual sessions it was clear that Emma was very angry with her parents and had had several arguments with them. They had retaliated by ignoring her and doing their own things. 'If you are going to behave like this, we have better things to do than taking all this abuse,' her mother had retorted. Evidently, Emma was not completely innocent and appeared to have antagonised her parents in trying to get them to take notice of her. When this was pointed out, Emma agreed to be co-operative and tactful. She said her mother liked shopping and could not object to Emma joining her; she could be more diplomatic and offer to join her in the weekly shopping trips to the supermarket before asking to go shopping in the nearby city. Both of them liked cooking and she could join her mother in cooking once a week. Considering the various pros and cons of the proposed solutions, Emma felt that the marital problems may stand in the way of trying to get them involved in the tasks. She wanted to know if the therapist could discuss marital issues with her parents. The therapist indicated that it was important to keep her problems and her parents' problems separate. If they needed help they could seek it elsewhere and it was their choice. The main issue for the therapist and Emma was to address the problems that they had already identified: non-involvement of parents and the invalidation she suffered at her mother's hands.

Family intervention: Mr and Mrs Day and Emma attended the family sessions. The therapist outlined Emma's 'symptom' and the various factors that contributed to it including her feeling of loneliness and boredom when she was at home on her own. He told them about the problem-solving approach and how Emma had made considerable improvements in getting her friends back. The therapist wondered how they could support Emma in overcoming her symptom. Initially her parents were defensive and attempted to blame Emma for her difficulties and divest themselves of any responsibility or part in it. They wanted Emma to 'kick the habit' and be a 'normal' teenager. This lead to an argument between Emma and her parents as each one kept blaming the other. The situation had to be defused by asking the parents about what sort of parents they wanted to be for Emma and what stood in the way of how they wanted to relate to her.

Her parents had felt that Emma was grown up and did not want to be dependent on them. Sean had always been independent and they *knew* that Emma was an independent girl. They were only giving her enough space so that she could be autonomous and self-sufficient. At this point Emma intervened and said that she missed them and wanted them to love her and be there for her. She felt distanced from them, not part of the family. More specifically she wanted to do things with them. This brought up the subject of how her father could help her by taking up with the school the issue of bulling. 'You are good at these sorts of things dad. If you take up the matter with the headteacher and the girls see you around school they won't dare bully me,' she said. She reminded him how effective he had been in dealing with a quarrelsome neighbour and pleaded with him to intervene at school. Her father said he had not known how bad things had been for Emma at school and agreed to take up the matter with the school authorities. As he spoke he became more animated and said that he would not hesitate to go to the local Member of Parliament or the press if the need be.

Her mother agreed to spend more time with her at home to help her overcome the 'habit'. But she wanted Emma to reciprocate by being civil and polite. Emma interrupted her to tell her that she would join in cooking with her at least once a week and would like to join her in the weekly shopping. There was much discussion about how the parents had assumed Emma to be grown up and not needing them. Her mother was prepared to sacrifice going out with her husband as often if only to improve her relationship with Emma. Mrs Day's relationship with her mother had been a stormy one and she had left home at 18 to get away from her, but a few years later her mother had died of cancer of the breast. Now she regretted not having made up with her before her death. She did not want Emma to ever lose touch with her. There were lots of tears shed during the session.

In a later family session they reported overall improvement in their relationships. The therapist brought up the topic of communication within the family and the need to validate the other person's feelings and actions even if one did not agree with them. Taking examples from children's common complaints such as crying after hurting themselves, the therapist discussed what an appropriate response would be. This led to a discussion about how they often responded to each other and they felt they were all culpable of not acknowledging each other's emotions and motivations. Mrs Day admitted that she had the habit of bypassing the stage of acknowledgement and getting on to the cause of the problem. Her husband said she could sound cold but he had got used to ignoring her on such occasions. For example, if he had met with an accident she would first ask about what caused it, who was at fault and what the damage to the car was, rather than find out if he was hurt. In a moment of self-reflection Mrs Day agreed that she was 'that sort of person'.

Course and outcome

Altogether Emma was seen for eight sessions of PST and the family was seen three times. During this period Emma reported improvement in her relationship with friends. She did have some disputes and setbacks with them but was able to take a long-term view of the relationships and ignore minor perturbations. 'I would be the loser, if I took each one of the disagreements seriously,' she explained. Her father kept his side of the bargain and had been to the school and spoken to the headteacher. The bullying stopped for a short period but soon resumed. He kept writing numerous letters to the school, local education authority and the papers. Emma was pleased that he was fighting her cause. Her mother stuck to her part of the agreement and stayed home on week days to keep Emma company. Emma joined her in cooking and baking cakes. They did the weekly shopping together. But Emma's social life did not improve a great deal. One positive development was that she got a boyfriend and was pleased to be with him. In many ways it made her feel better about herself.

Emma kept a record of the episodes of self-cutting. Although the frequency of self-injury got less, it took longer than expected to be abolished completely. This may have been because there was overall improvement in other areas of functioning and self-injury was not discussed much during the sessions. But midway through treatment Emma stopped self-cutting and never resorted to it again. At the beginning of treatment she had got rid of all sharp objects and instruments in her room as a precautionary measure. During the course of the treatment she was asked to take chances and not avoid sharp instruments. This she was able to achieve with ease. In parallel with the PST sessions she was requested to schedule enjoyable activities into her weekly timetable. Emma found this part of the treatment most difficult. Her boyfriend was not very helpful in this because he depended on her to unload his problems.

Nevertheless, Emma's symptom (self-cutting) ceased to exist and two of problems she had identified had shown considerable improvement. She reported that her mother continued to be dismissive of her problems, although she was making efforts to overcome her habitual way of responding. A sign of this was that she apologised, usually days after the event, for having been uncaring and insensitive.

Comments

Emma's case is quite typical of those with self-injurious behaviours seen in CAMHS. Her presentation at school with multiple cuts, oozing blood or the sight of numerous scars in the arms no doubt triggered alarm and panic among teachers and students. The spectacular way in which self-mutilation presents itself or is discovered usually has a dramatic effect among primary care professionals. Teachers and social workers who encounter self-injurious behaviour in adolescents feel paralysed and deskilled and usually seek urgent CAMHS involvement. Even among CAMHS workers there is a sense of unease and high anxiety when dealing with self-injurers. Once the uncommon, but serious, conditions described above have been excluded, careful consideration of the context of the behaviour is crucial to the management of such cases. In most instances the usual CAMHS practice of problem analysis and formulation is sufficient to manage most cases using simple interventions such as PST.

Emma's case could have been dealt with in a number of ways. In view of the many, significant family factors, many might have considered family therapy as the main method of treatment. However, most family therapists would agree that Emma needed some form of individual therapy. PST was chosen because of the evidence pointing to its effectiveness. Involvement of the family in the treatment was considered necessary to enable Emma to address problems not within her control. In CAMH practice it is important not to place the entire burden of, and responsibility for, change on the child.

Box 15.1 Research on self-injury shows that . . .

- Self-cutting as a form of deliberate self-harm is almost thrice as common in the community than self poisoning.
- Self-injury and its correlates are qualitatively different from self-poisoning.
- Self-cutting is most often impulsive and rarely carried out with suicidal intent.
- Self-injury provides a quick and dramatic release of physiological and emotional tension and is often employed as a method of coping with negative emotions.
- It may be fallacious to consider self-injury as a form of parasuicide.
- Problem solving therapy has been shown to be effective in self-harming behaviour.

References

Briere J, Gill E. Self-mutilation in clinical and general population samples: Prevalence, correlates and functions. *American Journal of Orthopsychiatry*. 1998; **68**: 609–20.

* D'Zurilla TJ. *Problem-solving Therapy: a social competence approach to clinical intervention*. New York: Springer; 1986.

Favazza AR. The coming of age of self-mutilation. *Journal of Nervous and Mental Diseases*. 1998; **186**: 259–68.

Ferreira de Castro E, Cunha MA, Pimenta F *et al*. Parasuicide and mental disorders. *Acta Psychiatrica Scandinavia*. 1998; **97**: 25–31.

Linehan M. *Cognitive-Behavioral Treatment of Borderline Personality Disorder*. New York: Guilford Press; 1993.

* Maynors-Wallis L. *Problem-solving Treatment for Anxiety and Depression: a practical guide*. Oxford: Oxford University Press; 2005.

Rodham K, Hawton K, Evans E. Reasons for deliberate self-harm: comparison of self-poisoners and self-cutters in a community sample of adolescents. *Journal of the American Academy of Child and Adolescent Psychiatry*. 2004; **43**: 80–87.

Townsend E, Hawton K, Altman DG *et al*. The efficacy of problem-solving treatments after deliberate self-harm: meta-analysis of randomized controlled trials with respect to depression, hopelessness and improvement in problems. *Psychological Medicine*. 2001; **31**: 979–88.

Chapter 16

Adolescent schizophrenia

Matt, a 15 years, 6 month old boy, was referred simultaneously by his General Practitioner and the crisis intervention team. He had been found in a park wandering and had been reported to the police by onlookers. When the police arrived on the scene and questioned him he had been unable to provide a satisfactory explanation for why he was not at school or what he was doing in the park. The police had searched him and found that he had a knife and a pair of scissors with him. He had been very anxious and agitated when he was brought home by the police. His behaviour had been odd at home. For example, he talked loudly in his room and been shouting out. He had been restless at nights and been walking around in his room. One night he had gone to the kitchen to prepare some food but left the cooker unattended. He was in another part of the house when the smoke alarm went off. Matt claimed that he had not used the cooker.

His parents had had to go to a funeral for two days. During this period he burst into his sister's room saying, 'You know what is going on.' His sister, Melanie (18 years), had telephoned her parents to say that Matt had been acting strange. On their return the parents made an appointment to see their GP. In the meantime, Matt wandered off from home and refused to come back. His mother and sister followed him down the street as far as they could. When they lost sight of him they came back home and informed the police. He was found the same day, sitting in a park, talking and singing to himself. With the help of the police, his parents contacted the Mental Health Crisis Team. He was seen at home the next day.

Clinical presentation and background

When Matt and his family were seen at home, his parents reported that his attendance at school had been erratic over the past 6 months. They felt that he was truanting and school was not taking any action. On a number of occasions he had set out to go to school but not attended and had been roaming around the streets. They were not sure what he was doing or how he spent the time. The school had reported to the parents that he was missing from school on a number of occasions. His mother had visited school and had been told that his schoolwork had been deteriorating and he went missing from school on a number of occasions. On questioning Matt, he had not been able to give a satisfactory explanation to his parents for his absence from school and had said that he had been away from school and been hanging around with his friends. His mother had spoken to his friends but they had said that they had no knowledge of his whereabouts. The parents had taken up the matter with Matt and wanted him to stop truanting and attend school regularly.

During this period they had noticed a change in his character. They found him to be restless and lacking in concentration. For example, Matt, who was a keen footballer, had not been able to sit through and watch a football match on television to the end. He had been a keen supporter of Manchester United and while the entire family had been watching an important football match in which Manchester United was playing a rival team, Matt had left the room soon after the match began and been found wandering around the house. The family considered this highly unusual for Matt because of his keen interest in football. They also noticed that he was in and out of the drawing room when he was at home but did nothing productive. At nights he could be heard pacing in his room or singing or talking out loud. At this time the parent's main concern was about loss of schoolwork. They felt that he was becoming a troublesome teenager, refusing to do as he was told and truanting from school. However, after the involvement of the police, they had started wondering about the possibility of something being wrong with him and wanted the GP to check him out.

When he was brought back home by the police he had claimed that everyone appeared different and that he himself had become different. He had been saying that he had a camera in his head and whatever he saw other people could see. At the time of examination he had not attended school for the past 4 weeks. The parents were sure that he was not taking any drugs. He had told his sister Melanie that she knew what he was thinking about and also had accused her of being an actress. He had said, 'You are not real, you are acting like Melanie.' He had been repeatedly saying, 'This is not real, it is a dream and I am going to wake up.' The parents felt that sometimes they could not understand his conversation. For example, he had been saying, 'Why are you asking me, you know what I am thinking. You know my thoughts, it is not fair.' They felt he was confused and said things that he did not mean.

Examination: When Matt walked into the room, he appeared somewhat suspicious and did not want to sit, preferring to stand close to the door. His parents reassured him and said that a doctor had come to see him and was there to help him to get better. Matt sat reluctantly on the edge of the chair, glancing around suspiciously. He was, however, co-operative and engaged in a conversation. He said he liked sports and had played football for the school team. He was also keen on cricket and described himself as a good bowler. Following further conversation about school and sporting activities, Matt felt more comfortable talking to the clinician. At one point he asked, 'Why are you asking me all these questions? You know what I know. You can see what I see.' He went on to say that other people knew about what he was thinking and what was in his head. He said he probably had a camera in his head which other people could see.

Other people knew that he was a 'freak' and that they put their head down whenever they saw him. He said there was a red car that passed their house frequently and that there were some people in it who were coming to get him. He got quite agitated and restless when talking about the 'red car'. At this point, he got up from his seat and looked out of the window and then turned back to the clinician and said, 'I feel different, something is wrong with me. I want to be well again.' When asked about whether things appeared different to him, he said that the world was different and things had changed and felt strange. He too had changed and his body felt different. The previous night he had thought he was God and had done 200 press-ups. While talking about his experiences he appeared incoherent, flitted from one subject to another without any rational connection or meaning. For example, he said, 'They look at me, I feel strange, like in Grange Hill. I feel I am 13. You know what happened to me at 13. Thirteen is unlucky. I am not going to be normal.' During the interview there were times when he laughed to himself quite inappropriately. He could not explain what he was laughing about. A number of times he repeated to himself, 'This is not real, it is a dream, I am going to wake up.'

Matt said that he heard voices in his head. Later he said the voices were out there in the street. He identified the voice as a man's voice and it was talking to him but he was not clear what the voice was telling him. Matt found it difficult to be in the room for too long and said that he wanted to go to his room and play music.

Mental state examination: His mental state was summarised as follows:

- Appearance and behaviour: Matt was a tall, well-built boy who appeared agitated and restless. He appeared somewhat perplexed and was obviously finding it difficult to explain some of his experiences. At times he appeared suspicious and at other times he was laughing to himself inappropriately.
- Speech: His speech was to a large extent coherent but at times he lost his train of thought and it was difficult to follow what he was saying. It appeared as if he wanted to say a lot of things but was finding it difficult to put them into words. At times he did not complete the sentence before going on to the next topic.
- Abnormalities in perception: Matt experienced occasional auditory hallucinations. This consisted of hearing another man's voice but he could not identify the person. There were no second person hallucinations.
- Mood: Matt appeared anxious and agitated; there was no evidence of depression or elation.
- Thinking: Matt admitted that he felt that his thoughts were 'mixed up' and found it difficult sometimes to relate his experiences. At times he stopped in mid-conversation as if he had lost the thought. At other times it was difficult to follow his train of thinking. He had persecutory delusions, such as people coming to get him in a red car. He also had ideas of reference, feeling that other people put their heads down when they saw him. More importantly, he felt his thoughts were audible and other people knew what he was thinking. Secondary elaboration of this was evident when he spoke of a camera in the head, although he was not sure in whose head the camera was. In addition he described feelings of derealisation (the world had changed) and depersonalisation (that he had changed).
- Cognitive functions: Matt's concentration and attention were poor. This was also evident during the interview. He had difficulties in watching television programmes, even the ones he was interested in.
- Insight: Matt was acutely aware that something was wrong with him but was unsure as to what it was. He felt that his experiences were in some way abnormal and that he was not going to get better.

Personal and family history: Matt was adopted by the Murray family when he was 6 months of age. In his family of origin there had been seven children and all of them had been removed from his mother because of neglect and placed with various carers by Social Services. The mother was said to have suffered from a psychotic illness, probably schizophrenia. He and his older brother, now in his 20s, were adopted by the Murray family, who had two girls of their own. At the time of examination, his older brother was in Brinsford Prison, having been convicted of theft and grievous bodily harm. His adoptive father, Mr Murray, was a credit collector and Mrs Murray was a full-time housewife. As far as the family could tell, Matt's development had been normal and there had been no particular setbacks. He had developed epilepsy at the age of 8 and had been on medication until the age of 13 years. The medication had been gradually withdrawn and he had been free of fits since. There was no other medical history of note. Matt was described as an average student at school, he did not particularly like school but was interested in football and cricket and played for the school football team. His family described him as a well behaved boy who had not caused them any problems in the past. He had no close friends but the family did not consider this a major problem. He had a number of acquaintances through his sporting activities but did not socialise with them outside school. He had turned down all invitations to join them in birthday parties or other activities.

Case conceptualisation and formulation

From the history and examination, it was clear that Matt was experiencing a psychotic episode. He appeared to be out of touch with reality, with evidence of thought disorder, auditory hallucinations, persecutory delusion and ideas of reference. He was agitated and perplexed. He had poor concentration and somewhat incoherent speech. In addition he had de-realisation and depersonalisation. He showed remarkable insight in that he knew that his experiences were abnormal and, from his point of view, unreal. In short he was showing the characteristic feature of a psychotic episode in which the boundary between internal experiences and external reality was breaking down. Four possible causes for the psychotic episode were considered. They were in order of likelihood: schizophrenia, manic depressive psychosis, drug misuse and temporal lone epilepsy.

Although he had some grandiose delusions ('being like God'), overall his mood was judged to be normal, thus excluding (for the moment) manic depressive psychosis. Given his age, drug misuse was a strong possibility, but on closer enquiry there was no evidence for it. A drug screen was carried out and proved to be negative. In temporal lobe epilepsy the psychotic symptoms are episodic and short-lived. Thus by a process of exclusion a diagnosis of schizophrenia was made.

However, the aetiology of the disorder was unclear. It was clear that Matt had a predisposition to schizophrenia by virtue of the strong family history. From the descriptions of his premorbid personality he appeared to have been a rather lonely and isolated individual. According to the stress-vulnerability model, schizophrenia is caused by an underlying psychobiological vulnerability, determined early in life by genetic and early environmental (e.g. perinatal) effects. Once the vulnerability is established, the onset of the illness and its course are determined by the interplay of various environmental and other stressors. In Matt's case there did not appear to be any specific stressful event that accounted for the occurrence of the disorder at this particular time.

Theoretical perspectives

Traditionally mental disorders have been classed into two broad groups, the neuroses and psychoses. The former includes anxiety-related problems such as OCD, PTSD, phobias, generalised anxiety and so on. Psychoses comprise schizophrenias, manic depressive disorders and related conditions. The main difference between the neuroses and psychoses is that in the psychoses the individual is believed to be out of touch with reality during the psychotic phase, whereas in neurotic disorders, in spite of the enormous suffering, the person's sense of reality remains intact. To the outside observer the psychotic person's thought processes and behaviours appear unusually irrational, illogical and incomprehensible. During a psychotic phase the person may experience hallucinations or delusions (see later). People with psychosis generally lack insight and are unaware that their experiences are not real.

The term 'psychotic disorder' is commonly used to mean major mental illness. The two main psychotic disorders are schizophrenia and manic depressive psychosis (bipolar disorder). Emile Kraepelin (1919), considered to be the father of psychiatry, was the first to differentiate between dementia precox (meaning schizophrenia) and manic depressive illness based on the natural history of the two illnesses. His observation that dementia precox (later named schizophrenia by Bleuler) was a chronic illness with poor prognosis as compared to the relatively non-deteriorating course of manic depressive illness has been borne out by all subsequent studies. In the following section first the general features of schizophrenia are discussed as it pertains to adults and this is followed by a description of the features unique to schizophrenia in children and adolescents.

Schizophrenia in adults: Schizophrenia is a relatively common form of psychotic disorder. The prevalence rates of schizophrenia are considered to be consistent worldwide. Its lifetime prevalence is nearly 1% and the annual incidence is about 10–15 per 100,000. It is a syndrome with various presentations and a variable, often relapsing, long-term course. The diagnosis has good reliability, even across ages and cultures, though there is no biological marker. Onset before the age of 30 is the norm, with men tending to present some 4 years younger than women. In 20% of the cases the onset of the illness is before the age of 18.

Schizophrenia is a chronic, severe and disabling mental illness. There are a number of distinguishing signs and symptoms of it. However, expression of these symptoms varies greatly from one individual to another. The characteristic symptoms of schizophrenia have been conceptualised as falling into three broad categories: positive symptoms, negative symptoms and cognitive or disorganised symptoms. The positive symptoms and signs are essentially excess or distortions of normal brain functions of thinking, perceiving, formation of ideas and sense of oneself, and include the following (*see* also Box 16.1).

Hallucinations: These are false perceptions in any of the senses that arise in the absence of any external stimulus. Although hallucinations can occur in any of the senses the most common are in the auditory modality, experienced as hearing voices. The voices are perceived as located in the external world and as actual and vivid. The hallmark of hallucinations in schizophrenia is that patients experience voices talking about him or her as 'he' or 'she' (third person auditory hallucinations), but second person hallucinations (voices talking to the person) are common, as are command hallucinations, olfactory, tactile, somatic and visual hallucinations. About 70% of people with schizophrenia experience hallucinations in one or more sensory modalities

Delusions: These are false personal beliefs held with absolute certainty and conviction in spite of obvious proof or evidence to the contrary dominating the patient's mind and untenable in terms of social or cultural background. The content of delusions often revolve around persecutory, religious, grandiose, somatic or referential themes. For instance, the person may believe they are being spied on, followed or tricked (paranoid delusions) or may believe that comments and actions of others, television or passages from books are directed specifically at them (referential delusions). Delusions may be realistic (e.g. being followed) or bizarre (e.g. believing that aliens have invaded earth). Delusions may be derived from attempts to make sense of other symptoms such as the experience of passivity (sensing that someone or something is controlling your body, emotions or thoughts). Typical experiences involve beliefs that thoughts are being taken out of one's head, or inserted into one's mind, or that thoughts are known to others (respectively termed thought withdrawal, thought insertion and thought broadcast).

Thought disorder: This refers to disorganised thinking expressed through abnormal spoken language. For example, the person jumps erratically from one topic to another during the conversation, grammatical structure of language breaks down and speech is generally speeded up and incoherent. Incoherent speech, disorganised thinking and derailment in the stream of thought and speech may occur. Patients with insight often say that their thoughts are mixed up and thinking is distorted. Patients with thought disorder may present with complaints of poor concentration or of their mind being blocked or emptied (thought block).

Negative symptoms: These are deficit symptoms that involve loss of personal ability, such as initiative, interest in others and sense of enjoyment. Blunted or fatuous emotions (flat affect), poverty of speech (alogia), withdrawal, loss of motivation and ambivalence (avolition) are typical behaviours. This may involve lack of energy, apathy or seeming absence of interest in activities they had been interested in (anhedonia).

Box 16.1 Key clinical features of schizophrenia

Positive symptoms

- Hallucinations: Most commonly auditory hallucination; voices talking to each other about the person or commenting on his or her actions or thoughts in the third person are characteristic of, but not exclusive to, schizophrenia.
- Delusions: False beliefs held with absolute conviction; the content of delusions may take several forms (persecutory, grandiose, reference and so on).
- Thought disorder: Thought insertion, withdrawal, broadcast; looseness of association; incoherent or disorganised speech, thought block, derailment of the stream of thought.

- Experiences of control: Feeling controlled by an alien force or power ('passivity' phenomena); 'made' feelings (e.g. bodily sensations being imposed), impulses and acts.

Negative symptoms

- Loss of motivation and initiative (avolition), poverty of speech and thought (alogia), loss of emotional expressiveness (flattening of affect), apathy, anhedonia (loss of ability to enjoy), loss of interest and social withdrawal.

The prognosis in adult schizophrenia depends on presentation, response to treatment and the quality of aftercare. Early and continued medication remains the key to good management. Acute onset over several weeks rather than many months, a supportive family, personal intelligence and insight, positive rather than negative symptoms, later age of onset (over 25 years) and a good response to low dose drugs are indicative of better outcome. By contrast, the worst-case scenario could be an insidious onset illness over several years in a teenager from a disrupted family who shows possible brain damage or additional learning difficulties.

Differential diagnosis: The presentation of schizophrenia may evolve over time, from non-specific depression or anxiety into psychotic states with typical symptoms. Differential diagnosis is limited but other conditions need to be excluded. These include temporal lobe epilepsy, manic-depressive psychosis and drug-induced states. Psychotic symptoms, often indistinguishable from those seen in schizophrenia, occur in manic depressive illness. Mania typically presents with hyperactivity, an elevated or excessive irritable mood, sleep loss, pressure of speech and a tendency to jump from topic to topic (flight of ideas). The latter may mimic forms of thought disorder, while grandiose beliefs (often delusional) may generate excess spending or a chaotic lifestyle. Hypomania is the term applied to a less severe form without psychotic features.

Schizophrenia can sometimes be triggered by heavy use of stimulant or hallucinogenic drugs. There is increasing evidence that cannabis use can be a contributing trigger to developing schizophrenia. Some studies suggest that cannabis is neither a sufficient nor a necessary factor for schizophrenia, but that cannabis may significantly increase the risk of developing schizophrenia and may be, among others, a significant causal factor. A recent review of studies from which a causal contribution to schizophrenia can be assessed has suggested that cannabis doubles the risk of developing schizophrenia on an individual level and may be responsible for up to 8% of cases in the population (Arseneault *et al.*, 2004). Drug intoxication and withdrawal may present with psychotic symptoms. Thus in illegal drug use, symptoms may mimic or precipitate a psychotic episode.

Aetiology: The causes of schizophrenia are not known. However, interplay of genetic, biological, environmental and psychological factors are thought to be involved. Schizophrenia is known to run in families. Evidence for a genetic aetiological cause grows stronger: up to 50% of identical (mono-zygotic) twins will share a diagnosis, compared to about 15% of non-identical (dizygotic) twins. The strength of genetic factors varies across families, but some 10% of a person's first degree relatives (parents, siblings and children) will also be schizophrenic, as will 50% of the children of two schizophrenic parents.

Schizophrenia in children and adolescence: Thankfully, psychotic disorders are not common in children and adolescents, but when they do occur it causes severe disruption and disability in the young person and family. The majority of episodes of psychotic disorder in adolescence would be the first such episode of the illness and there is bound to be considerable diagnostic uncertainty, as the natural history of the disorder is yet to unfold. It may be the first episode of a lifelong disorder such as schizophrenia or the manifestation of the other major mental illness, manic-depressive psychosis (also called bipolar affective disorder). It may be a psychotic disorder secondary to an organic disorder (particularly temporal lone epilepsy), substance misuse or it may be a brief psychotic episode to be followed by full recovery and no further episodes of illness.

The diagnostic criteria for children and adolescents is little different from those in adulthood, albeit with a recognition that a lack of progress or development in a teenager maybe the equivalent of deterioration in an adult. Child and adolescent onset schizophrenia may be divided into two classes: the very early onset (occurring before 13) and early or adolescent onset (occurring between 13 and 19) schizophrenia. The frequency of schizophrenia rises very rapidly during adolescence and beyond, reaching a peak between 25 and 30. The very early onset variety is rare. Around adolescence the prevalence rises rapidly to give a rate of 2–3 per 1000 in the teenage population.

Early onset adolescent schizophrenia has been shown to be associated with poor premorbid functioning and early developmental delays. Studies show that about 20% of adolescents with schizophrenia show language and reading delays and in about one third of cases there has been significant difficulties in social development affecting the ability to make and keep friends. Below average IQ, around 85, appears to be the norm in those with adolescent schizophrenia. Adolescent schizophrenia frequently presents with an insidious as opposed to an acute onset. It is characterised both by more prominent negative symptoms (e.g. flattened and inappropriate affect and bizarre manneristic behaviour) and by relatively fewer well-informed systematised delusions and auditory hallucinations when compared with adult schizophrenia. Some studies have found that the disorganised and undifferentiated sub-types were predominantly of adolescent onset, whereas the paranoid sub-type was most frequently first diagnosed in adult life. Although all sub-types can occur in adolescence, there is a relative predominance of the disorganised sub-type, which in earlier systems of classification would have been described as hebephrenia. A positive family history of schizophrenia amongst first relatives was found in 20% of adolescent probands with schizophrenia. This is about double the rate reported in comparable studies in adult onset schizophrenia.

Adolescent schizophrenia tends to run a chronic course, with only a small minority of cases making a full symptomatic recovery from the first psychotic episode. Adolescent schizophrenia is associated with a severe and unrelenting clinical course. In general, studies on outcomes in adolescent onset schizophrenia show that:

- in 25% the onset is insidious and they rarely recover
- in 25% no further episodes occur

- in 50% the prognosis is very poor with frequent relapses, marked disability and cognitive decline.

The main predictors of poor outcome in adolescent schizophrenia are poor premorbid functioning, negative symptoms and disorganised thought pattern. Progress in the first six months appears to be a good indicator of the eventual outcome (Hollis, 2000).

Choice of treatment and management

Management of schizophrenia requires pharmacological, psychological and social approaches, depending on the stage of the illness. Currently the mainstay of treatment is the use of anti-psychotic medication. Other forms of intervention are not possible without anti-psychotic medication. The newer atypical anti-psychotic medications (such as risperidone, olanzapine, and clozapine) are preferred over older typical anti-psychotic medications (such as chlorpromazine and haloperidol) due to their favourable side effect profile. Hospitalisation may be required with severe episodes. In contrast with their dramatic effect on positive symptoms, antipsychotics have more modest effects on negative symptoms and cognitive impairment. NICE (2002) has produced guidelines for the treatment of schizophrenia.

Education about the nature of the disorder is essential for the family and the young person. Psychological interventions have centred on work with individual patients to develop social skills, cope with symptoms and identify relapse early. Relapse in schizophrenia seems closely associated with the level of the family's emotional expression as measured by formal assessments of critical comments or expressed hostility in family interviews. There is a close relationship between high arousal in the family and early relapse; this can be lowered by structured family education, reducing face-to-face contact through attendance at a day centre, and formal behavioural family therapy. Recently cognitive therapy to reduce the impact of delusional beliefs or hallucinations has shown promise.

In adults with schizophrenia a key worker can help with adherence to medication and aid with disability benefits and housing needs. Day care, with an active rehabilitation unit aimed at developing job skills or simply support with low-key activities, can improve personal functioning (for example hygiene, conversation and friendships), as well as ensuring early detection of relapse. There is evidence that targeted community support may reduce the need for respite, crisis or compulsory admissions. A recently innovation is early intervention teams that target early detection and treatment in people between 14 and 35 years by providing rapid comprehensive pharmacological and psychosocial treatment packages.

Management plan for Matt

Matt was willing to take treatment and his family was very supportive. He was judged to be not requiring inpatient care. He was commenced on a low dose of risperidone beginning with 2 mg daily. He was visited at home initially on a twice weekly and later on a weekly basis. The dose was gradually increased to 4 mg daily. There was good response to medication and the hallucinations and delusions disappeared almost completely. Initially Matt did not show any prominent side effects. The family was pleased that he was retuning to his normal self. He was taking an interest in watching his favourite programmes on television. He went out with the family on shopping trips. His uncle had come to reside with the family and took a special interest in Matt and they went out on walks and did bowling and snooker.

The family was given information about schizophrenia but found it difficult to understand the extent and seriousness of the illness. They and Matt were given leaflets on schizophrenia (Royal College of Psychiatrists, 2004a and 2004b) and encouraged to join the local national schizophrenia association. At the beginning of the illness they expected it to be a brief episode and felt that Matt would make a good recovery and be able to peruse his education in college.

He was visited by the specialist child and adolescent mental health nurse to discuss methods of coping and early signs of relapse and help the family understand Matt's illness. Family meetings were held regularly to discuss how best to manage Matt at home. Fortunately, the family was very supportive and helpful. However, Matt was judged to be unfit to attend school and unfortunately the local education authority was slow in making alternative arrangements. Once he turned 16 he was deemed not to be of 'school-going age'. Attempts to arrange occupational therapy were not successful because it was not available for his age group. Attempts to get other agencies involved met with little success. Social services were informed but provided no help because there was no mental health social worker for his age group. He was assessed by a voluntary agency to provide him with a 'buddy', but they felt he was 'too good' for such a service.

Course and outcome

Matt remained at home during the next six months. He was free of psychotic symptoms but went out very little. He had lost all his friends and felt isolated. His self-confidence plummeted and he was reluctant to meet with young people of his age. This had a disastrous effect on his level of personal functioning. During this period he complained of tiredness and lethargy and was not motivated to do much at home. In particular, he refused to go out with his parents claiming that he was too tired. Over the months he spent most of the time in his room and lost interest in things he did previously. Attempts were made to get him to attend college for a life skills course. With support from the specialist nurse and his tutor at college he attended the course for one week and then gave up.

At this point Matt's symptoms had changed. He had no active psychotic symptoms but he was lethargic, unmotivated and was housebound. He had lost interest in watching football matches on television and spent most of the time in his room. He was reluctant to go out with the family and avoided meeting family friends and visitors. He claimed that he had lost interest in things and was content to spend most of the time doing nothing. All attempts by his parents and uncle to take him out met with resistance. On examination he was apathetic, his movements and speech were slow and he appeared to be have lost interest in almost everything but he did not admit to feeling depressed. He was unconcerned about his appearance and was observed to be neglecting himself. His level of hygiene was poor and his parents had to exhort him to clean and bathe himself. He was found to be laughing inappropriately.

At this time there were a number of possibilities for his deterioration:

- side effect of drugs
- appearance of negative symptoms of schizophrenia
- onset of an episode of clinical depression
- lack of stimulation.

A second opinion was sought from the regional Tier 4 CAMHS. The consultant psychiatrist who saw him felt that he needed active rehabilitation. Unfortunately no services were available. On the advice of the regional unit the medication was changed to olanzapine but there was little improvement. The family were getting frustrated with Matt and started, for the first time, to blame him for being lazy and not trying enough to help himself. He was considered for admission to the regional psychiatric Tier 4 service but there were no beds available at the time of the reviews. At the age of 16 and a half he was referred to an adult consultant psychiatrist interested in rehabilitation. She felt that he would benefit from a change of medication. Consequently he was admitted to an adult psychiatric ward to start him on clozapine, an atypical anti-psychotic drug used in resistant schizophrenia and because of its potentially serious side effects his care was transferred to the adult service.

He was in hospital for a week. He did not have any side effects with clozapine. The adult community mental health team (CMHT) became involved in his care. He had a community psychiatric nurse (CPN) as his key worker. He went out with Matt often and helped him with basic skills in managing himself. He was reported to be more animated and have regained his interest in sports. However, he lacked confidence to go out on his own and was dependent on the CPN to go out. The social worker from the CMHT helped the family in accessing all the benefits. He was engaged in various activities with the occupational therapist. He joined a group for young people with psychosis run by the occupational therapist. He was said to have interacted well with the young people and contributed to the discussion with enthusiasm.

Matt is now 21 and attends the outpatient psychiatric clinic regularly. He continues to live at home and continues to be severely disabled. The last entry in his clinic notes read as follows: 'Matt attended clinic with his CPN and was neatly dressed and appeared more relaxed and settled. He feels that he is doing well. He said he had his good days and bad days. His CPN says that Matt has slipped back in some areas, such as keeping his room tidy and going out on his own. I am pleased that he has resumed playing football. He has made some friends and plays pool with them. He can also watch television without feeling agitated. On the whole we feel that he has made good progress over the years despite a few setbacks. He is on clozapine 150 mg in the morning and 200 mg at night. He is receiving input from occupational therapy and also has a support worker in addition to the CPN. He has been encouraged to join a vocational training course of his choice. However, he is reluctant to take the next step. We will keep him under review.'

Comments

Six years after the onset of his psychotic episode Matt remains severely disabled. Although the CMHT that cares for him feels that he is doing well compared to the other patients, Matt, now 21, lives at home, goes out very little on his own and has no career plans. He has been symptom-free since the change of medication to clozapine at the age of 17 and has not had any relapses. However, despite the attempts by the CMHT to rehabilitate him, he is functionally severely disabled and is heavily dependent on his parents and psychiatric services. Matt's case illustrates most vividly the devastating effect of schizophrenia in adolescents. The chronic and disabling course of the illness over the last 6 years appears to have transformed an active and vibrant schoolboy into an invalid who is homebound and dependent.

His case also illustrates one of the most prominent features in the natural history of schizophrenia, the symptom–disability gap. This refers to the onset and persistence of personal and social disabilities in spite of improvement in symptoms, as illustrated in Figure 16.1. While symptoms may be controlled by antipsychotic medication, the disability that accompanies schizophrenia is persistent and needs other psychosocial interventions. It is important to point out that the disability in schizophrenia is an intrinsic part of the illness.

This case also shows up the weakness in the services that young people with schizophrenia receive. Unlike in adults, the availability of support services for this age group is badly lacking. Educational services bowed out of his life when he was 16; the locality had no mental health social workers for this age group; there was no occupational therapy or other supports and the family and Matt had to cope with the problem all by themselves. The local CAMHS was not geared to care for those with psychoses; there were no Assertive Community Treatment Teams (ACTT) and no occupational therapy and no day hospital was available. Adolescent inpatient beds were not there when an admission was considered necessary (for commencing clozapine). Consequently, and most inappropriately, his treatment with clozapine was delayed and when he was admitted he was admitted to an adult psychiatric ward.

For the CAMHS clinicians who worked with him, the experience was frustrating and time-consuming. Non-availability of resources meant they had to manage him as best as they could, including the treatment, family work and provision of support. Many fruitless hours were spent on *attempting to find out* what was available 'out there' in the community for him in education, social services and the voluntary sector. The early intervention team was helpful but in the absence of other support services found their role to be limited.

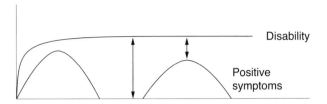

Figure 16.1 Symptoms and disability in Matt. His disabilities persisted despite good symptom control. Arrows indicate the symptom–disability gap.

Box 16.2 Research on adolescent (early onset) schizophrenia says that . . .

- In about 20% of the cases of schizophrenia the onset of the illness is before the age of 18 years.
- Early onset schizophrenia is a severe illness and in about 80% of cases it follows an unremitting course.
- It is associated with poor premorbid functioning, below average IQ and a strong family history of psychosis.
- The extent of disability often persists despite symptom reduction; hence the need for active psychosocial interventions.
- Pharmacotherapy with newer antipsychotic medication is the mainstay treatment, without which psychosocial interventions would not be possible.
- Psychosocial and family interventions (support, education and reducing high EE) are necessary to reduce disability and decrease the risk of relapse.

Note

The author wishes to thank Liane Patel, Clinical Nurse Specialist, for sharing the care of Matt.

References

Arseneault L, Cannon M, Witton J. Causal association between cannabis and psychosis: examination of the evidence. *British Journal of Psychiatry*. 2004; **184**: 110–17.

* Hollis C. Adult outcomes of child and adolescent-onset schizophrenia: diagnostic stability and predictive validity. *American Journal of Psychiatry*. 2000; **157**: 1652–9.

National Institute for Clinical Excellence (NICE). *Schizophrenia. Core interventions in the treatment and management of schizophrenia in primary and secondary care*. London: NICE; 2002. Available at www.nice.org.uk/pdf/cg1niceguideline.pdf.

Royal College of Psychiatrists. Mental health and growing up. 3rd edn. Schizophrenia. Fact sheet 21. For parents and teachers. London: Royal College of Psychiatrists; 2004a.

Royal College of Psychiatrists. Mental health and growing up. 3rd edn. Psychotic illness. Fact sheet 33. For young people. London: Royal College of Psychiatrists; 2004b.

Index

Page numbers in *italic* refer to figures or tables.